Heart Diseases & Disorders
Sourcebook, 2nd Edition

Household Safety Sourcebook

Immune System Disorders Sourcebook

Infant & Toddler Health Sourcebook

Injury & Trauma Sourcebook

Kidney & Urinary Tract Diseases &
Disorders Sourcebook

Learning Disabilities Sourcebook,
2nd Edition

Leukemia Sourcebook

Liver Disorders Sourcebook

Lung Disorders Sourcebook

Medical Tests Sourcebook, 2nd Edition

Men's Health Concerns Sourcebook,
2nd Edition

Mental Health Disorders Sourcebook,
2nd Edition

Mental Retardation Sourcebook

Movement Disorders Sourcebook

Obesity Sourcebook

Osteoporosis Sourcebook

Pain Sourcebook, 2nd Edition

Pediatric Cancer Sourcebook

Physical & Mental Issues in Aging
Sourcebook

Podiatry Sourcebook

Pregnancy & Birth Sourcebook,
2nd Edition

Prostate Cancer

Public Health Sourcebook

Reconstructive & Cosmetic Surgery
Sourcebook

Rehabilitation Sourcebook

Respiratory Diseases & Disorders
Sourcebook

Sexually Transmitted Diseases
Sourcebook, 2nd Edition

Skin Disorders Sourcebook

Sleep Disorders Sourcebook

Sports In[juries]

Stress-Related Disorders Sourcebook

Stroke Sourcebook

Substance Abuse Sourcebook

Surgery Sourcebook

Transplantation Sourcebook

Traveler's Health Sourcebook

Vegetarian Sourcebook

Women's Health Concerns Sourcebook,
2nd Edition

Workplace Health & Safety Sourcebook

Worldwide Health Sourcebook

Teen Health Series

Cancer Information for Teens

Diet Information for Teens

Drug Information for Teens

Mental Health Information
for Teens

Sexual Health Information
for Teens

Skin Health Information
for Teens

Sports Injuries Information
for Teens

Alzheimer's Disease
SOURCEBOOK

Third Edition

Health Reference Series

Third Edition

Alzheimer's Disease SOURCEBOOK

*Basic Consumer Health Information about Alzheimer's
Disease, Other Dementias, and Related Disorders,
Including Multi-Infarct Dementia, AIDS Dementia
Complex, Dementia with Lewy Bodies, Huntington's
Disease, Wernicke-Korsakoff Syndrome (Alcohol-Related
Dementia), Delirium, and Confusional States*

*Along with Information for People Newly Diagnosed
with Alzheimer's Disease and Caregivers, Reports
Detailing Current Research Efforts in Prevention,
Diagnosis, and Treatment, Facts about Long-Term Care
Issues, and Listings of Sources for Additional Information*

Edited by
Karen Bellenir

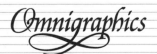

Omnigraphics

615 Griswold Street • Detroit, MI 48226

Bibliographic Note

Because this page cannot legibly accommodate all the copyright notices, the Bibliographic Note portion of the Preface constitutes an extension of the copyright notice.

Edited by Karen Bellenir

Health Reference Series

Karen Bellenir, *Managing Editor*
David A. Cooke, MD, *Medical Consultant*
Elizabeth Barbour, *Permissions Associate*
Dawn Matthews, *Verification Assistant*
Laura Pleva Nielsen, *Index Editor*
EdIndex, Services for Publishers, *Indexers*

* * *

Omnigraphics, Inc.

Matthew P. Barbour, *Senior Vice President*
Kay Gill, *Vice President—Directories*
Kevin Hayes, *Operations Manager*
Leif Gruenberg, *Development Manager*
David P. Bianco, *Marketing Consultant*

* * *

Peter E. Ruffner, *Publisher*

Frederick G. Ruffner, Jr., *Chairman*

Copyright © 2003 Omnigraphics, Inc.

ISBN 0-7808-0666-2

Library of Congress Cataloging-in-Publication Data

Alzheimer's disease Sourcebook : basic consumer health information about Alzheimer's disease, other dementias, and related disorders, including multi-infarct dementia, AIDS dementia complex, dementia with Lewy bodies, Huntington's disease, Wernicke-Korsakoff syndrome (alcohol-related dementia), delirium, and confusional states; along with information for people newly diagnosed with Alzheimer's disease and caregivers, reports detailing current research efforts in prevention, diagnosis, and treatment, facts about long-term care issues, and listings of sources for additional information / edited by Karen Bellenir.--3rd ed.
    p. cm. -- (Health reference series)
    ISBN 0-7808-0666-2 (lib. bdg. : alk. paper)
    1. Alzheimer's disease--Popular works. 2. Dementia--Popular works. I. Bellenir, Karen. II. Health reference series (Unnumbered)

RC523.2.A45 2003
616.8'31--dc22

2003060930

This book is printed on acid-free paper meeting the ANSI Z39.48 Standard. The infinity symbol that appears above indicates that the paper in this book meets that standard.

Printed in the United States

Table of Contents

Part III: Diagnosing and Treating Dementias

Part IV: Coping with Alzheimer's Disease: Information for the Newly Diagnosed

Part V: Coping with Alzheimer's Disease: Information for Caregivers

Part VI: Alzheimer's Disease Research

Part VII: Additional Help and Information

Preface

About This Book

Alzheimer's disease is a degenerative disorder in which certain brain functions, including memory and judgement, are impaired and then lost. Alzheimer's disease currently affects 4 million Americans. Because the risk for developing Alzheimer's disease increases as a person ages and because the U.S. population as a whole is aging, the estimated number of affected people will grow dramatically—to 14 million by the year 2050—unless a prevention or cure is found. Although Alzheimer's disease remains an elusive and devastating disorder, medical researchers have begun to discover many of its secrets.

This *Sourcebook* provides updated information about Alzheimer's disease and other types of dementia, including multi-infarct dementia, frontotemporal dementia, Binswanger's disease, Huntington's disease, dementia with Lewy bodies, and Wernicke-Korsakoff syndrome. It explains recent advances made in understanding the causes of dementing disorders, improvements made in diagnostic procedures, and discoveries that have helped identify potential treatments. For newly diagnosed Alzheimer's patients, it explains what to expect. For people involved in long-term caregiving, it offers information about commonly experienced challenges and coping strategies. A glossary and directories of resources provide additional help and information.

How to Use This Book

This book is divided into parts and chapters. Parts focus on broad areas of interest. Chapters are devoted to single topics within a part.

Part I: Understanding Alzheimer's Disease explains normal brain function and describes the changes associated with Alzheimer's disease. It reviews known, theoretical, and controversial factors that may play a role in the development of Alzheimer's disease, and it reports on the typical stages often experienced as the disease progresses.

Part II: Other Dementias and Related Disorders includes information about Binswanger's disease, Creutzfeldt-Jakob disease, dementia with Lewy bodies (DLB), frontotemporal dementia, multi-infarct dementia, Wernicke-Korsakoff syndrome (alcohol-related Dementia) and other common forms of non-Alzheimer's dementia.

Part III: Diagnosing and Treating Dementias highlights important facts about mental changes during aging and the warning signs that may accompany early Alzheimer's disease or other dementia. It explains screening tests and other tools that may be used in making a diagnosis. Treatments that may help delay the worsening of Alzheimer's disease symptoms are also explained.

Part IV: Coping with Alzheimer's Disease: Information for the Newly Diagnosed discusses the early stages of the disease and describes what to expect. It offers strategies for slowing mental declines and maintaining health through adequate nutrition. It also addresses personal issues such as depression, driving, and advance planning for long-term care.

Part V: Coping with Alzheimer's Disease: Information for Caregivers provides suggestions for family members and friends of Alzheimer's disease patients. It offers ideas for ensuring home safety and coping with some of the most frequently encountered caregiving challenges, including sleep problems, wandering, and inappropriate behaviors. It also offers practical suggestions for dealing with caregiver stress, evaluating housing options, and coping with the final stages of the disease.

Part VI: Alzheimer's Disease Research includes information about some of the most promising areas of current study. It explains recent findings related to mental functioning and describes new tools being developed to fight Alzheimer's disease.

Part VII: Additional Help and Information provides a glossary of terms related to Alzheimer's disease and suggestions for additional reading. The Safe Return Program, which can help when dementia patients wander and become lost, is described. Several directories list sources for Alzheimer's disease information, discount medications, and caregiver resources. A chapter explaining what to do and who to contact if you suspect elder abuse is also included.

Bibliographic Note

This volume contains documents and excerpts from publications issued by the following U.S. government agencies: Alzheimer's Disease Education and Referral (ADEAR) Center; National Center for Health Statistics; National Institute of Neurological Disorders and Stroke (NINDS); National Institute on Aging; National Institutes of Health (NIH); National Women's Health Information Center; and the U.S. Administration on Aging (AOA).

In addition, this volume contains copyrighted documents from the following organizations and individuals: A.D.A.M., Inc.; AgeNet, Inc.; Alzheimer Scotland - Action on Dementia; Alzheimer Society of Canada; Alzheimer's Association; Alzheimer's Association of Los Angeles, Riverside, and San Bernardino Counties; Alzheimer's Australia NSW; Alzheimer's Society (UK); American Academy of Family Physicians; American Academy of Neurology; American Association of Retired Persons (AARP); American Federation for Aging Research; American Geriatrics Society; American Psychological Association; Baylor College of Medicine, Department of Neurology; Cleveland Clinic Foundation; Clinicians Group/Jobson Publishing's *Neurology Reviews*; Peggy Eastman; eMedicine; Family Caregiver Alliance; Fisher Center for Alzheimer's Research; Greater East Ohio Area Alzheimer's Association; Huntington's Disease Society; Medical College of Wisconsin's *MCW HealthLink*; Merck & Co., Inc.'s *The Merck Manual*; Northwestern University Medical School's Cognitive Neurology and Alzheimer's Disease Center; Pick's Disease Support Group; Project Inform; Penelope Roques; Dorothy Seman, MS, RN; Stanford/VA Alzheimer's Research Center of California; University of Florida, College of Health and Human Performance; and the Washington University School of Medicine in St. Louis.

Acknowledgements

In addition to the organizations, agencies, and individuals listed above, special thanks go to many others who have worked hard to help bring this book to fruition. They include editorial assistant Michael Bellenir, permissions associate Liz Barbour, indexer Edward J. Prucha, and eagle-eyed noticer of final details Barry Puckett.

Note from the Editor

This book is part of Omnigraphics' *Health Reference Series*. The series provides basic information about a broad range of medical concerns. It is not intended to serve as a tool for diagnosing illness, in prescribing treatments, or as a substitute for the physician/patient relationship. All persons concerned about medical symptoms or the possibility of disease are encouraged to seek professional care from an appropriate health care provider.

Our Advisory Board

The *Health Reference Series* is reviewed by an Advisory Board comprised of librarians from public, academic, and medical libraries. We would like to thank the following board members for providing guidance to the development of this series:

Dr. Lynda Baker,
Associate Professor of Library and Information Science,
Wayne State University, Detroit, MI

Nancy Bulgarelli,
William Beaumont Hospital Library, Royal Oak, MI

Karen Imarisio,
Bloomfield Township Public Library, Bloomfield Township, MI

Karen Morgan,
Mardigian Library, University of Michigan-Dearborn,
Dearborn, MI

Rosemary Orlando,
St. Clair Shores Public Library, St. Clair Shores, MI

Medical Consultant

Medical consultation services are provided to the *Health Reference Series* editors by David A. Cooke, MD. Dr. Cooke is a graduate of Brandeis University, and he received his M.D. degree from the University of Michigan. He completed residency training at the University of Wisconsin Hospital and Clinics. He is board-certified in Internal

Medicine. Dr. Cooke currently works as part of the University of Michigan Health System and practices in Brighton, MI. In his free time, he enjoys writing, science fiction, and spending time with his family.

Health Reference Series *Update Policy*

The inaugural book in the *Health Reference Series* was the first edition of *Cancer Sourcebook* published in 1989. Since then, the *Series* has been enthusiastically received by librarians and in the medical community. In order to maintain the standard of providing high-quality health information for the layperson the editorial staff at Omnigraphics felt it was necessary to implement a policy of updating volumes when warranted.

Medical researchers have been making tremendous strides, and it is the purpose of the *Health Reference Series* to stay current with the most recent advances. Each decision to update a volume will be made on an individual basis. Some of the considerations will include how much new information is available and the feedback we receive from people who use the books. If there is a topic you would like to see added to the update list, or an area of medical concern you feel has not been adequately addressed, please write to:

Editor
Health Reference Series
Omnigraphics, Inc.
615 Griswold Street
Detroit, MI 48226
E-mail: editorial@omnigraphics.com

Part One

Understanding
Alzheimer's Disease

Chapter 1

Alzheimer's Disease: An Overview

Introduction

Dementia is a brain disorder that seriously affects a person's ability to carry out daily activities. The most common form of dementia among older people is Alzheimer's disease (AD), which involves the parts of the brain that control thought, memory, and language. Although scientists are learning more every day, right now they still do not know what causes AD, and there is no cure.

Scientists think that up to 4 million Americans suffer from AD. The disease usually begins after age 60, and risk goes up with age. While younger people also may get AD, it is much less common. About 3 percent of men and women ages 65 to 74 have AD, and nearly half of those age 85 and older may have the disease. It is important to note, however, that AD is not a normal part of aging.

AD is named after Dr. Alois Alzheimer, a German doctor. In 1906, Dr. Alzheimer noticed changes in the brain tissue of a woman who had died of an unusual mental illness. He found abnormal clumps (now called amyloid plaques) and tangled bundles of fibers (now called

Text in this chapter is from "Alzheimer's Disease Fact Sheet," National Institute on Aging, NIH Pub. No. 03-3431, February 2003. The section "Statistics about Alzheimer's Disease," is reprinted with permission of the Alzheimer's Association. For additional information, call the Alzheimer's Association national toll-free number, 800-272-3900, or visit their website at www.alz.org. © 2003 Alzheimer's Association. All rights reserved.

neurofibrillary tangles). Today, these plaques and tangles in the brain are considered signs of AD.

Scientists also have found other brain changes in people with AD. Nerve cells are lost in areas of the brain that are vital to memory and other mental abilities. There also are lower levels of chemicals in the brain that carry complex messages back and forth between nerve cells. AD may disrupt normal thinking and memory by blocking these messages between nerve cells.

Table 1.1. Alzheimer's Disease in the U.S.

Deaths Annually	49,558
Age-Adjusted Death Rate	18.0 deaths per 100,000
Cause of Death Rank Among Americans:	8th

Source: Based on figures for 2000, *National Vital Statistics Reports*, Vol. 50, No. 15, National Center for Health Statistics, Centers for Disease Control and Prevention.

What Causes AD?

Scientists do not yet fully understand what causes AD. There probably is not one single cause, but several factors that affect each person differently. Age is the most important known risk factor for AD. The number of people with the disease doubles every 5 years beyond age 65.

Family history is another risk factor. Scientists believe that genetics may play a role in many AD cases. For example, familial AD, a rare form of AD that usually occurs between the ages of 30 and 60, is inherited. However, in the more common form of AD, which occurs later in life, no obvious inheritance pattern is seen. One risk factor for this type of AD is a gene that makes a protein called apolipoprotein E (apoE). Everyone has apoE, which helps carry cholesterol in the blood. The apoE gene has three forms. One seems to protect a person from AD, and another seems to make a person more likely to develop the disease. It is likely that other genes also may increase the risk of AD or protect against AD, but they remain to be discovered.

4

Scientists still need to learn a lot more about what causes AD. In addition to genetics and apoE, they are studying education, diet, environment, and viruses to learn what role they might play in the development of this disease.

What Are the Symptoms of AD?

AD begins slowly. At first, the only symptom may be mild forgetfulness. In this stage, people may have trouble remembering recent events, activities, or the names of familiar people or things. They may not be able to solve simple math problems. Such difficulties may be a bother, but usually they are not serious enough to cause alarm.

However, as the disease goes on, symptoms are more easily noticed and become serious enough to cause people with AD or their family members to seek medical help. For example, people in the middle stages of AD may forget how to do simple tasks, like brushing their teeth or combing their hair. They can no longer think clearly. They begin to have problems speaking, understanding, reading, or writing. Later on, people with AD may become anxious or aggressive, or wander away from home. Eventually, patients need total care.

How Is AD Diagnosed?

An early, accurate diagnosis of AD helps patients and their families plan for the future. It gives them time to discuss care while the patient can still take part in making decisions. Early diagnosis also offers the best chance to treat the symptoms of the disease.

Today, the only definite way to diagnose AD is to find out whether there are plaques and tangles in brain tissue. To look at brain tissue, however, doctors must wait until they do an autopsy, which is an examination of the body done after a person dies. Therefore, doctors can only make a diagnosis of "possible" or "probable" AD while the person is still alive.

At specialized centers, doctors can diagnose AD correctly up to 90 percent of the time. Doctors use several tools to diagnose "probable" AD, including:

- Questions about the person's general health, past medical problems, and any difficulties the person has carrying out daily activities.

- Medical tests—such as tests of blood, urine, or spinal fluid.

- Tests of memory, problem solving, attention, counting, and language.

- Brain scans.

These test results help the doctor find other possible causes of the person's symptoms. For example, thyroid problems, drug reactions, depression, brain tumors, and blood vessel disease in the brain can cause AD-like symptoms. Some of these other conditions can be treated successfully.

Recently, scientists have focused on a type of memory change called mild cognitive impairment (MCI), which is different from both AD and normal age-related memory change. People with MCI have ongoing memory problems, but they do not have other losses like confusion, attention problems, and difficulty with language. Scientists funded by the National Institute on Aging (NIA) are studying information collected from the Memory Impairment Study to learn whether early diagnosis and treatment of MCI might prevent or slow further memory loss, including the development of AD.

How Is AD Treated?

AD is a slow disease, starting with mild memory problems and ending with severe brain damage. The course the disease takes and how fast changes occur vary from person to person. On average, AD patients live from 8 to 10 years after they are diagnosed, though the disease can last for as many as 20 years.

No treatment can stop AD. However, for some people in the early and middle stages of the disease, the drugs tacrine (Cognex), donepezil (Aricept), rivastigmine (Exelon), or galantamine (Reminyl) may help prevent some symptoms from becoming worse for a limited time. Also, some medicines may help control behavioral symptoms of AD such as sleeplessness, agitation, wandering, anxiety, and depression. Treating these symptoms often makes patients more comfortable and makes their care easier for caregivers.

Developing new treatments for AD is an active area of research. Scientists are testing a number of drugs to see if they prevent AD, slow the disease, or help reduce symptoms.

There is evidence that inflammation in the brain may contribute to AD damage. Some scientists believe that drugs such as nonsteroidal anti-inflammatory drugs (NSAIDs) might help slow the progression of AD, although recent studies of two of these drugs, rofecoxib

(Vioxx) and naproxen (Aleve), have shown that they did not delay the progression of AD in people who already have the disease. Scientists are now testing other NSAIDs to find out if they can slow the onset of the disease.

Research has shown that vitamin E slows the progress of some consequences of AD by about 7 months. Scientists now are studying vitamin E to learn whether it can prevent or delay AD in patients with MCI.

Recent research suggests that ginkgo biloba may be of some help in treating AD symptoms. There is no evidence that ginkgo will cure or prevent AD. Scientists now are trying to find out whether ginkgo biloba can delay or prevent dementia in older people.

Research also is under way to see if estrogen reduces the risk of AD or slows the disease. One study showed that estrogen does not slow the progression of already diagnosed disease, but more research is needed to find out if it may play another role. For example, scientists now are trying to find out whether estrogen can prevent development of AD in women with a family history of the disease.

People with AD and those with MCI who want to help scientists test possible treatments may be able to take part in clinical trials, which are studies to find out whether a new treatment is both safe and effective. Healthy people also can help scientists learn more about the brain and AD. The NIA and the Food and Drug Administration (FDA) are working together to maintain the AD Clinical Trials Database, which lists AD clinical trials sponsored by the Federal government and private companies. To find out more about these studies, contact the NIA's Alzheimer's Disease Education and Referral (ADEAR) Center at 800-438-4380, or visit the ADEAR Center Website at www. alzheimers.org. You also can sign up for e-mail alerts on new clinical trials that have been added to the database.

Many of these studies are being done at NIA-supported Alzheimer's Disease Centers located throughout the United States. These centers carry out a wide range of research, including studies of the causes, diagnosis, treatment, and management of AD. To get a list of these centers, contact the ADEAR Center.

Is There Help for Caregivers?

Most often, spouses or other family members provide the day-to-day care for people with AD. As the disease gets worse, people often need more and more care. This can be hard for caregivers and can affect their physical and mental health, family life, job, and finances.

The Alzheimer's Association has chapters nationwide that provide educational programs and support groups for caregivers and family members of people with AD. For more information, contact the Alzheimer's Association (800-272-3900; website: www.alz.org).

Research

Scientists have come a long way in their understanding of AD. Findings from years of research have begun to clarify differences between normal age-related memory changes, MCI, and AD. Scientists also have made great progress in defining the changes that take place in the AD brain, which allows them to pinpoint possible targets for treatment. These advances are the foundation for the National Institutes of Health (NIH) Alzheimer's Disease Prevention Initiative, which is designed to:

- understand why AD occurs and who is at greatest risk of developing it
- improve the accuracy of diagnosis and the ability to identify those at risk
- discover, develop, and test new treatments
- discover treatments for behavioral problems in patients with AD

Statistics about Alzheimer's Disease

Alzheimer's disease (AD) is a progressive, degenerative disease of the brain, and the most common form of dementia. Some things you should know about Alzheimer's disease:

- Approximately 4 million Americans have AD.
- 14 million Americans will have AD by the middle of this century (2050) unless a cure or prevention is found.
- One in 10 persons over 65 and nearly half of those over 85 have AD. A small percentage of people as young as their 30's and 40's get the disease.
- A person with AD will live an average of eight years and as many as 20 years or more from the onset of symptoms.
- U.S. society spends at least $100 billion a year on AD. Neither Medicare nor most private health insurance covers the long-term care most patients need.

- Alzheimer's disease is costing American business $61 billion a year—$36.5 billion is the cost to business of care giving (lost productivity from absenteeism of employees who care for family members with Alzheimer's); the rest is the business share of the costs of health and long-term care.

- More than 7 of 10 people with Alzheimer's disease live at home. Almost 75% of the home care is provided by family and friends. The remainder is "paid" care costing an average of $12,500 per year. Families pay almost all of that out-of-pocket.

- Half of all nursing home residents suffer from AD or a related disorder. The average cost for nursing home care is $42,000 per year but can exceed $70,000 per year in some areas of the country.

- The average lifetime cost per patient is $174,000.

- The Alzheimer's Association has granted nearly $120 million dollars in research grants (since 1982).

- The federal government estimates spending approximately $598.9 million for Alzheimer disease research in FY2002.

Chapter 2

Age-Related Memory Loss: What Is Normal?

Age-Related Memory Changes

Understanding Memory Loss

From time to time, everyone experiences memory losses over seemingly simple tasks like finding a set of keys or remembering names or important appointments. The fact is that people of all ages occasionally have trouble remembering things.

Contrary to many myths and stereotypes about memory associated with age, memory loss is not inevitable for older people. Scientists have found that barring illness or disease, our minds can stay healthy and strong well into old age. In fact, long-term memory seems to remain intact with advancing age, and intellectual capacity can expand.

As people grow older, however, difficult with memory may trigger concern that something serious is wrong. An unspoken fear among

---

This chapter begins with a document titled "Age-Related Memory Changes." This information is reprinted with permission from the Alzheimer's Association of Los Angeles, Riverside, and San Bernardino Counties. © 1999. For more information, call the Helpline at (800) 660-1993, or visit www.alzla. org. Text under the heading "'Normal' Older Adult Forgetfulness Versus Dementia," is reprinted with permission from a document by the same title, © 2002 Alzheimer's Disease and Related Disorders Association of NWS (New South Wales), Inc. (www. alznsw.asn.au). Text under the heading "Memory Loss—Should I Be Concerned," is by Margaret Winker, MD. It is reprinted with permission from a document by the same title, © 2001 The American Geriatrics Society (www.americangeriatrics.org).

many older persons is that forgetting things may signal a disease such as Alzheimer's. Most older people do not get Alzheimer's; only five to eight percent of the population over age 65 are likely to become afflicted with the disease. The memory changes they notice may be caused by temporary and treatable conditions. As a general rule, the more concerned an older adult is about memory loss, the less likely they are to have Alzheimer's Disease. Individuals with Alzheimer's Disease are often unaware of their own loss of function.

Memory Changes Associated with Aging

As people age, they may mistakenly assume their memories will fail. Although researchers have identified some memory changes that are associated with normal aging, the large majority of older people will not face severe memory loss. Rather, older adults generally experience memory reduction only in certain areas.

Some of the normal age-related memory changes are:

- **Slower thinking:** All body systems become less efficient with age, including thinking and problem solving abilities. The speed of learning and recall decreases, so it may require more time to learn new things and/or retrieve information. Short-term memory doesn't necessarily fade with age; it just takes longer to function.

- **Difficulty in paying attention:** Many memory changes are due to problems of attention, not retention. Reduction in the ability to concentrate as a person ages makes it harder to remember. Distractions are more difficult to ignore and interruptions may cause forgetfulness.

- **More memory cues required for recall:** As people age, more memory aids or cues are needed, and more often, to retrieve information from memory. A cue can be a word, picture, smell, rhyme, or anything associated with information or events to be remembered.

"Normal" Older Adult Forgetfulness Versus Dementia

- "Normal" older adult forgetfulness: "Sometimes I walk into the kitchen and can't remember what I came in there for. So, I go out of the room and later on I remember what I needed in the kitchen."

- A person with dementia: Loses car keys and then happens to find them but doesn't remember what they are for.

Table 2.1. Forgetfulness vs. Dementia

Description	Person With Dementia	"Normal" Older Adult
Forgets	whole experience	parts of an experience
Forgets words or names for things or objects	progressive	occasional (tip-of-the-tongue)
Delayed recall of names	often	rarely
Follows written or verbal directions	gradually unable	usually able
Ability to use notes, reminders, cues from environment	gradually unable	usually able
Follow a story on TV, in a movie or in a book	gradually loses ability	usually able
Calculations	gradually loses ability	may be slower than before
Self-care capacity (dressing, bathing, cooking etc.)	gradually unable	usually able

Tips for Keeping Your Brain Fit and Memory Sharp

As yet there is no prevention or cure for Alzheimer's disease and other forms of forgetfulness. The following are a few tips for keeping your brain more "fit" and memory sharp.

- **Avoid harmful substances:** Excessive drinking and drug abuse damage brain cells.

- **Challenge yourself:** Read widely, keeping mentally active and learning new skills strengthens brain connections and promotes new ones.

- **Trust yourself more:** If people feel they have control over their lives, their brain chemistry actually improves.

These strategies can help keep your memory sharp, regardless of your schooling and years:

- Relax. Tension may prolong a memory lapse.
- Pay attention. Concentrate on what you want to remember.
- Minimize and restrict distractions.
- Take your time.
- Organize belongings. Designate a place for "unforgettables."
- Repeat names of new acquaintances in conversation.
- Use a notepad and carry a calendar. This may not keep your memory sharp, but will compensate for memory problems.

Debunking Memory Myths

Dr. Barry Gordon, U.S. author of *Memory: Remembering and Forgetting in Everyday Life*, debunks some popular misconceptions about aging and memory.

Myth. Forgetfulness is a sign that something is wrong with your brain.

Fact. If we didn't have the capacity to forget, we'd all go crazy. The ability to remember what is important and discard the rest is a skill to be treasured.

Myth. You lose 10,000 brain cells a day, and one day you just run out.

Fact. An exaggerated fear. Some parts of the brain do lose nerve cells, but not where the process of thinking takes place. You lose some nerve connections, but it's possible to grow new ones or maintain the connections you have by exercising your mind.

Myth. To tell if your memory is normal, compare yourself to others.

Fact. A huge range of ability exists across the general population. Even a single individual experiences variations in memory over the course of a lifetime. Just as certain people have a talent for music and others do not, some of us are naturally more gifted at various types of remembering.

Memory Loss—Should I Be Concerned?

Problems with memory can have many causes. If you have trouble with your memory, you should discuss the problem with your doctor.

I can't remember things like I used to. Should I be concerned?

Although problems with memory become increasingly common as people age, most people will never develop significant memory impairment. Some people may experience mild problems with word finding and remembering names; others will develop more substantial memory problems with inability to remember conversations or difficulty functioning in unfamiliar circumstances.

What causes memory problems?

Some mild memory problems can occur in normal older adults, but sometimes memory problems can be a sign of temporary confusion, called delirium, or more persistent memory loss, called dementia. It is difficult to predict whether a person who has mild problems with memory will go on to develop more severe memory loss, because dementia becomes more common as people age. Problems with memory can have many causes, including medication side effects, strokes, infections, depression, thyroid disease, and vitamin B_{12} deficiency, so it is important to be aware of problems with memory and identify causes that can be treated or prevented. Often, caregivers are the first to notice that a family member is having problems with memory.

Should I see a doctor if I have trouble with my memory?

If you have trouble with your memory, you should discuss the problem with your doctor. Tell the doctor the specific problems, when they occur, any recent changes in your home environment, and all the medicines you are taking, including nonprescription and herbal or "natural" remedies; also let him or her know if you drink alcohol. Tell your doctor about when the problems first started, and whether the problems have been the same, worse, or better over time. Any fever, chills, pain, weight loss or gain, or recent changes in other medical conditions should be discussed with your doctor. Any problems with depressed mood should be discussed, including problems with appetite or sleep disturbance. Be sure to tell your doctor if you have had any falls or blackout spells or if you are no longer able to care for yourself or socialize or do errands like you have in the past.

What will the doctor do?

After discussing these issues and performing a physical examination, your doctor may perform a screening memory test that includes

15

basic questions regarding memory. The result of the screening test may be normal, borderline, or abnormal.

What if I complete a screening test and the results are normal or borderline?

If the memory test is normal or low-normal, the doctor may suggest that you keep track of any memory problems over the next few months and repeat the test after six months or so. Or the doctor may suggest another type of memory testing called neuropsychological testing. This type of testing is similar to the memory screen but includes many more questions and tasks. The purpose of this test is to find out if the problems with memory are not severe enough to show up on the screening test, but are apparent in the more in-depth test. If the neuropsychological testing is normal, then the problems with memory are likely the very mild memory problems that may occur with aging. If the test is borderline, the results can help the doctor decide if additional testing might be important to look for a cause of memory loss.

What if the test is abnormal?

If the memory test is abnormal, the doctor will talk with the person and caregiver, if involved, about evaluating possible causes of memory loss. Longer-term memory loss may be caused by a number of conditions including Alzheimer's disease and vascular disease in the brain (small strokes in the brain), and less commonly, by thyroid disease, a low vitamin B_{12} level, or inadequately treated syphilis. In addition to the history of the memory problems and the physical examination, blood tests, and sometimes imaging studies of the brain, such as CT (computerized tomographic) or MRI (magnetic resonance imaging) are necessary to detect most of these illnesses.

If no other explanation for the memory loss is found, the most common cause for memory loss is Alzheimer's disease. With the tests currently available, the only way to know for certain that a person has Alzheimer's disease is by taking a small sample of the brain, called a biopsy. This test is very rarely done, so Alzheimer's disease can only be presumed in most people. Researchers are trying to develop new tests to diagnose Alzheimer's disease, but so far no tests are reliable enough to use for diagnosis.

What if I have probable Alzheimer's disease?

If Alzheimer's disease is the most likely diagnosis, you and your family members may benefit from information provided by organizations about what to expect with Alzheimer's disease and about the support services that are available. No treatments that we know of will cure Alzheimer's disease. One treatment may help some of the symptoms of memory loss, but the drugs, called acetylcholinesterase inhibitors (tacrine [Cognex], donepezil, [Aricept]) have common side effects of nausea and diarrhea, and one drug, tacrine can cause reversible liver damage. These drugs can improve memory equal to about four to six months of memory decline, but memory will nonetheless continue to decline after the drug is started, and if the drug is stopped, the memory loss will become as severe as if the drug had never been started.

Many researchers are studying ways to detect, treat and prevent Alzheimer's disease. If you would like to participate in a study of Alzheimer's disease, or would like more information, you can contact the Alzheimer's Association, the Alzheimer's Disease Education and Referral Center at the National Institute on Aging, or speak with your doctor about researchers in your area.

—Section by Margaret Winker, MD

Chapter 3

Inside the Human Brain

A Walking Tour through the Brain

The brain is a remarkable organ. Seemingly without any effort, it allows us to carry out every element of our daily lives. It manages many of the body functions that happen without our knowledge or direction, such as breathing, blood circulation, and digestion. It also directs all the functions we carry out consciously. We can speak, move, see, remember, feel emotions, and make decisions because of the complicated mix of chemical and electrical processes that take place in our brains.

Our brains are made of nerve cells and lots of other cell types. Nerve cells are also called neurons. The neurons of all animals function in basically the same way, even though animals can be very different from each other. What sets people apart from other animals is the huge number of nerve cells we have in the cerebral cortex, regions of which are proportionally much larger in humans than in any other animals. These regions are the parts of the brain where cognitive functions, like thinking, learning, speaking, remembering, and making decisions, take place. The many interconnections among the nerve cells in these regions also make us different from other animals.

From "A Walking Tour Through the Brain," excerpted from "Alzheimer's Disease: Unraveling the Mystery," Alzheimer's Disease Education and Referral (ADEAR) Center, a service of the National Institute on Aging, NIH Pub. No. 02-3782, October 2002. The full text of this document is available online at www.alzheimers.org/unraveling/index.htm.

19

To understand Alzheimer's disease, it's important to know a bit about the brain. This chapter gives an inside view of the normal brain, how it works, and what happens during aging.

The Brain's Vital Statistics

- Adult weight: about 3 pounds

- Adult size: a medium cauliflower

- Number of neurons: 100,000,000,000 (1 billion)

- Number of synapses (the gap between neurons): 100,000,000,000,000 (100 trillion)

The Human Brain

The Three Main Players

The cerebral hemispheres account for 85 percent of the brain's weight. The billions of neurons in the two hemispheres are connected by a thick bundle of nerves called the corpus callosum. Scientists now think that the two hemispheres differ not so much in what they focus on (the "logical versus artistic" notion), but how they process information. The left hemisphere appears to focus on the details (such as recognizing a particular face in a crowd). The right hemisphere focuses on the broad background (such as understanding the relative position of objects in a space). The cerebral hemispheres have an outer layer called the cerebral cortex. This is where the brain processes sensory information received from the outside world, controls voluntary movement, and regulates conscious thought and mental activity.

The cerebellum takes up a little more than 10 percent of the brain. It's in charge of balance and coordination. The cerebellum also has two hemispheres. They are always receiving information from the eyes, ears, and muscles and joints about the body's movements and position. Once the cerebellum processes the information, it works through the rest of the brain and spinal cord to send out instructions to the body. The cerebellum's work allows us to walk smoothly, maintain our balance, and turn around without even thinking about it.

The brain stem sits at the base of the brain. It connects the spinal cord with the rest of the brain. Even though it's the smallest of the three main players, its functions are crucial to survival. The brain stem controls the functions that happen automatically to keep us alive—our heart rate, blood pressure, and breathing. It also relays information between the brain and the spinal cord, which then sends out messages to the muscles, skin, and other organs. Sleep and dreaming are also controlled by the brain stem.

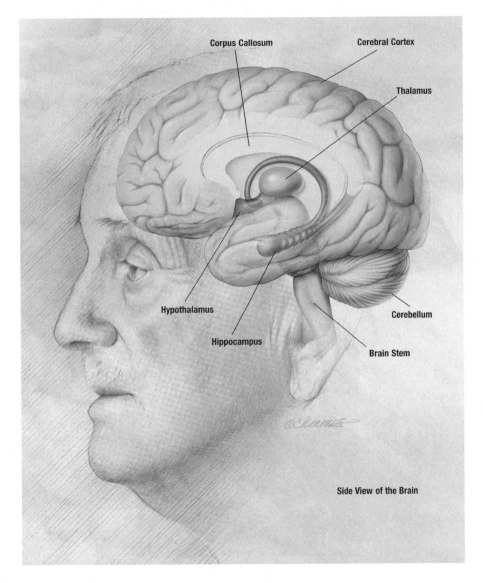

Figure 3.1. *Side view of the brain.*

Other Crucial Parts

Several other essential parts of the brain lie deep inside the cerebral hemispheres:

- The limbic system links the brain stem with the higher reasoning elements of the cerebral cortex. It controls emotions and instinctive behavior. This is also where the sense of smell is located.

- The hippocampus is important for learning and short-term memory. This part of the brain is considered to be the site where short-term memories are converted into long-term memories for storage in other brain areas.

- The thalamus receives sensory and limbic information, processes it, and then sends it to the cerebral cortex.

- The hypothalamus is a structure under the thalamus that monitors activities like body temperature and food intake. It issues instructions to correct any imbalances. The hypothalamus also controls the body's internal clock.

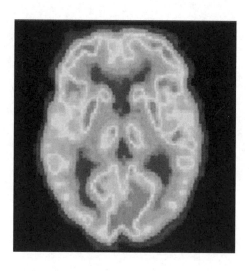

Figure 3.2. PET scan of 20-year old brain.

The Brain in Action

New imaging techniques allow scientists to monitor brain function in living people. This is opening up worlds of knowledge about normal brain function and how it changes with age or disease.

One of these techniques is called positron emission tomography, or PET scanning. PET scans measure blood flow and glucose metabolism throughout the brain. When nerve cells in a region of the brain become active, blood flow and metabolism in that region increase. These increases are usually shown as red and yellow colors on a PET scan. Shades of blue and black indicate decreased or no activity within a brain region. In essence, a PET scan produces a "map" of the active brain.

Scientists use PET scans to see what happens in the brain when a person is engaged in a physical or mental activity, at rest, or even sleeping or dreaming. Scientists can also inject chemicals tagged with a tracer that will "light up" on PET scans. These tracers can track the activity of brain chemicals, for example neurotransmitters such as dopamine and serotonin. Some of these neurotransmitters are altered with age, disease, and drug treatment.

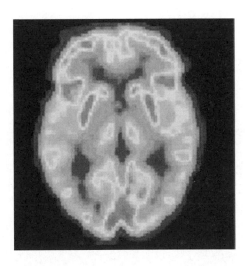

Figure 3.3. PET scan of 80-year old brain.

23

The Aging Brain

As a person gets older, changes occur in all parts of the body, including the brain:

- Some neurons shrink, especially large ones in areas important to learning, memory, planning, and other complex mental activities.

- Tangles and plaques develop in neurons and surrounding areas, though in much smaller amounts than in Alzheimer's disease.

- Damage by free radicals increases (free radicals are a kind of molecule that reacts easily with other molecules).

What is the impact of these changes? Healthy older people may notice a modest decline in their ability to learn new things and retrieve information, such as remembering names. They may perform worse on complex tasks of attention, learning, and memory. However, if given enough time to perform the task, the scores of healthy people in their 70s and 80s are often the same as those of young adults. As they age, adults often improve their vocabulary and other forms of verbal knowledge.

Chapter 4

The Life and Death of a Neuron

Introduction

Until recently, most neuroscientists thought we were born with all the neurons we were ever going to have. As children we might produce some new neurons to help build the pathways—called neural circuits—that act as information highways between different areas of the brain. But scientists believed that once a neural circuit was in place, adding any new neurons would disrupt the flow of information and disable the brain's communication system.

In 1962, scientist Joseph Altman challenged this belief when he saw evidence of neurogenesis (the birth of neurons) in a region of the adult rat brain called the hippocampus. He later reported that newborn neurons migrated from their birthplace in the hippocampus to other parts of the brain. In 1979, another scientist, Michael Kaplan, confirmed Altman's findings in the rat brain, and in 1983 he found neural precursor cells in the forebrain of an adult monkey.

These discoveries about neurogenesis in the adult brain were surprising to other researchers who didn't think they could be true in humans. But in the early 1980s, a scientist trying to understand how birds learn to sing suggested that neuroscientists look again at neurogenesis in the adult brain and begin to see how it might make sense. In a series of experiments, Fernando Nottebohm and his research

"The Life and Death of a Neuron," National Institute of Neurological Disorders and Stroke, Prepared by Office of Communications and Public Liaison, NIH Publication No. 02-3440d, September 2002, reviewed October 10, 2002.

team showed that the numbers of neurons in the forebrains of male canaries dramatically increased during the mating season. This was the same time in which the birds had to learn new songs to attract females.

Why did these bird brains add neurons at such a critical time in learning? Nottebohm believed it was because fresh neurons helped store new song patterns within the neural circuits of the forebrain, the area of the brain that controls complex behaviors. These new neurons made learning possible. If birds made new neurons to help them remember and learn, Nottebohm thought the brains of mammals might too.

Other scientists believed these findings could not apply to mammals, but Elizabeth Gould later found evidence of newborn neurons in a distinct area of the brain in monkeys, and Fred Gage and Peter Eriksson showed that the adult human brain produced new neurons in a similar area.

For some neuroscientists, neurogenesis in the adult brain is still an unproven theory. But others think the evidence offers intriguing possibilities about the role of adult-generated neurons in learning and memory.

The Architecture of the Neuron

The central nervous system (which includes the brain and spinal cord) is made up of two basic types of cells: neurons and glia. Glia outnumber neurons by a substantial amount—some scientists have estimated it to be as large as nine to one—but in spite of their smaller numbers, neurons are the key players in the brain.

Neurons are information messengers. They use electrical impulses and chemical signals to transmit information between different areas of the brain, and between the brain and the rest of the nervous system. Everything we think and feel and do would be impossible without the work of neurons and their support cells, the glial cells called astrocytes and oligodendrocytes.

Neurons have three basic parts: a cell body and two extensions called an axon and a dendrite. Within the cell body is a nucleus, which controls the cell's activities and contains the cell's genetic material. The axon looks like a long tail and transmits messages from the cell. Dendrites look like the branches of a tree and receive messages for the cell. Neurons communicate with each other by sending chemicals, called neurotransmitters, across a tiny space, called a synapse, between the axons and dendrites of adjacent neurons.

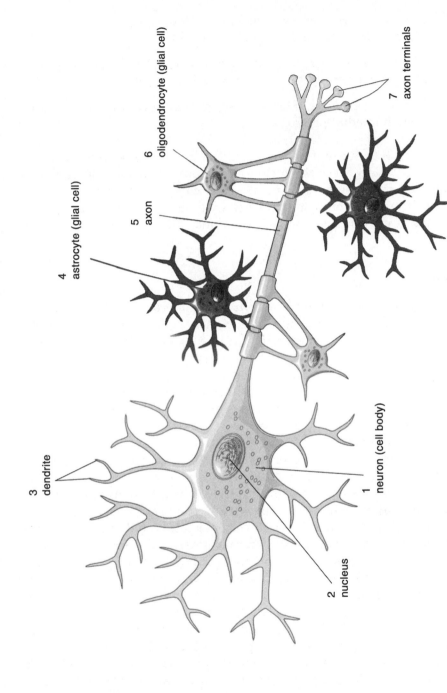

Figure 4.1. The architecture of the neuron.

There are three classes of neurons:

1.   Sensory neurons carry information from the sense organs (such as the eyes and ears) to the brain.

2.   Motor neurons have long axons and carry information from the central nervous system to the muscles and glands of the body.

3.   Interneurons have short axons and communicate only within their immediate region.

Scientists think that neurons are the most diverse kind of cell in the body. Within these three classes of neurons are hundreds of different types, each with specific message-carrying abilities.

How these neurons communicate with each other by making connections is what makes each of us unique in how we think, and feel, and act.

Birth

The extent to which new neurons are generated in the brain is a controversial subject among neuroscientists. Although the majority of neurons are already present in our brains by the time we are born, there is evidence to support that neurogenesis (the scientific word for the birth of neurons) is a lifelong process.

Neurons are born in areas of the brain that are rich in concentrations of neural precursor cells (also called neural stem cells). These cells have the potential to generate most, if not all, of the different types of neurons and glia found in the brain.

Neuroscientists have observed how neural precursor cells behave in the laboratory. Although this may not be exactly how these cells behave when they are in the brain, it gives us information about how they could be behaving when they are in the brain's environment.

The science of stem cells is still very new, and could change with additional discoveries, but researchers have learned enough to be able to describe how neural stem cells generate the other cells of the brain. They call it a stem cell's lineage and it is similar in principle to a family tree.

Neural stem cells increase by dividing in two and producing either two new stem cells, or two early progenitor cells, or one of each.

When a stem cell divides to produce another stem cell, it is said to self-renew. This new cell has the potential to make more stem cells.

When a stem cell divides to produce an early progenitor cell, it is said to differentiate. Differentiation means that the new cell is more specialized in form and function. An early progenitor cell does not have the potential of a stem cell to make many different types of cells. It can only make cells in its particular lineage.

Early progenitor cells can self-renew or go in either of two ways. One type will give rise to astrocytes. The other type will ultimately produce neurons or oligodendrocytes.

Migration

Once a neuron is born it has to travel to the place in the brain where it will do its work.

How does a neuron know where to go? What helps it get there?

Scientists have seen that neurons use at least two different methods to travel:

1.   Some neurons migrate by following the long fibers of cells called radial glia. These fibers extend from the inner layers to the outer layers of the brain. Neurons glide along the fibers until they reach their destination.

2.   Neurons also travel by using chemical signals. Scientists have found special molecules on the surface of neurons—adhesion molecules—that bind with similar molecules on nearby glial cells or nerve axons. These chemical signals guide the neuron to its final location.

Not all neurons are successful in their journey. Scientists think that only a third reach their destination. The rest either never differentiate, or die and disappear at some point during the two to three week phase of migration.

Some neurons survive the trip, but end up where they shouldn't be. Mutations in the genes that control migration create areas of misplaced or oddly formed neurons that can cause disorders such as childhood epilepsy or mental retardation. Some researchers suspect that schizophrenia and the learning disorder dyslexia are partly the result of misguided neurons.

Differentiation

Once a neuron reaches its destination, it has to settle in to work. This final step of differentiation is the least well-understood part of neurogenesis.

Neurons are responsible for the transport and uptake of neurotransmitters—chemicals that relay information between brain cells.

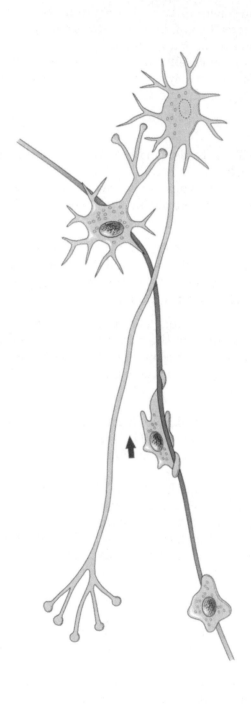

Figure 4.2. Some neurons migrate by riding along extensions (radial glia) until they reach their final destinations.

Depending on its location, a neuron can perform the job of a sensory neuron, a motor neuron, or an interneuron, sending and receiving specific neurotransmitters.

In the developing brain, a neuron depends on molecular signals from other cells, such as astrocytes, to determine its shape and location, the kind of transmitter it produces, and to which other neurons it will connect. These freshly born cells establish neural circuits—or information pathways connecting neuron to neuron—that will be in place throughout adulthood.

But in the adult brain, neural circuits are already developed and neurons must find a way to fit in. Researchers suspect that astrocytes play a similar role in the adult brain, actively regulating the function and synapse formation of new neurons.

As a new neuron settles in, it starts to look like surrounding cells. It develops an axon and dendrites and begins to communicate with its neighbors.

Death

Although neurons are the longest living cells in the body, large numbers of them die during migration and differentiation.

The lives of some neurons can take abnormal turns. Some diseases of the brain are the result of the unnatural deaths of neurons.

- In Parkinson's disease, neurons that produce the neurotransmitter dopamine die off in the basal ganglia, an area of the brain that controls body movements. The brain can no longer control the body and people shake and jerk in spasms.

- In Huntington's disease, a genetic mutation causes over-production of a neurotransmitter called glutamate, which kills neurons in the basal ganglia. As a result, people twist and writhe uncontrollably.

- In Alzheimer's disease, unusual proteins build up in and around neurons in the neocortex and hippocampus, parts of the brain that control memory. When these neurons die, people lose their capacity to remember and their ability to do everyday tasks. Physical damage to the brain and other parts of the central nervous system can also kill or disable neurons.

- Blows to the brain, or the damage caused by a stroke, can kill neurons outright or slowly starve them of the oxygen and nutrients they need to survive.

31

- Spinal cord injury can disrupt communication between the brain and muscles when neurons lose their connection to axons located below the site of injury. These neurons may still live, but they lose their ability to communicate.

Hope Through Research

Scientists hope that by understanding more about the life and death of neurons they can develop new treatments, and possibly even cures, for brain diseases and disorders that affect the lives of millions of Americans.

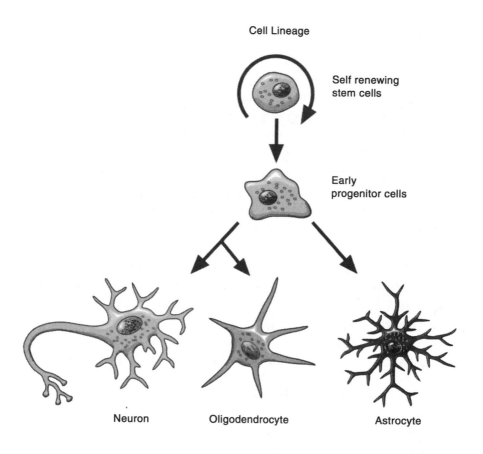

Figure 4.3. *Stem cells differentiate to produce different types of nerve cells.*

The most current research suggests that neural stem cells can generate many, if not all, of the different types of neurons found in the brain and the nervous system. Learning how to manipulate these stem cells in the laboratory into specific types of neurons could produce a fresh supply of brain cells to replace those that have died or been damaged.

Therapies could also be created to take advantage of growth factors and other signaling mechanisms inside the brain that tell precursor cells to make new neurons. This would make it possible to repair, reshape, and renew the brain from within.

For information on other neurological disorders or research programs funded by the National Institute of Neurological Disorders and Stroke, contact the Institute's Brain Resources and Information Network (BRAIN) at:

BRAIN
P.O. Box 5801
Bethesda, Maryland 20824
Phone: 800-352-9424
Website: http://www.ninds.nih.gov

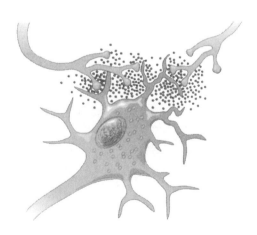

Figure 4.4. *One method of cell death results from the release of excess glutamate.*

Chapter 5

Plaques and Tangles: The Hallmarks of Alzheimer's Disease

Alzheimer's disease disrupts each of the three processes that keep neurons healthy: communication, metabolism, and repair. This disruption causes certain nerve cells in the brain to stop working, lose connections with other nerve cells, and finally, die. The destruction and death of nerve cells causes the memory failure, personality changes, problems in carrying out daily activities, and other features of the disease.

The brains of AD patients have an abundance of two abnormal structures—beta amyloid plaques and neurofibrillary tangles. This is especially true in certain regions of the brain that are important in memory. Plaques are dense, mostly insoluble (cannot be dissolved) deposits of protein and cellular material outside and around the neurons. Tangles are insoluble twisted fibers that build up inside the nerve cell. Though many older people develop some plaques and tangles, the brains of AD patients have them to a much greater extent. Scientists have known about plaques and tangles for many years, but recent research has shown much about what they are made of, how they form, and their possible roles in AD.

From "Plaques and Tangles: The Hallmarks of AD," excerpted from "Alzheimer's Disease: Unraveling the Mystery," Alzheimer's Disease Education and Referral (ADEAR) Center, a service of the National Institute on Aging, NIH Pub. No. 02-3782, October 2002. The full text of this document is available online at www.alzheimers.org/unraveling/index.htm.

Amyloid Plaques

Plaques are made of beta-amyloid, a protein fragment snipped from a larger protein called amyloid precursor protein (APP). These fragments clump together and are mixed with other molecules, neurons, and non-nerve cells. In AD, plaques develop in the hippocampus, a structure deep in the brain that helps to encode memories, and in other areas of the cerebral cortex that are used in thinking and making decisions. We still don't know whether beta-amyloid plaques themselves cause AD or whether they are a by-product of the AD process. We do know that changes in APP structure can cause a rare, inherited form of AD.

From APP to Beta-Amyloid

APP is a protein that appears to be important in helping neurons grow and survive. APP may help damaged neurons repair themselves and may help parts of neurons grow after brain injury. In AD, something causes APP to be snipped into fragments, one of which is called beta-amyloid; the beta-amyloid fragments eventually clump together into plaques.

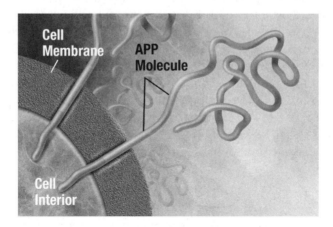

Figure 5.1. APP is associated with the cell membrane, the thin barrier that encloses the cell. After it is made, APP sticks through the neuron's membrane, partly inside and partly outside the cell.

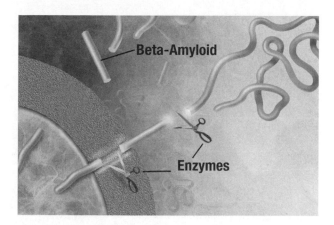

Figure 5.2. *Enzymes (substances that cause or speed up a chemical re-action) act on the APP and cut it into fragments of protein, one of which is called beta-amyloid.*

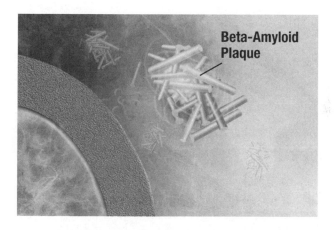

Figure 5.3. *The beta-amyloid fragments begin coming together into clumps outside the cell, then join other molecules and non-nerve cells to form in-soluble plaques.*

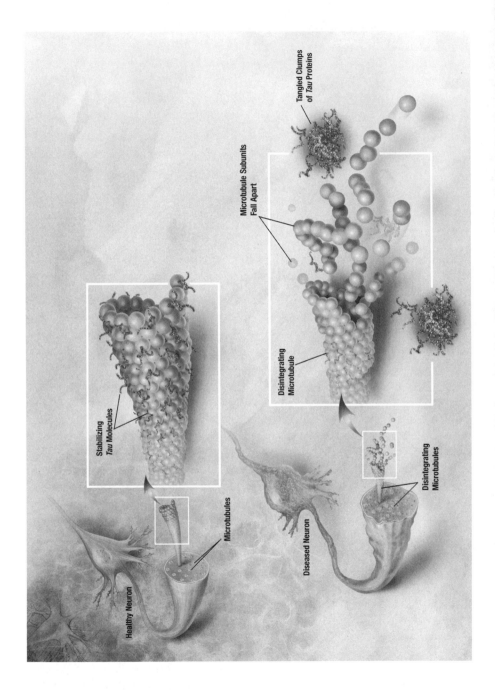

Figure 5.4. *Neurofibrillary tangles.*

APP is associated with the cell membrane, the thin barrier that encloses the cell. After it is made, APP sticks through the neuron's membrane, partly inside and partly outside the cell. Enzymes (substances that cause or speed up a chemical reaction) act on the APP and cut it into fragments of protein, one of which is called beta-amyloid. The beta amyloid fragments begin coming together into clumps outside the cell, then join other molecules and non-nerve cells to form insoluble plaques.

Neurofibrillary Tangles

Healthy neurons have an internal support structure partly made up of structures called microtubules. These microtubules act like tracks, guiding nutrients and molecules from the body of the cell down to the ends of the axon and back. A special kind of protein, tau, makes the microtubules stable. In AD, tau is changed chemically. It begins to pair with other threads of tau and they become tangled up together. When this happens, the microtubules disintegrate, collapsing the neuron's transport system. This may result first in malfunctions in communication between neurons and later in the death of the cells.

Chapter 6

Risk Factors for Alzheimer's Disease

What are risk factors?

Many diseases have specific causes; for example, a virus causes measles. However, for many chronic disorders (long-lasting conditions such as Alzheimer's disease), the causes remain uncertain. In their search for answers, scientists look for factors that appear to be linked to the development of a disease. These are "risk factors"—if they are present, there is an increased chance, but not a certainty, that the disease will develop.

Risk factors are characteristics or exposures that appear to have some relationship to the development of a disease. They can include family background, work history, or exposures to a substance or product. Some risk factors can be modified (for example, lowering blood pressure reduces the risk of stroke); other risk factors cannot be modified (for example, age or family history).

It is important to note that risk factors are not necessarily causes of a disease. No single study can verify a link between a disease and a specific factor; repeated studies are necessary before a causal link can be established.

How are risk factors determined?

Two types of studies are used to determine risk factors. One approach is to study people who already have the disease (such as Alzheimer's disease) and compare them with persons without the disease, who are otherwise similar in age, gender and other characteristics. This is known as a case-control study. Information is gathered on their personal and family characteristics, as well as on past exposures that may have occurred through lifestyle and work. Risk factors that are more frequent in the diseased than the non-diseased group can be identified. This method was used in the first analysis of risk factors for Alzheimer's disease from the Canadian Study of Health and Aging (CSHA).[1]

The second approach is to monitor a group of healthy people over a long period of time; this is known as a cohort study. From this group, people who have a particular characteristic or who were exposed to a particular substance are compared to those without the characteristic or exposure to detect any difference in the rate at which the two groups develop a disease. Lifestyle factors (such as diet) as well as family and work histories are examined in the diseased and non-diseased groups. Factors known to be associated with a specific disease are of particular interest. In this way, characteristics and exposures that are associated with the occurrence of the disease can be identified. This approach was used in the second analysis of risk factors for Alzheimer's disease from the CSHA (CSHA-2).[2]

Recent data from CSHA-2 have been published identifying new areas of reduced risk for Alzheimer's disease. These preliminary findings are important because they indicate lifestyle choices that can be made that would help protect against Alzheimer's disease.

What are the risk factors associated with Alzheimer's disease?

Age. The CSHA provides evidence to support age as a risk factor.

Family history. Many studies indicate that people with a relative (parent, brother or sister) with Alzheimer's disease have a greater chance of developing the disease than those with no family history.

The more common form of Alzheimer's disease is called sporadic Alzheimer's disease and accounts for 90 to 95 per cent of all cases. The role of heredity in sporadic Alzheimer's disease is unclear and continues to be the subject of intense research.

A rare form of the disease, familial autosomal dominant Alzheimer's disease (FAD), accounts for approximately 5 to 10 per cent of all cases and is known to be inherited—the disease will occur if the disease gene is present. (Each chromosome carries many genes that are strung together like beads on a string. These genes are the basic units that allow specific characteristics to be passed from one generation to the next.)

In certain families, FAD is passed directly from one generation to another through a dominant inheritance pattern. This means that if a parent is affected, each child has a 50 per cent chance of inheriting the disease gene and will develop Alzheimer's disease in adulthood.

ApoE gene. Chromosome 19 has the apolipoprotein E gene (apoE) that affects cell activity. The apoE gene has three alleles: apoE e2, apoE e3 and apoE e4. Alleles are copies of a gene. A person inherits two alleles of a gene, one from the mother and one from the father. The presence of the e4 allele is associated with an increased risk of Alzheimer's disease with an earlier age of onset (that is, before age 70). The apoE gene cannot predict Alzheimer's disease, but it may be useful in confirming diagnosis. It should be noted that the absence of the e4 allele reduces the risk of Alzheimer's disease.

Down syndrome. Almost all individuals with Down syndrome over the age of 40 have changes to brain cells typical of Alzheimer's disease. In these individuals, dementia usually develops in their 50's or 60's.[4]

Cognitive impairment with no dementia (CIND) or mild cognitive impairment (MCI). In the CSHA, a group of participants was identified as having mild cognitive impairment, but did not meet the clinical definition of having dementia. This group was followed for several years, and recent evidence has indicated that of the survivors, 5 to 6 percent of the group developed Alzheimer's disease annually.[5] Research into the progression of CIND or MCI is ongoing.

Head injury. Some studies have shown that people who have had a head injury with loss of consciousness have an increased chance of developing Alzheimer's disease. To prevent head injury and therefore possibly prevent dementia, it would be prudent to use helmets for sports activities, such as cycling, and safety belts when driving in a vehicle.

Education. Several studies have shown that people who have less than six years of formal education appear to have a higher risk of developing Alzheimer's disease. Low education may reflect early experiences that were not beneficial to brain development. Or, higher education may delay the onset of symptoms of Alzheimer's disease possibly due to greater brain reserve or educational activities that may stimulate brain activity. Education as a protective factor requires more study to determine whether it is education that makes a difference or other factors related to it (for example, income level).

Anti-inflammatory medications. Researchers have noticed signs of inflammation in the regions of the brain of people with Alzheimer's disease. While inflammation can be a normal immune system response to injury or disease, chronic inflammation can cause damage. Thus, inflammation in the brain may contribute to nerve damage. Other research, such as the CSHA, showed that people with arthritis have a lesser chance of developing Alzheimer's disease than those without it. People with arthritis usually take non-steroidal anti-inflammatory drugs (NSAIDs) to alleviate symptoms. At this time, NSAIDs cannot be recommended for the treatment or prevention of Alzheimer's disease. Research is ongoing in this area.

Aluminum. The connection between Alzheimer's disease and aluminum is still under debate in the scientific community. Some studies have indicated that exposure to aluminum in drinking water increased the chances of individuals developing Alzheimer's disease.

Physical activity. Recent data from the CSHA-2 indicate that regular physical activity was associated with reduced risk of Alzheimer's disease. This information supports previous clinical trials showing exercise to benefit cognitive function. Identifying the protective effect of regular physical activity is an important finding as it may represent a relatively safe and available strategy to help prevent Alzheimer's disease, as well as many other chronic conditions. The CSHA-2 recommends that further research should be conducted in this area.

What other factors are being investigated?

Other factors being investigated by researchers in relation to Alzheimer's disease include:

- existing diseases or conditions that a person may have (such as heart disease, high cholesterol or high homocysteine levels in the blood)
- toxins in the environment (such as fertilizers or pesticides)
- antioxidants (such as vitamin E)

- lifestyle choices (such as wine and coffee consumption, and diet)

What is our current understanding of risk factors?

In general, scientists today believe that Alzheimer's disease is caused by several factors, including those that are inherited and those that are not.

Additional risk factors may be identified as more studies are carried out. Uncovering risk factors increases our understanding of the disease and is a step towards solving the Alzheimer puzzle.

Notes

1. Canadian Study of Health and Aging: Risk factors for Alzheimer's Disease in Canada. *Neurology* 1994; 44:2073-2080.

2. Risk Factors for Alzheimer's Disease: A Prospective Analysis from the Canadian Study of Health and Aging, *American Journal of Epidemiology* 2002; Vol. 156, No. 5, 445-453.

3. Canadian Study of Health and Aging Working Group. Canadian Study of Health and Aging: study methods and prevalence of dementia. *Canadian Medical Association Journal* 1994; 150:899-913, and personal communication, CSHA.

4. Preventing Dementia, S.E. Black, C. Patterson, J. Feightner, *The Canadian Journal of Neurological Sciences* 2001; 28: Suppl. 1-S56-S66.

5. Management of Dementing Disorders: Conclusions from the Canadian Consensus Conference on Dementia, Supplement to *CMAJ* 1999; 160 (12 Suppl), S5.

Chapter 7

The Role of Genes in Alzheimer's Disease

Introduction

Scientists do not yet fully understand what causes Alzheimer's disease (AD). However, the more they learn about AD, the more they become aware of the important function genes play in the development of this devastating disease.

Genes

All living things are made up of basic units called cells, which are so tiny that you can only see them through the lens of a strong microscope. Most of the billions of cells in the human body have one nucleus that acts as a control center, housing our 46 chromosomes. A chromosome is a thread-like structure found in the cell's nucleus, which can carry hundreds, sometimes thousands, of genes. In humans, a set of 23 chromosomes is inherited from each parent. The genetic material on these 23 chromosomes is collectively referred to as the human genome. Through research, scientists now believe the human genome is made up of about 30,000 genes. Genes direct almost every aspect of the construction, operation, and repair of all living things. For example, genes contain information that determines eye and hair color and other traits inherited from our parents. In addition, genes

"Alzheimer's Disease Genetics Fact Sheet," Alzheimer's Disease Education and Referral Center (ADEAR), National Institute on Aging, NIH Pub. No. 03-4012, February 2003.

ensure that we have two hands and can use them to do things, like play the piano.

Genes alone are not all-powerful. Most genes can do little until spurred on by other substances. Although they are necessary in their own right, genes basically wait inside the cell's nucleus for other molecules to come along and read their messages. These messages provide the cell with instructions for building a specific protein.

Proteins are an important building block in all cells. Bones and teeth, muscles and blood, for example, are formed from different proteins. They help our bodies grow, work properly, and stay healthy. Amino acids are the building blocks of proteins. A gene provides the code, or blueprint, for the type and order of amino acids needed to build a specific protein. Sometimes a genetic mutation (or defect) can occur, leading to the production of a faulty protein. In addition to gene mutations, the environment (the food we eat, the air we breath, or chemicals we are exposed to) can affect the production of a protein by interrupting the translation of the genetic message. Faulty proteins can cause cell malfunction, disease, and death.

Scientists are studying genes to learn more about the proteins they make and what these proteins actually do in the body. They also hope to discover what illnesses are caused when genes don't work right.

The Genetics of Alzheimer's Disease

Diseases such as cystic fibrosis, muscular dystrophy, and Huntington's disease are single-gene disorders. If a person inherits the gene that causes one of these disorders, he or she will usually get the disease. AD, on the other hand, is not caused by a single gene. More than one gene mutation can cause AD, and genes on multiple chromosomes are involved.

The two basic types of AD are familial and sporadic. Familial AD (FAD) is a rare form of AD, affecting less than 10 percent of AD patients. All FAD is early-onset, meaning the disease develops before age 65. It is caused by gene mutations on chromosomes 1, 14, and 21. Even if one of these mutated genes is inherited from a parent, the person will almost always develop early-onset AD. This inheritance pattern is referred to as autosomal dominant inheritance. In other words, all offspring in the same generation have a 50/50 chance of developing FAD if one of their parents had it.

ApoE in Sporadic Alzheimer's Disease

The majority of AD cases are sporadic, meaning they have no known cause. Because this type of AD usually develops after age 65, it often is referred to as late-onset AD. Sporadic AD shows no obvious inheritance pattern; however, in some families, clusters of cases have been seen. Although a specific gene has not been identified as the cause of sporadic AD, genetics does appear to play a role in the development of this form of AD. Researchers have identified an increased risk of developing sporadic AD related to the apolipoprotein E (apoE) gene found on chromosome 19. This gene codes for a protein that helps carry cholesterol in the bloodstream. ApoE comes in several different forms, or alleles, but three occur most frequently: apoE2 (E2), apoE3 (E3), and apoE4 (E4).

People inherit one apoE allele from each parent. Having one or two copies of the E4 allele increases a person's risk of getting AD. That is, having the E4 allele is a risk factor for AD, but it does not mean that AD is certain. Some people with two copies of the E4 allele (the highest risk group) do not develop the disease while others with no E4s do. The rarer E2 allele appears to be associated with a lower risk of AD. The E3 allele is the most common form found in the general population and may play a neutral role in AD. The exact degree of risk of AD for any given person cannot be determined based on apoE status.

ApoE Testing in Research or Diagnosis

A blood test is available that can identify which apoE alleles a person has. However, because the apoE4 gene is only a risk factor for AD, this blood test cannot tell whether a person will develop AD or not. Instead of a yes or no answer, the best information a person can get from this genetic test for apoE is maybe or maybe not. Although some people want to know whether they will get AD later in life, this type of prediction is not yet possible. In fact, some researchers believe that screening measures may never be able to predict AD with 100 percent accuracy.

In a research setting, apoE testing may be used to identify study volunteers who may be at a higher risk of getting AD. In this way, researchers can look for early brain changes in some patients. This test also helps researchers compare the effectiveness of treatments for patients with different apoE profiles. Most researchers believe that the apoE test is useful for studying AD risk in large groups of people but not for determining one person's individual risk. Predictive screening in otherwise healthy people will be useful if an accurate/reliable test is developed and effective ways to treat or prevent AD are available.

In diagnosing AD, apoE testing is not a common practice. The only definite way to diagnose AD is by viewing a sample of a person's brain tissue under a microscope to determine if there are plaques and tangles present. This is usually done after the person dies. However, through a complete medical evaluation (including a medical history, laboratory tests, neuropsychological tests, and brain scans), doctors can diagnose AD correctly up to 90 percent of the time. Doctors look to rule out other diseases and disorders that can cause the same symptoms of Alzheimer's disease. If no cause is identified, a person is said to have "probable" or "possible" AD. In some cases, apoE testing may be used in combination with these other medical test to strengthen a suspected case of AD. Currently, there is no medical test to establish if a person without the symptoms of AD is going to develop the disease. ApoE testing as a patient screening (predictive) method is not recommended.

Concerns about Confidentiality

ApoE testing, and indeed all genetic testing, raises ethical, legal, and social questions for which we have few answers. Generally, confidentiality laws protect apoE information gathered for research purposes. On the other hand, information obtained in apoE testing may not remain confidential if it becomes part of a person's medical records. Thereafter, employers, insurance companies, and other health care organizations could find out this information, and discrimination could result. For example, employment opportunities or insurance premiums could be affected.

Genetic Counseling

Depending on the study, research volunteers may have the opportunity, during genetic counseling, to learn the results of their apoE testing. The meaning of these results is complex. Since the results of apoE testing can be hard to understand, and more importantly, devastating to those tested, the National Institute on Aging (NIA) and the Alzheimer's Association recommend that research volunteers and their families receive genetic counseling before and after testing.

People who learn through testing that they have an increased risk of getting AD may experience emotional distress and depression about the future because there is not yet an effective way to prevent or cure the disease. Through counseling, families can learn about the genetics of AD, the tests themselves, and possible meanings of the results. Due to privacy, emotional, and health care issues, the primary goal of genetic counseling is to help people with AD and their families explore and cope with the consequences of such knowledge.

Experts still do not know how limited information about AD risk can benefit people. Among the issues are privacy and confidentiality policies related to genetic information and AD, and the small number of genetic counselors now trained in neurodegenerative disorders. In addition, little is known about how stigma associated with an increased risk for AD may affect people's families and their lives.

Research Questions

Learning more about the role of apoE in the development of AD may help scientists identify who would benefit from prevention and treatment efforts. Age, still the most important known risk factor for AD, continues to be associated with the disease even when no known genetic factors are present. Research focusing on advancing age may help explain the role that other genes play in most AD cases. Scores of AD researchers are studying the genetics of AD. In addition, researchers, ethicists, and health care providers are developing policies about the appropriate use of genetic testing and counseling for AD.

Recent research suggests that certain alleles of other as yet unidentified genes also may increase risk in late-onset cases. The National Institute on Aging (NIA) has launched a major initiative focused on discovering remaining genetic risk factors for late-onset AD. Together with commercial researchers, geneticists from the NIA's Alzheimer's Disease Centers are working to create a genetic sampling of families affected by multiple cases of late-onset AD. Researchers are seeking large families with more than one living relative with late-onset AD. Families interested in participating in this study can contact the National Cell Repository for Alzheimer's Disease at 1-800-526-2839 or 1-317-274-7360. Information may also be requested through their website, www.iupui.edu/~medgen/research/alz/alzheimer.html.

For More Information

Accurate, current information about AD and its risk factors is important to patients and their families, health professionals, and the public. The Alzheimer's Disease Education and Referral (ADEAR) Center is a service of the NIA and is funded by the Federal Government. The ADEAR Center offers information and publications about diagnosis, treatment, patient care, caregiver needs, long-term care, education and training, and research related to AD. Staff respond to telephone, e-mail, and written requests and make referrals to local and national resources.

ADEAR Center
P.O. Box 8250
Silver Spring, MD 20907-8250
Phone: 1-800-438-4380
Fax: 301-495-3334
Website: www.alzheimers.org
E-mail: adear@alzheimers.org

For the free fact sheet, "Genetic Counseling: Valuable Information for You and Your Family," write, fax, or e-mail the National Society for Genetic Counselors (NSGC). Their address is: NSGC, Executive Office, 233 Canterbury Drive, Wallingford, PA 19086-6617, Website: www.nsgc.org, 610-872-7608 (voice mail), 610-872-1192 (fax), e-mail: nsgclistQ@aol.com. The NSGC does not provide information about specific genetic disorders.

Additional Internet information about AD and genetics is available from the National Human Genome Research Institute (NHGRI), part of the National Institutes of Health. Visit the NHGRI Website at www. genome.gov.

The National Library of Medicine (NLM) National Center for Biotechnology Information (NCBI) has produced a gene map of the human genome, which can be viewed at www.ncbi.nlm.nih.gov/genemap99/.

Key Terms

Alleles—different forms of the same gene. Two or more alleles can shape each human trait. Each person receives two alleles, one from each parent. This combination is one factor among many that influences a variety of processes in the body. On chromosome 19, the apolipoprotein E (apoE) gene has three common forms or alleles: E2, E3, and E4. Thus, the possible combinations in one person are E2/2, E2/3, E2/4, E3/3, E3/4, or E4/4.

ApoE Gene—a gene on chromosome 19 involved in making apoE, a substance that helps carry cholesterol in the bloodstream. ApoE is considered a "susceptibility" gene for AD and appears to influence the age of onset of the disease. However, it is not the sole cause of AD. No cause and effect relationship exists between a person's apoE status and the development of AD.

Chromosomes—thread-like structures in every cell of the human body. Chromosomes carry genes. All healthy people have 46 chromosomes in 23 pairs. Usually, people receive one chromosome in each pair from each parent.

Genes—basic units of heredity that direct almost every aspect of the construction, operation, and repair of living organisms. Each gene is a set of biochemical instructions that tells a cell how to assemble one of many different proteins. Each protein has its own highly specialized role to play in the body.

Genetic Mutations—permanent changes to genes. Once such change occurs, it can be passed on to children. The relatively rare, early-onset familial AD is associated with mutations in genes on chromosomes 1, 14, and 21.

Human Genome—the total genetic information found on the 23 chromosomes inherited from a parent. Through research decoding the human genome scientists believe humans have between 30,000 to 35,000 genes.

Proteins—Cells translate genetic information into specific proteins. Proteins determine the physical and chemical characteristics of cells and therefore organisms. Proteins are essential to all life processes.

Chapter 8

Environmental Factors in Alzheimer's Disease

Researchers do not know the exact cause of Alzheimer's disease, but it likely is due to a variety of genetic and environmental factors. The most studied of the environmental factors are aluminum, zinc, food-borne poisons, and viruses.

Aluminum

One of the most publicized and controversial theories concerns aluminum, which became a suspect in Alzheimer's disease when researchers found traces of this metal in the brains of patients with Alzheimer's disease. Many studies since then have either not been able to confirm this finding or have had questionable results.

Aluminum does turn up in higher amounts than normal in some autopsy studies of Alzheimer's patients, but not in all. Further doubt about the importance of aluminum stems from the possibility that the aluminum found in some studies did not all come from the brain tissues being studied. Instead, some could have come from the special substances used in the laboratory to study brain tissue.

Aluminum is a common element in the Earth's crust and is found in small amounts in numerous household products and in many foods.

As a result, there have been fears that aluminum in the diet or absorbed in other ways could be a factor in Alzheimer's. One study found that people who used antiperspirants and antacids containing aluminum had a higher risk of developing Alzheimer's. Others have also reported an association between aluminum exposure and Alzheimer's disease.

On the other hand, various studies have found that groups of people exposed to high levels of aluminum do not have an increased risk. Moreover, aluminum in cooking utensils does not get into food and the aluminum that does occur naturally in some foods, such as potatoes, is not absorbed well by the body. On the whole, scientists can say only that it is still uncertain whether exposure to aluminum plays a role in Alzheimer's disease.

Zinc

Zinc has been implicated in Alzheimer's disease in two ways. Some reports suggest that too little zinc is a problem, others that too much zinc is at fault. Too little zinc was suggested by autopsies that found low levels of zinc in the brains of Alzheimer's disease patients, especially in the hippocampus.

On the other hand, a recent study suggests that too much zinc might be the problem. In this laboratory experiment, zinc caused soluble beta amyloid from cerebrospinal fluid to form clumps similar to the plaques of Alzheimer's disease. Current experiments with zinc are pursuing this lead in laboratory tests that more closely mimic conditions in the brain.

Food-Borne Poisons

Toxins in foods have come under suspicion in a few cases of dementia. Two amino acids found in seeds of certain legumes in Africa, India and Guam may cause neurological damage. Both enhance the action of the neurotransmitter glutamate, also implicated in Alzheimer's disease.

In Canada, an outbreak of a neurological disorder similar to Alzheimer's occurred among people who had eaten mussels contaminated with domoic acid. This chemical, like the legume amino acids, is a glutamate stimulator. While these toxins may not be a common cause of dementia, they could eventually shed some light on the mechanisms that lead to neuron degeneration.

Viruses

In some neurological diseases a virus is the culprit, lurking in the body for decades before a combination of circumstances stirs it to action.

For years researchers have sought a virus or other infectious agent in Alzheimer's disease.

This line of research has yielded little in the way of hard evidence so far, although one study in the late 1980s did provide some data that have kept the possibility alive. A larger investigation is now under way.

Chapter 9

Alzheimer's Disease and Down Syndrome

What is Down syndrome?

Down syndrome is a genetic disorder in which a person has extra chromosome 21 material. The syndrome causes delays and limitations in physical and intellectual development. The extra chromosome material can be inherited from either parent.

Common characteristics of the syndrome include:

* low muscle tone
* flat face (low nasal bridge and small nose)
* eye openings that slant downwards and inwards
* single crease across the centre of the palm
* smaller than normal size
* the delay of both physical and intellectual development

The incidence of Down syndrome is approximately one in every 700 births. The condition is not related to sex, race, nationality, religion or socioeconomic status. The exact cause of Down syndrome is not known.

The age of the mother at the time of child bearing is currently the only known risk factor for Down syndrome. As a mother's age increases so do her chances of having a child with Down syndrome. There is about a one in 1000 chance of having an affected child if the mother is under age 30; this increases to one in 100 if the mother is over age 40. However, it is important to understand that many children with Down syndrome are born to younger women.

Children with Down syndrome may have:

- congenital heart disease
- respiratory infections
- visual problems
- poor hearing
- poorly functioning thyroid

How is Down syndrome associated with Alzheimer's disease?

Many individuals with Down syndrome who live past the age of 35 develop the characteristic markers for Alzheimer's disease. The markers are plaques and/or tangles in the brain. Not all individuals who have these markers develop symptoms of Alzheimer's disease. Studies show that as people with Down syndrome age, they are more likely to develop Alzheimer's disease, as in the general population.

What considerations are there when making a diagnosis of Alzheimer's disease when Down syndrome is present.

Making a diagnosis of Alzheimer's disease is more difficult when an individual has Down syndrome for the following reasons:

- People with Down syndrome have a wide range of health problems associated with aging and these may mimic or mask the presence of Alzheimer's disease.

- The usual skill tests used for diagnosis do not take into account the existing disabilities of the person with Down syndrome.

- The limited verbal and other communication skills of some people with Down syndrome may affect the assessment.

When people have Down syndrome, physicians rely heavily on caregivers for details of their medical history. Their reports can assist in separating pre-existing disabilities from Alzheimer's disease symptoms.

Caregivers can also verify whether or not there has been a decrease in intellectual function or life skills.

Is providing Alzheimer's disease care different when Down syndrome is involved?

There are no real differences in providing care, but there are a number of factors to consider:

- As with anyone with Alzheimer's disease, it is essential that all caregivers are educated to understand the disease and its effects on the individual.

- Caregivers may need additional support because of the new needs of the individual and the length of time they may have already been providing care.

- The techniques used by caregivers to cope with behavior exhibited by some people with Down syndrome may become ineffective as abilities decline.

Chapter 10

The Changing Brain in Alzheimer's Disease

No one knows exactly what causes the Alzheimer's disease (AD) process to begin or why some of the normal changes associated with aging become so much more extreme and destructive in patients with the disease. We do know a lot, however, about what happens in the brain once AD takes hold and about the physical and mental changes that occur over time. The time from diagnosis to death varies—as little as 3 years if the patient is over 80 when diagnosed, as long as 10 or more years if the patient is younger. Although the course of AD is not the same in every patient, symptoms seem to develop over the same general stages.

Preclinical AD

AD begins in the entorhinal cortex, which is near the hippocampus and has direct connections to it. It then proceeds to the hippocampus, the structure that is essential to the formation of short-term and long-term memories. Affected regions begin to atrophy (shrink). These brain changes probably start 10 to 20 years before any visible signs and symptoms appear. Memory loss, the first visible sign, is the main feature of mild cognitive impairment (MCI). Many scientists

From "The Changing Brain in Alzheimer's Disease," excerpted from "Alzheimer's Disease: Unraveling the Mystery," Alzheimer's Disease Education and Referral (ADEAR) Center, a service of the National Institute on Aging, NIH Pub. No. 02-3782, October 2002. The full text of this document is available online at www.alzheimers.org/unraveling/index.htm.

think MCI is often an initial, transitional phase between normal brain aging and AD.

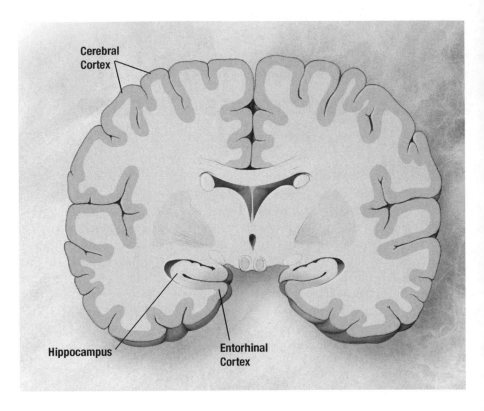

Figure 10.1. *Preclinical Alzheimer's Disease.*

Mild AD

As the disease begins to affect the cerebral cortex, memory loss continues and changes in other cognitive abilities emerge. The clinical diagnosis of AD is usually made during this stage. Signs of mild AD can include:

• Memory loss

- Confusion about the location of familiar places (getting lost begins to occur)
- Taking longer to accomplish normal daily tasks
- Trouble handling money and paying bills
- Poor judgment leading to bad decisions
- Loss of spontaneity and sense of initiative
- Mood and personality changes, increased anxiety

The growing number of plaques and tangles first damage areas of brain that control memory, language, and reasoning. It is not until later in the disease that physical abilities decline. This leads to a situation in mild AD in which a person seems to be healthy, but is actually having more and more trouble making sense of the world around him or her. The realization that something is wrong often comes gradually because the early signs can be confused with changes that can

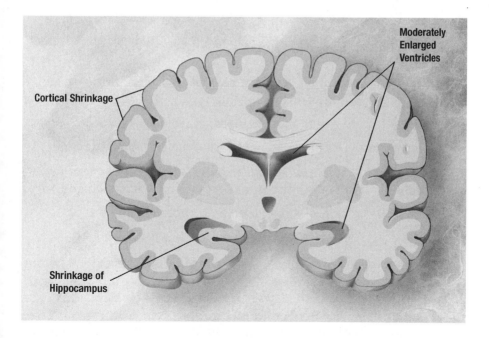

Figure 10.2. Mild Alzheimer's Disease.

happen normally with aging. Accepting these signs and deciding to go for diagnostic tests can be a big hurdle for patients and families to cross.

Moderate AD

By this stage, AD damage has spread further to the areas of the cerebral cortex that control language, reasoning, sensory processing, and conscious thought. Affected regions continue to atrophy and signs and symptoms of the disease become more pronounced and widespread. Behavior problems, such as wandering and agitation, can occur. More intensive supervision and care become necessary, and this can be difficult for many spouses and families. The symptoms of this stage can include:

- Increasing memory loss and confusion
- Shortened attention span
- Problems recognizing friends and family members
- Difficulty with language; problems with reading, writing, working with numbers
- Difficulty organizing thoughts and thinking logically
- Inability to learn new things or to cope with new or unexpected situations
- Restlessness, agitation, anxiety, tearfulness, wandering—especially in the late afternoon or at night
- Repetitive statements or movement, occasional muscle twitches
- Hallucinations, delusions, suspiciousness or paranoia, irritability
- Loss of impulse control (shown through sloppy table manners, undressing at inappropriate times or places, or vulgar language)
- Perceptual-motor problems (such as trouble getting out of a chair or setting the table)

Behavior is the result of complex brain processes, all of which take place in a fraction of a second in the healthy brain. In AD, many of these processes are disturbed, and this is the basis for many distressing or inappropriate behaviors. For example, a person may angrily refuse to take a bath or get dressed because he does not understand what his caregiver has asked him to do. If he does understand, he may not remember how to do it. The anger is a mask for his confusion and anxiety. Or, a person with AD may constantly follow her husband or caregiver and fret when the person is out of sight. To a person who cannot remember the past or anticipate the future, the world around her can be strange and frightening. Sticking close to a trusted and familiar caregiver may be the only thing that makes sense and provides security. Taking off clothes may seem reasonable to a person with AD who feels hot and doesn't understand or remember that undressing in public is not acceptable.

Severe AD

In the last stage of AD, plaques and tangles are widespread throughout the brain, and areas of the brain have atrophied further. Patients cannot recognize family and loved ones or communicate in any way. They are completely dependent on others for care. All sense of self seems to vanish. Other symptoms can include:

- Weight loss
- Seizures, skin infections, difficulty swallowing

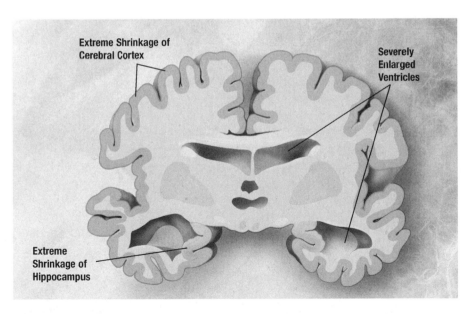

Figure 10.3. Severe Alzheimer's Disease.

- Groaning, moaning, or grunting
- Increased sleeping
- Lack of bladder and bowel control

At the end, patients may be in bed much or all of the time. Most people with AD die from other illnesses, frequently aspiration pneumonia. This type of pneumonia happens when a person is not able to swallow properly and breathes food or liquids into the lungs.

Chapter 11

The Stages of Alzheimer's Disease

Although every Alzheimer's patient is different, there are some general stages that most every patient goes through: forgetfulness, confusion, disorientation, and dependency.

Please keep in mind that your loved one may display symptoms from several stages and may move from stage to stage, and back again. Also, he may not display all of the symptoms described:

Stage 1: Forgetfulness

Symptoms

- recent memory loss begins to affect job performance
- vague complaints
- less tolerant
- angry
- less energy
- no initiative
- slow to react and learn
- forgets what he/she was just told to do

From "Overview: Stages." This information is reprinted with permission from the Greater East Ohio Area Alzheimer's Association, Akron office. © 2003. For more information, call 800-441-3322 or visit their website at www.tri countyalz.org.

- loss of spontaneity, spark, or zest for life
- loss of initiative, can't start anything
- mood/personality changes, anxious about his symptoms, keeps to himself
- poor judgment, makes bad decisions
- takes longer with routine chores
- trouble handling money, paying bills

Examples

- forgets which bills are paid
- forgets which cards are played in bridge
- forgets phone numbers and items on grocery list
- difficulty driving a car
- difficulty cooking, following recipes
- difficulty maintaining a checkbook
- loses things
- forgets to take grocery list
- arrives at wrong time or place or constantly rechecks calendar
- *"Mother's not the same—she's withdrawn, disinterested"*
- appears less outgoing, hides things, gets upset easily
- spends all day making dinner and forgets three courses
- pays the bills three times over or doesn't pay for three months

Care

- try to understand the person's anger and confusion (and your own)
- offer support in times of frustration
- begin to organize and simplify daily routines; structure the home environment for safety

Stage 2: Confusion

Symptoms

- needs assistance to manage

- can't calculate, understand, concentrate, plan, or decide
- slow to react or overreacts
- can't cope with failure
- self-absorbed
- increasing memory loss and confusion

Examples

- not performing activities of daily living such as bathing and cooking
- giving money to strangers

Care

- be prepared to offer supervision
- provide help but treat as an adult
- give one-step directions
- limit choices
- set routines
- remind and repeat gently
- encourage strengths
- accept some withdrawal

Stage 3: Disorientation

Symptoms

- obviously disabled
- lethargic
- disoriented to time and place
- uncertain how to react
- poor recent memory
- inappropriate behavior problems
- problems recognizing close friends and/or family
- repetitive statements and/or movements
- restless, especially in late afternoon and at night

- occasional muscle twitches or jerking
- perceptual-motor problems
- problems organizing thoughts and/or thinking logically
- can't find right words, makes up stories to fill in
- problems with reading, writing, and numbers
- may be suspicious, irritable, fidgety, teary, or silly
- loss of impulse control, sloppy, won't bathe or afraid to bathe, trouble dressing
- gains and then loses weight, may see or hear things that are not there: *"My daddy is waiting for me outside. I'm going home."*
- may have fixed ideas that are not real (delusions)
- needs full-time supervision

Examples

- can't remember visits immediately after you leave
- repetitive movements, statements, tapping, or folding
- sleeps often and awakens frequently at night and may try to jump up and "go to work"
- perceptual-motor problems such as having difficulty getting into a chair or setting a table
- can't find right words: *"I used to be a boss big man and now I'm an old big dummy..."*
- problems with reading numbers; can't follow written signs, write name, add or subtract
- suspicious, may accuse spouse of hiding things or of infidelity, may act childish or finger clothes constantly
- loss of impulse control such as forgetting table manners
- may forget proper place to dress/undress
- huge appetite for junk food or other people's food
- forgets when last meal occurred, then gradually loses interest in food
- examples of perceptual losses or hallucinations: *"There are babies in this house;" "The police are after me;" "I want to go home"*

Care

- devise and use memory aids
- offer reassurance
- approach slowly
- explain before doing a task
- decipher meanings
- relate to feelings, not to words
- use touch to communicate

Stage 4: Dependency

Symptoms

- can't recognize family or self in mirror
- needs assistance with simple tasks
- appears apathetic
- perception is distorted
- physical disabilities:
  - loss of coordination
  - inability to feed himself or to swallow
  - greater immobility (may be unable to walk)
  - seizures
  - skin breakdown
  - infections
  - loss of bowel and bladder control
- loses weight even with an adequate diet
- little capacity for self care
- can't communicate with words
- may put everything into mouth or touch everything

Examples

- looks in the mirror and talks to own image
- needs help with bathing, dressing, eating, or toileting
- may groan, scream, or make grunting sounds

73

Care

- assist with daily needs
- remember that the behavior is not intentional
- understand the disease is affecting the patient
- ask for support in both practical and emotional matters
- look to the community for resources/respite care
- nursing home placement may need to be considered

Part Two

Other Dementias and Related Disorders

Chapter 12

AIDS Dementia Complex

Dementia is a brain disorder that affects a person's ability to think clearly and can impact his or her daily activities. AIDS dementia complex (ADC)—dementia caused by HIV infection—is a complicated syndrome made up of different nervous system and mental symptoms. These symptoms are somewhat common in people with HIV disease.

The frequency of ADC increases with advancing HIV disease and as CD4+ cell counts decrease. It is fairly uncommon in people with early HIV disease, but it's more common in people with severely weakened immune systems and symptoms of advanced disease. Severe ADC is almost exclusively seen only in people with advanced HIV disease.

ADC consists of many conditions that can be of varying degrees and may progressively worsen. These conditions can easily be mistaken for symptoms of other common HIV-associated problems including depression, drug side effects or opportunistic infections that affect the brain like toxoplasmosis or lymphoma. Symptoms of ADC may include poor concentration, forgetfulness, loss of short- or long-term memory, social withdrawal, slowed thinking, short attention span, irritability, apathy (lack of caring or concern for oneself or others), weakness, poor coordination, impaired judgment, problems with vision and personality change.

Reprinted with permission from "AIDS Dementia Complex," © April 2002. From Project Inform. For more information, contact the National HIV/AIDS Treatment Hotline 800-822-7422, or visit our website, www.projectinform.org.

Because ADC varies so much from person to person, it is poorly understood and has been reported and described in many conflicting ways. This chapter will shed light on some of these issues as well as the available treatments for ADC.

Possible Symptoms of Early Stage ADC

- Difficulty concentrating
- Difficulty remembering phone numbers or appointments
- Slowed thinking
- Longer time needed to complete complicated tasks
- Reliance on list keeping to help track daily activities
- Mental status tests and other mental capabilities may be normal
- Irritability
- Unsteady gait (walk) or difficulty keeping balance
- Poor hand coordination and change in writing
- Depression

Possible Symptoms of Middle Stage ADC

- Symptoms of motor dysfunction, like muscle weakness
- Poor performance on regular tasks
- More concentration and attention required
- Slow responses and frequently dropping objects
- General feelings of indifference or apathy
- Slowness in normal activities, like eating and writing
- Walking, balance and coordination requires a great deal of effort

Possible Symptoms of Late Stage ADC

- Loss of bladder or bowel control
- Spastic gait, making walking more difficult
- Loss of initiative or interest
- Withdrawing from life
- Psychosis or mania
- Confinement to bed

What Is ADC?

ADC is characterized by severe changes in four areas: a person's ability to understand, process and remember information (cognition); behavior; ability to coordinate muscles and movement (motor coordination); or emotions (mood). These changes are called ADC when they're believed to be related to HIV itself rather than other factors that might cause them, like other brain infections, drug side effects, etc.

In ADC, cognitive impairment is often characterized by memory loss, speech problems, inability to concentrate and poor judgment. Cognitive problems are often the first symptoms a person with ADC will notice. These include the need to make lists in order to remember routine tasks or forgetting, in mid-sentence, what one was talking about.

Behavioral changes in ADC are the least understood and defined. They can be described as impairments in one's ability to perform common tasks and activities of daily living. These changes are found in 30–40% of people with early ADC.

Motor impairment is often characterized by a loss of control of the bladder; loss of feeling in and loss of control of the legs; and stiff, awkward or obviously slowed movements. Motor impairment is not common in early ADC. Early symptoms may include a change in handwriting.

Mood impairments are defined as changes in emotional responses. In ADC, this impairment is associated with conditions, such as severe depression, severe personality changes (psychosis) and, less commonly, intense excitability (mania).

The Symptoms of ADC

Properly diagnosing ADC is heavily dependent on the keen judgment of doctors, often together with specialists like psychiatric, brain or neurology experts. It's easy to imagine how difficult it is to determine impairments in mood and behavior since there's no standard or common course of ADC. In one person it may be very mild with periods of varying severity of symptoms. In another it can be abrupt, severe and progressive. Currently, there is no way to tell how a person will progress with ADC.

Sometimes symptoms of ADC are overlooked or dismissed by caregivers, who may believe the symptoms are due to advanced HIV disease. In fact, people with advanced disease generally do not have symptoms of ADC but do have fairly normal mental functioning as long as they also have no other neurological problems. At the other end of the spectrum, ADC should be carefully distinguished from severe depression—common among people with HIV that may result in symptoms similar to ADC.

ADC occurs more commonly in children with HIV than with adults. It presents similarly and is often more severe and progressive.

How Does HIV Cause ADC?

While it is clear that HIV can cause serious nervous system disease, how it causes ADC is unclear. In general, nervous system and mental disorders are caused by the death of nerve cells. While HIV does not directly infect nerve cells, it's thought that HIV can somehow kill them indirectly.

Macrophages—white cells that are prevalent in the brain and act as large reservoirs for HIV—appear to be HIV's first target in the central nervous system. HIV-infected macrophages can carry HIV into the brain from the bloodstream. Test tube studies offer these hypotheses about how macrophages may help destroy nerve cells:

- An infected macrophage in the brain may shed a particle on HIV's outer coat (called gp120), causing damage to nerve cells.

- HIV's TAT gene, which helps produce new virus, detaches from HIV and circulates in the blood, causing toxic effects in nerve cells.

- The macrophage itself releases a number of substances that, in excess, can be toxic to the brain. Some examples are quinolinic acid and nitric oxide, among an array of other signal molecules. These can bind to nerve cells and cause cell dysfunction or death. Research has found higher levels of quinolinic acid and other markers of cell activation in the CSF of people with ADC.

- HIV infection of other brain cells, including astrocytes.

Incidence

Anecdotal reports indicate that there are fewer people with ADC since anti-HIV therapy became standard. People who develop ADC today tend to be "sicker" than those who developed it before the use of anti-HIV therapy. One early study from England supports this theory.

The British study found that only 2% of people with AIDS taking AZT developed ADC from 1982–1988, compared to 20% of those not on AZT. The incidence of ADC dropped from 53% in 1987 (before the arrival of AZT) to 3% in 1988 (after the arrival of AZT).

Early in the epidemic, many new AIDS cases were attributed to ADC. These newly diagnosed people often had ADC but no other AIDS-related condition. Many doctors report that they are no longer seeing people who have just ADC. It has increasingly become a disease of late-stage AIDS when people suffer from multiple infections.

Diagnosing ADC

Three tests are required to diagnose ADC accurately: a mental status exam, one of the standard scans (CT and/or MRI), and a spinal tap. These may also help tell ADC apart from other brain disorders like toxoplasmosis, PML (progressive multifocal leukoencephalopathy) or lymphoma. Care should be taken, however, as ADC may occur along with the symptoms of other brain disorders. Diagnosing both conditions at the same time can be more difficult.

The main way to detect and evaluate ADC is through a mental status exam. The examination is designed to reveal problems like short- or long-term memory loss, problems with orientation, concentration and abstract thinking as well as swings in mood. Imaging of the brain with scans (like an x-ray) is also used. Certain lab tests can also be useful like examining cerebrospinal fund (CSF), obtained by a spinal tap (also called lumbar puncture).

CT and MRI scans are routinely used in the detection of ADC. CT scans are x-rays that use special beams to produce detailed images of organs and structures within the body. In people with ADC these scans usually show signs of destroyed brain tissue. MRI, or Magnetic Resonance Imaging, is a sensitive brain scan that is used when CT findings are not conclusive. Results from both of these tests are helpful in ruling out other causes for the symptoms.

Tests of CSF may help determine if someone has ADC, but they are not conclusive. Mostly they're used to rule out other causes of the symptoms of ADC, and that's why they're important. Many people with ADC have higher levels of certain proteins or white blood cells in their CSF. However, not everyone with these levels turn out to have ADC. Also, people with advanced ADC are generally more likely to have higher HIV levels in their CSF, although people with no symptoms of brain disorders sometimes have high HIV levels in their CSF.

What If I Think I Have ADC?

- Don't be afraid to tell your doctor or any other providers that you suspect something is wrong. If you don't have a doctor or need help finding one, contact local AIDS organizations for help in getting one. They can also help you find a doctor for a second opinion if you need one.

- Keep a small notepad with you and write down your symptoms whenever they occur. This information will greatly help your doctor to help you.

- Build as much support as possible, including friends, family and professionals. Although it's possible to treat ADC successfully, it may take awhile for some symptoms to go away.

Treating ADC

The best therapies to treat ADC appear to be anti-HIV drugs, and high-dose AZT is the most studied drug for it. However, many specialists contend that how well a potent regimen controls HIV reproduction overall is more important than the actual drugs used in the regimen. This may or may not include using standard, or even high-dose, AZT as part of the regimen.

Generally speaking, creating an anti-HIV regimen with the extra goal of treating ADC follows three basic principals:

1. Start a potent regimen (usually 3 drugs) to decrease HIV levels to below the limit of detection of viral load tests;

2. In people who have used anti-HIV therapy before, consider the prior therapy history as well as information from anti-HIV resistance tests;

3. If possible, use anti-HIV drugs that cross the blood-brain barrier as part of a combination therapy regimen.

It's believed—based on findings that high-dose AZT (1,000–1,200 mg/daily) can cross the blood-brain-barrier and effectively treat ADC—that an anti-HIV drug that crosses the blood-brain barrier might help prevent or treat ADC. To date, AZT is the best understood treatment available for ADC. Several groups have reported improvements in cognitive functions with AZT as well as prevention of HIV infection of the brain. Larger doses (1,000 mg compared to the now-standard 600 mg per day) of AZT appear to be necessary for treating ADC. However, high-dose AZT may present problems since many people with HIV, particularly those who are the sickest, are often unable to tolerate its side effects.

While AZT may be the most researched drug for treating ADC, other anti-HIV drugs that cross the blood-brain barrier may be equally useful. These include AZT, d4T (stavudine, Zerit), abacavir (Ziagen), nevirapine (Viramune), amprenavir (Agenerase) and to a lesser degree indinavir (Crixivan) and 3TC (lamivudine, Epivir). Efavirenz (Sustiva) has not been shown to cross this barrier to a significant degree, but some experts speculate that it may be useful in treating ADC.

Anti-HIV therapies are best used in combinations. It may also be important to consider a drug's ability to cross into the brain when constructing an effective regimen. For information on developing long-term strategies and creating potent anti-HIV therapy regimen, call Project Inform's hotline.

Treating the Symptoms of ADC

Psycho-active drugs are often used to treat the symptoms of ADC. These include anti-psychotics, anti-depressants, anxiolytics, psycho-stimulants, anti-manics, and anti-convulsants. These drugs do not treat the underlying cause of ADC, or even stop its progression. However, they may ease some of its symptoms. Haloperidol (Haldol) is often used for easing ADC symptoms, though it has many side effects. People with ADC are sensitive to Haldol, so small doses of 5–10 mg daily should be used to avoid severe side effects.

Ritalin (methylphenidate) has been used with success in people with ADC to ease apathy and to increase energy, concentration and appetite. Daily doses of 5–10 mg are often sufficient.

In cases of severe behavior disorders, anti-psychotics like Thorazine and Mellaril can be used to control agitation. Lorazepam (Ativan) and diazepam (Valium) may also be used for sedation and controlling anxiety. Other drugs include perphenazine (Trilafon), thiothixene (Navane), molindone (Moban), and fluoxetine (Prozac) with bupropion (Wellbutrin).

Many of the therapies listed here may have potential drug interaction with commonly used anti-HIV therapies as well as therapies to treat or prevent HIV-related conditions. For more information about drug interactions, call Project Inform's hotline.

What If Someone I Care for Has Symptoms or Was Diagnosed with ADC?

- Help them access the proper diagnosis and treatment.

- Understand that loss of mental and emotional control is terribly frightening for most people, even if it's only moderate or short-term. However, be honest about their symptoms as you offer support and encouragement to establish trust.

- Because mood changes and memory problems are common with ADC, you may encounter resistance while trying to help. Helping the person you care for to write down their symptoms in their own handwriting, as they experience them, can sometimes encourage them to seek medical care.

- Professional caregivers, like home health aides, are sometimes needed to care for people with severe ADC or ADC that doesn't respond to treatment. Seeking this kind of support is sometimes the best way to help those you love.

- Caregiving for someone with memory and behavioral problems can be overwhelming, especially if it's over a long period of time. There are support services in many cities for those who care for others with life-threatening illnesses.

Conclusion

New treatments for ADC are desperately needed. It's also important that new anti-HIV drugs be fully evaluated for their usefulness in treating ADC. At the same time, promising drugs that may work to treat the underlying causes of ADC also need to be investigated.

This material has been produced as a result of a collaboration between Project Inform and Gay Men's Health Crisis. For more information about Project Inform, call the Project Inform hotline at 1-800-822-7422. For more information about Gay Men's Health Crisis in New York, call 212-367-1451. Special thanks goes to Dr. Richard Price of University of California's San Francisco General Hospital, Neurology Services and Dr. Justin McArthur, Professor of Neurology and Epidemiology at John Hopkins University in Baltimore for their editorial support.

Chapter 13

Binswanger's Disease

What is Binswanger's disease?

Binswanger's disease, sometimes referred to as subcortical dementia, is a rare form of dementia characterized by cerebrovascular lesions in the deep white-matter of the brain, loss of memory and cognition, and mood changes. Patients usually show signs of abnormal blood pressure, stroke, blood abnormalities, disease of the large blood vessels in the neck, and disease of the heart valves. Other prominent features of the disease include urinary incontinence, difficulty walking, clumsiness, slowness of conduct, lack of facial expression, and speech difficulty. These symptoms, which tend to begin after the age of 60, are not always present in all patients and may sometimes appear only as a passing phase.

Is there any treatment?

There is no specific course of treatment for Binswanger's disease. Treatment is symptomatic, often involving the use of medications to control high blood pressure, depression, heart arrhythmias and low blood pressure.

What is the prognosis?

Binswanger's disease is a slowly progressive condition for which there is no cure. The disorder is often marked by strokes and partial recovery.

"NINDS Binswanger's Disease Information Page," National Institute of Neurological Disorders and Stroke (NINDS), reviewed November 2002. For more information from NINDS visit www.ninds.nih.gov.

What research is being done?

The National Institute of Neurological Disorders and Stroke (NINDS) conducts and supports a wide range of research on dementing disorders, and scientists are currently re-evaluating the definitions for certain dementias, including Binswanger's disease/subcortical dementia. The goals of research are to improve the diagnosis of dementias and to find ways to treat and prevent them. The National Institute on Aging and the National Institute of Mental Health also support research related to the dementias.

Chapter 14

Cerebral Atrophy

What is cerebral atrophy?

Cerebral atrophy is a condition characterized by a decrease in the size or a wasting away of brain cells and tissues. It may result from malnutrition, abnormal cell or hormonal changes, or stroke. Symptoms include muscle weakness, vision or speech impairments, and dementia. Neuroimaging techniques such as magnetic resonance imaging (MRI), computed tomography (CT), positron emission tomography (PET), and single-photon emission computed tomography (SPECT), are used to diagnose the disorder. Cerebral atrophy may be a feature of numerous disorders, and may affect only part of the brain.

Is there any treatment?

Generally, treatment—which is symptomatic and supportive—depends upon the specific disorder of which cerebral atrophy is a component. In some cases, drug therapy may relieve some symptoms. Care that maintains and stimulates individuals with the disorder improves their quality of life.

What is the prognosis?

The prognosis for individuals with the disorder varies. Progressive cerebral atrophy is fatal because the atrophy spreads to all parts of

"NINDS Cerebral Atrophy Information Page," National Institute of Neurological Disorders and Stroke (NINDS), reviewed July 2001. For more information from NINDS, visit www.ninds.nih.gov.

87

the brain. Cerebral atrophy that is limited to a specific area of the brain affects normal functioning, however, it is not necessarily fatal.

What research is being done?

The National Institute of Neurological Disorders and Stroke (NINDS) conducts and supports research on conditions of the brain and spinal cord, including cerebral atrophy. Much of this research focuses on learning more about the cause(s) of these conditions, and finding ways to prevent and treat them.

Chapter 15

Creutzfeldt-Jakob Disease (CJD)

What is Creutzfeldt-Jakob disease?

Creutzfeldt-Jakob disease (CJD) is a rare, degenerative, invariably fatal brain disorder. It affects about one person in every one million people per year worldwide; in the United States there are about 200 cases per year. CJD usually appears in later life and runs a rapid course. Typically, onset of symptoms occurs about age 60, and about 90 percent of patients die within one year. In the early stages of disease, patients may have failing memory, behavioral changes, lack of coordination and visual disturbances. As the illness progresses, mental deterioration becomes pronounced and involuntary movements, blindness, weakness of extremities, and coma may occur.

There are three major categories of CJD:

- In sporadic CJD, the disease appears even though the person has no known risk factors for the disease. This is by far the most common type of CJD and accounts for at least 85 percent of cases.

- In hereditary CJD, the person has a family history of the disease and/or tests positive for a genetic mutation associated with CJD. About 5 to 10 percent of cases of CJD in the United States are hereditary.

"Creutzfeldt-Jakob Disease Fact Sheet," National Institute of Neurological Disorders and Stroke (NINDS), reviewed March 15, 2002. For more information from NINDS, visit www.ninds.nih.gov.

- In acquired CJD, the disease is transmitted by exposure to brain or nervous system tissue, usually through certain medical procedures. There is no evidence that CJD is contagious through casual contact with a CJD patient. Since CJD was first described in 1920, fewer than one percent of cases have been acquired CJD.

CJD belongs to a family of human and animal diseases known as the transmissible spongiform encephalopathies (TSEs). Spongiform refers to the characteristic appearance of infected brains, which become filled with holes until they resemble sponges under a microscope. CJD is the most common of the known human TSEs. Other human TSEs include kuru, fatal familial insomnia (FFI), and Gerstmann-Straussler-Scheinker disease (GSS). Kuru was identified in people of an isolated tribe in Papua New Guinea and has now almost disappeared. Fatal familial insomnia and GSS are extremely rare hereditary diseases, found in just a few families around the world. Other TSEs are found in specific kinds of animals. These include bovine spongiform encephalopathy (BSE), which is found in cows and often referred to as "mad cow" disease, scrapie, which affects sheep and goats, mink encephalopathy, and feline encephalopathy. Similar diseases have occurred in elk, deer, and exotic zoo animals.

What are the symptoms of the disease?

CJD is characterized as a rapidly progressive dementia. Initially, patients experience problems with muscular coordination; personality changes, including impaired memory, judgment, and thinking; and impaired vision. People with the disease also may experience insomnia, depression, or unusual sensations. CJD does not cause a fever or other flu-like symptoms. As the illness progresses, the patients' mental impairment becomes severe. They often develop involuntary muscle jerks called myoclonus, and they may go blind. They eventually lose the ability to move and speak and enter a coma. Pneumonia and other infections often occur in these patients and can lead to death.

There are several known variants of CJD. These variants differ somewhat in the symptoms and course of the disease. For example, a variant form of the disease—called new variant or variant (nv-CJD, v-CJD), described in Great Britain and France—begins primarily with psychiatric symptoms, affects younger patients than other types of CJD, and has a longer than usual duration from onset of symptoms to death. Another variant, called the panencephalopathic form, occurs primarily in Japan and has a relatively long course, with symptoms often progressing for several years. Scientists are trying to learn what causes these variations in symptoms and course of the disease. Some symptoms of CJD can be similar to symptoms of other progressive neurological disorders, such as Alzheimer's or Huntington's disease. However, CJD causes unique changes in brain tissue which can be seen at autopsy. It also tends to cause more rapid deterioration of a person's abilities than Alzheimer's disease or most other types of dementia.

How is CJD diagnosed?

There is currently no single diagnostic test for CJD. When a doctor suspects CJD, the first concern is to rule out treatable forms of dementia such as encephalitis (inflammation of the brain) or chronic meningitis. A neurological examination will be performed and the doctor may seek consultation with other physicians. Standard diagnostic tests will include a spinal tap to rule out more common causes of dementia and an electroencephalogram (EEG) to record the brain's electrical pattern, which can be particularly valuable because it shows a specific type of abnormality in CJD. Computerized tomography of the brain can help rule out the possibility that the symptoms result from other problems such as stroke or a brain tumor. Magnetic resonance imaging (MRI) brain scans also can reveal characteristic patterns of brain degeneration that can help diagnose CJD.

The only way to confirm a diagnosis of CJD is by brain biopsy or autopsy. In a brain biopsy, a neurosurgeon removes a small piece of tissue from the patient's brain so that it can be examined by a neuropathologist. This procedure may be dangerous for the patient, and the operation does not always obtain tissue from the affected part of the brain. Because a correct diagnosis of CJD does not help the patient, a brain biopsy is discouraged unless it is needed to rule out a treatable disorder. In an autopsy, the whole brain is examined after death. Both brain biopsy and autopsy pose a small, but definite, risk that the surgeon or others who handle the brain tissue may become accidentally infected by self-inoculation. Special surgical and disinfection procedures can minimize this risk. A fact sheet with guidance on these procedures is available from the National Institute of Neurological Disorders and Stroke (NINDS) and the World Health Organization.

Scientists are working to develop laboratory tests for CJD. One such test, developed at NINDS, is performed on a person's cerebrospinal fluid and detects a protein marker that indicates neuronal degeneration.

This can help diagnose CJD in people who already show the clinical symptoms of the disease. This test is much easier and safer than a brain biopsy. The false positive rate is about 5 to 10 percent. Scientists are working to develop this test for use in commercial laboratories. There have been reports of other ways of diagnosing the disease, including tonsil biopsies, which may lead to other tests.

How is the disease treated?

There is no treatment that can cure or control CJD. Researchers have tested many drugs, including amantadine, steroids, interferon, acyclovir, antiviral agents, and antibiotics. However, none of these treatments has shown any consistent benefit.

Current treatment for CJD is aimed at alleviating symptoms and making the patient as comfortable as possible. Opiate drugs can help relieve pain if it occurs, and the drugs clonazepam and sodium valproate may help relieve myoclonus. During later stages of the disease, changing the person's position frequently can keep him or her comfortable and helps prevent bedsores. A catheter can be used to drain urine if the patient cannot control bladder function, and intravenous fluids and artificial feeding also may be used.

What causes Creutzfeldt-Jakob disease?

Some researchers believe an unusual "slow virus" or another organism causes CJD. However, they have never been able to isolate a virus or other organism in people with the disease. Furthermore, the agent that causes CJD has several characteristics that are unusual for known organisms such as viruses and bacteria. It is difficult to kill, it does not appear to contain any genetic information in the form of nucleic acids (DNA or RNA), and it usually has a long incubation period before symptoms appear. In some cases, the incubation period may be as long as 40 years. The leading scientific theory at this time maintains that CJD and the other TSEs are caused not by an organism but by a type of protein called a prion.

Prions occur in both a normal form, which is a harmless protein found in the body's cells; and in an infectious form, which causes disease. The harmless and infectious forms of the prion protein are nearly identical, but the infectious form takes a different folded shape than the normal protein. Sporadic CJD may develop because some of a person's normal prions spontaneously change into the infectious form of the protein and then alter the prions in other cells in a chain reaction.

Once they appear, abnormal prion proteins stick together and form fibers and/or clumps called plaques that can be seen with powerful microscopes. Fibers and plaques may start to accumulate years before symptoms of CJD begin to appear. It is still unclear what role these abnormalities play in the disease or how they might affect symptoms.

About 5 to 10 percent of all CJD cases are inherited. These cases arise from a mutation, or change, in the gene that controls formation of the normal prion protein. While prions themselves do not contain genetic information and do not require genes to reproduce themselves, infectious prions can arise if a mutation occurs in the gene for the body's normal prions. If the prion gene is altered in a person's sperm or egg cells, the mutation can be transmitted to the person's offspring. Several different mutations in the prion gene have been identified. The particular mutation found in each family affects how frequently the disease appears and what symptoms are most noticeable. However, not all people with mutations in the prion gene develop CJD. This suggests that the mutations merely increase susceptibility to CJD and that other, still-unknown factors also play a role in the disease.

How is CJD transmitted?

CJD is not a contagious disease. Although it can be transmitted to other people, the risk of this happening is extremely small. CJD cannot be transmitted through the air or through touching or most other forms of casual contact. Spouses and other household members of sporadic CJD patients have no higher risk of contracting the disease than the general population. However, direct or indirect contact with brain tissue and spinal cord fluid from infected patients should be avoided to prevent transmission of the disease through these materials.

In a few very rare cases, CJD has spread to other people from grafts of dura mater (a tissue that covers the brain), transplanted corneas, implantation of inadequately sterilized electrodes in the brain, and injections of contaminated pituitary growth hormone derived from human pituitary glands taken from cadavers. Doctors call these cases that are linked to medical procedures iatrogenic cases. Since 1985, all human growth hormone used in the United States has been synthesized by recombinant DNA procedures, which eliminates the risk of transmitting CJD by this route.

The appearance of the new variant of CJD (nv-CJD or v-CJD) in several younger than average people in Great Britain and France has led to concern that BSE may be transmitted to humans through consumption of contaminated beef. Although laboratory tests have shown a strong similarity between the prions causing BSE and v-CJD, there is no direct proof to support this theory. Furthermore, BSE has never been found in the United States, and importation of cattle and beef from countries with BSE has been banned in the United States since 1989 to reduce the risk that it will occur in this country.

Many people are concerned that it may be possible to transmit CJD through blood and related blood products such as plasma. Some animal studies suggest that contaminated blood and related products may transmit the disease, although this has never been shown in humans. If there are infectious agents in these fluids, they are probably in very low concentrations. Scientists do not know how many abnormal prions a person must receive before he or she develops CJD, so they do not know whether these fluids are potentially infectious or not. They do know that, even though millions of people receive blood transfusions each year, there are no reported cases of someone contracting CJD from a transfusion. Even among hemophiliacs, who sometimes receive blood plasma concentrated from thousands of people, there are no reported cases of CJD. This suggests that, if there is a risk of transmitting CJD through blood or plasma, it is extremely small.

How can people avoid spreading the disease?

To reduce the already very low risk of CJD transmission from one person to another, people should never donate blood, tissues, or organs if they have suspected or confirmed CJD, or if they are at increased risk because of a family history of the disease, a dura mater graft, or other factor.

Normal sterilization procedures such as cooking, washing, and boiling do not destroy prions. Caregivers, health care workers, and undertakers should take the following precautions when they are working with a person with CJD:

- Wash hands and exposed skin before eating, drinking, or smoking.

- Cover cuts and abrasions with waterproof dressings.

- Wear surgical gloves when handling a patient's tissues and fluids or dressing the patient's wounds.

- Avoid cutting or sticking themselves with instruments contaminated by the patient's blood or other tissues.

- Use disposable bedclothes and other cloth for contact with the patient. If disposable materials are not available, regular cloth should be soaked in undiluted chlorine bleach for an hour or more, then washed in a normal fashion after each use.

- Use face protection if there is a risk of splashing contaminated material such as blood or cerebrospinal fluid.

- Soak instruments that have come in contact with the patient in undiluted chlorine bleach for an hour or more, then use an autoclave (pressure cooker) to sterilize them in distilled water for at least one hour at 132–134 degrees Centigrade.

A fact sheet listing additional precautions for healthcare workers and morticians is available from the NINDS and the World Health Organization.

What research is taking place?

Many researchers are studying CJD. They are examining whether the transmissible agent is, in fact, a prion or a product of the infection, and are trying to discover factors that influence prion infectivity and how the disorder damages the brain. Using rodent models of the disease and brain tissue from autopsies, they are also trying to identify factors that influence susceptibility to the disease and that govern when in life the disease appears. They hope to use this knowledge to develop improved tests for CJD and to learn what changes ultimately kill the neurons so that effective treatments can be developed.

How can I help research?

Scientists are conducting biochemical analyses of brain tissue, blood, spinal fluid, urine, and serum in hope of determining the nature of the transmissible agent or agents causing Creutzfeldt-Jakob disease. To help with this research, they are seeking biopsy and autopsy tissue, blood, and cerebrospinal fluid from patients with CJD and related diseases. A list of investigators interested in receiving such material is available online at www.ninds.nih.gov/health_and_ medical/pubs/creutzfeldt-jakob_disease_fact_sheet.htm.

Where can I get help?

The following organization can provide information and support for people and families affected by Creutzfeldt-Jakob disease:

Creutzfeldt-Jakob Disease Foundation
P.O. Box 611625
North Miami, FL 33261-1625
Toll-Free: 800-659-1991 (Help Line)
Website: http://www.cjdfoundation.org

If you are interested in learning more about steps taken to ensure the safety of beef and other agricultural products in the United States, contact:

United States Department of Agriculture (USDA)
National Agricultural Library
10301 Baltimore Avenue
Beltsville, MD 20705-2351
Phone: 301-504-5755
Website: http://www.usda.gov

For information on the safety of medical products and procedures, contact:

Food and Drug Administration
Office of Consumer Affairs, Room 1685
5600 Fishers Lane
Rockville, MD 20857
Toll Free: 888-463-6332
Website: http://www.fda.gov

Chapter 16

Delirium and Confusional States

Delirium (Acute Confusional State)

Definition: A clinical state characterized by fluctuating disturbances in cognition, mood, attention, arousal, and self-awareness, which arises acutely, either without prior intellectual impairment or superimposed on chronic intellectual impairment.

Some practitioners use the terms delirium and acute confusional state synonymously; others use delirium to refer to a subset of confused people with hyperactivity. Still others use delirium to refer to full-blown confusion and confusional state to refer to mild disorientation.

A person who is less alert (with clouding of consciousness) and has difficulty paying attention also has difficulty accurately perceiving and interpreting data from the environment and acquiring or remembering new information; he may misinterpret factual information or have illusions. As a result, the person does not reason logically, has difficulty manipulating symbolic data (for example, performing arithmetic or explaining proverbs), becomes anxious and agitated or withdraws from the environment, and may think in paranoid and delusional ways.

Etiology

Delirium may occur in persons with a normal brain but is more common in those with underlying brain disease, such as dementia. It is more common in the elderly, probably due to changes in neurotransmitters, geriatric cerebral cell loss, and concomitant disease. Delirium may be due to primary brain diseases or diseases elsewhere in the body that affect the brain; causes are usually metabolic, toxic, structural, or infectious. Regardless of cause, the cerebral hemispheres or the arousal mechanisms of the thalamus and reticular activating system of the brain stem become physiologically impaired. Disruption of sleep and extreme stress superimposed on acute disease may worsen symptoms of delirium (as in intensive care psychosis).

Metabolic or toxic causes: Virtually any metabolic disorder can cause delirium. Some important metabolic and toxic causes of delirium are listed in Table 16.1. In elderly persons, drug side effects are the most common cause.

Structural causes: Structural lesions that can precipitate delirium include vascular occlusion and cerebral infarction, subarachnoid hemorrhage, cerebral hemorrhage, primary or metastatic brain tumors,

Table 16.1. Metabolic and Toxic Causes of Delirium

Disorders	Drugs with Anti-cholinergic Properties	Other Drugs
Anoxia	Antiemetics	Alcohol
Hyperkalemia	Antihistamines (e.g.,	Antihypertensives
Hyperparathyroidism	diphenhydramine)	Benzodiazepines
Hyperthyroidism	Antiparkinsonian drugs	Cimetidine
Hypoglycemia	Antipsychotics	Digoxin
Hypokalemia	Antispasmodics	Narcotics
Hypothyroidism	Muscle relaxants	Other CNS depres-
Metabolic acidosis	Tricyclic antidepressants	sants
Postconcussion		
Postictal state		
Transient ischemia		

subdural hematomas, and brain abscesses. Most structural lesions can be detected by CT (computed tomography) or MRI (magnetic resonance imaging), and many produce focal neurologic signs observable during physical examination.

Infectious causes: Delirium may be caused by acute meningitis or encephalitis or by infections outside the brain, perhaps through the elaboration of toxins or production of fever. Pneumonia (even without impaired oxygenation), urinary tract infections, sepsis, or fever from viral infections can produce confusion in the vulnerable brain. Slower-developing embolic abscesses or opportunistic infections are difficult to diagnose clinically and, in some cases, require brain biopsies for proper evaluation.

Symptoms and Signs

The symptoms of delirium often fluctuate rapidly, even within a matter of minutes, and tend to be worse late in the day (sundowning). The most prominent is a clouding of consciousness accompanied by disorientation to time, place, or person. The ability to pay attention is poor. Confusion regarding day-to-day events and daily routines is common. Changes in personality and affect are common. Symptoms include irritability, inappropriate behavior, fearfulness, excessive energy, or even frankly psychotic features, such as delusions, hallucinations (commonly visual), or paranoia. Some persons become quiet, withdrawn, or apathetic, whereas others become agitated or hyperactive; physical restlessness is often expressed by pacing. A person may display contradictory emotions within a short time span. Thinking becomes disorganized, and speech is often disordered, with prominent slurring, rapidity, neologisms, aphasic errors, or chaotic patterns. Normal patterns of sleeping and eating are usually grossly distorted. Some persons experience dizziness.

Diagnosis

A rapid medical evaluation is imperative because delirium can have a grave prognosis and the underlying condition is often treatable. According to some estimates, 18% of hospitalized elderly persons with delirium die, and hospitalization is twice as long for those who develop confusion as for those who do not.

The diagnosis rests almost entirely on clinical grounds. Diagnostic criteria are listed in Table 16.2. Laboratory tests should include full chemistries, CBC (complete blood count) with differential, a test for syphilis such as the Venereal Disease Research Laboratories (VDRL) test, urinalysis with culture, blood cultures, thyroid function tests, vitamin B_{12} levels, and a toxicology screening. Unless status epilepticus (an extremely rare finding in the elderly) or encephalitis is suspected, EEGs (electroencephalograms), lumbar punctures, single

Table 16.2. Diagnostic Criteria for Delirium

Disturbance of consciousness (reduced clarity of awareness of the environment) with reduced ability to focus, sustain, or shift attention.

Change in cognition (for example, memory deficit, disorientation, language disturbance) or development of a perceptual disturbance that is not better accounted for by preexisting, established, or evolving dementia.

The disturbance develops over a short time (usually hours or days) and tends to fluctuate during the course of the day.

For delirium due to a general medical condition:

Evidence from the history, physical examination, or laboratory tests that the disturbance is due to the direct physiologic consequences of a general medical condition.

For substance intoxication delirium:

Evidence from the history, physical examination, or laboratory tests that either

1. Symptoms listed in the first two criteria developed during substance intoxication
2. Drug use is etiologically related to the disturbance.

For substance withdrawal delirium:

Evidence from the history, physical examination, or laboratory tests that the symptoms listed in the first two criteria developed during or shortly after a withdrawal syndrome.

For delirium due to multiple etiologies:

Evidence from the history, physical examination, or laboratory test that the delirium has more than one etiology (for example, more than one general medical condition, a general medical condition plus substance intoxication or a drug side effect).

Source: Modified from American Psychiatric Association: *Diagnostic and Statistical Manual of Mental Disorders*, fourth edition, Washington, DC, American Psychiatric Association, 1994, pp. 129, 131–133; reprinted with permission. Copyright, 1994 American Psychiatric Association.

photon emission computed tomography, and positron emission tomography are not useful. A single CT scan with contrast can detect old or recent infarctions or subdural hematomas.

Delirium with apathy must be differentiated from depression, especially in the elderly, although the two often occur together. Similarly, agitation and hallucinations associated with delirium must be distinguished from those of a functional psychosis—a psychiatric disorder that almost always lacks the disorientation, memory loss, and cognitive impairment found in delirious (or intoxicated) patients. A history of manic illness or schizophreniform disorders suggests a diagnosis of psychiatric disease.

Systemic medical diseases may precipitate delirium and should be sought to guide treatment; an example is the Wernicke-Korsakoff syndrome, which is marked by confusion, disorientation, and memory loss. Hypothermia, tachycardia, hypotension, tremor, and ophthalmoplegia strongly suggest alcohol-related disease. Status epilepticus consisting of absence or complex partial seizures can produce a confused state that is hard to distinguish from delirium. The seizure states, however, produce a steadier but less intense pattern of bewilderment and less drowsiness than does delirium. Despite a confused appearance, affected epileptic patients usually have a surprisingly good sense of direction compared with most delirious patients. Nonconvulsive status epilepticus can be readily detected by EEG. EEG recordings with spike and wave or sharp wave discharges are diagnostic. Delirium alone seldom precipitates convulsive status epilepticus, but a generalized tonic-clonic seizure often results in a state of delirium for up to a day or more. In encephalopathy, the EEG shows a rhythm slower than alpha from both hemispheres. Triphasic waves may appear in hepatic or renal encephalopathy.

Treatment

Symptoms are usually reversible when the underlying cause is identified quickly and managed properly, particularly if the cause is hypoglycemia, an infection, an iatrogenic factor, drug toxicity, or an electrolyte imbalance. However, recovery may be slow (days to even weeks or months), especially in the elderly.

All unnecessary drugs should be stopped. Identifiable disease should be treated, and fluids and nutrients should be given. A patient suspected of alcohol abuse or withdrawal should be given thiamine 100 mg IM (intramuscular) daily for at least 5 days, to ensure absorption. During hospitalization, such patients should be monitored for

signs of withdrawal, which can be manifested by autonomic disturbances and worsening confusion.

The environment should be as quiet and calm as possible, prefer-
ably with low lighting but not total darkness. Staff and family members should reassure the patient, reinforce orientation, and explain
proceedings at every opportunity. Additional drugs should be avoided
unless needed to reverse the underlying condition. However, sometimes agitation must be treated symptomatically, particularly when
it threatens the well-being of the patient, a caregiver, or a staff member. Restraints used judiciously can help prevent the patient from
pulling out IV (intravenous) and other lines. Restraints should be
applied by someone trained in their use, released at least every 2 hours
to prevent injury, and discontinued as soon as possible.

Few scientific data are available to guide the choice of drugs to treat
delirium. Low doses of haloperidol (as little as 0.25 mg po, IM, or IV)
or thioridazine (5 mg po) can help in managing the delirious patient.
Larger doses (haloperidol 2 to 5 mg or thioridazine 10 to 20 mg) are
sometimes needed. Newer drugs, such as risperidone, can be used
instead of haloperidol for oral therapy but are not available IM or IV.
Short- or intermediate-acting benzodiazepines (for example, alprazolam, triazolam) can control agitation over the short term; benzodiazepines may worsen confusion, but if required, the smallest effective
dose should be used. All psychoactive drugs should be reduced and
then eliminated as soon as possible so that recovery can be assessed.

Confusional States and Acute Memory Disorders

Background

Confusion (encephalopathy) is defined as the inability to maintain
a coherent stream of thought or action. The hallmark of acute confusional states is impairment in attention and/or arousal or acute
changes in perception or other higher order behaviors. Delirium is a
more specific syndrome, defined as an impairment of attention or
arousal. The usage of the two terms overlaps considerably. *The Diagnostic and Statistical Manual of Mental Disorders, Fourth Edition
(DSM-IV)* differentiates delirium as including impaired perceptions
and attention, but adds that delirium should have an acute or subacute onset (unlike dementia) and be associated with disruptions of
the sleep-wake cycles (diurnal fluctuations) and evidence of a general
medical condition causing the condition. Dementia may consist of a
nonacute confusional state, which may or may not be reversible with
treatment and may or may not be due to a progressive condition.

Pathophysiology

Acute confusion is a symptom rather than a disease, so the pathophysiology depends upon the etiology of the syndrome. The syndrome can be attributable to numerous causes, which include pulmonary disease (for example, hypoxia); other abnormal systemic metabolic conditions (for example, hepatic or renal disease); ingestion of toxins or medications; electrolyte abnormalities (especially sodium, BUN [blood urea nitrogen], creatinine, glucose, calcium, magnesium, phosphorus); sepsis or systemic infections (including simple urinary tract infections); nutritional deficiencies (for example, thiamine, cobalamin, niacin); endocrine disorders (for example, thyroid or adrenal hypofunction or hyperfunction); and acute psychiatric disorders (especially affective disorders).

Specific neurological pathophysiology may include diffuse disorders such as seizures, postictal states, progressive dementias, central nervous system (CNS) infections such as human immunodeficiency virus (HIV) infection or chronic cryptococcal meningitis, other types of meningoencephalomyelitis (including herpes simplex encephalitis), and paraneoplastic disorders. Focal CNS disorders also can cause confusion if strategically placed. Lesion loci that can cause confusional states include the basal forebrain (for example, infarction as complication of surgery to repair an anterior communicating artery aneurysm), the caudate nucleus, and thalamic lesions that affect both Papez circuit (anterior nucleus, fornix, mammillothalamic tract) and basolateral circuit (dorsomedial nuclei, intermediolateral nuclei). In addition, Wernicke aphasia and mirror-image lesions of the Wernicke area affecting the right hemisphere also can present with acute confusion or agitation. Infectious and inflammatory disorders of the CNS, including vasculitis and others, also need to be considered.

Mortality/Morbidity

Confusional states may have extremely high rates of mortality and morbidity, especially if they are undiagnosed. The morbidity and mortality rates depend heavily on the underlying disease.

Age

- Age is an important factor in the consideration of confusional states. Mild toxic or metabolic insults, such as medication side effects, electrolyte imbalances, thyroid disease, or many other conditions, may affect the elderly more severely than they

103

would affect a younger individual. Physicians should consider the age of the patient when prescribing medication or assessing its adverse effects.

- For example, elderly patients may have exaggerated responses to over-the-counter and prescription medications with anticholinergic activity. These include agents such as diphenhydramine (Benadryl, Tylenol PM) and atropine sulfate (for example, Lomotil). Mellaril, a prescription antipsychotic medication, also has high anticholinergic activity. These drugs may cause exaggerated adverse effects, including sundowning.

Causes

Potential causes of acute confusional states are numerous. A good clinician is thorough and systematic in the evaluation.

- Intoxication
  - Intoxicants can include prescription and over-the-counter medications, as well as alcohol and illegal drugs. Although these causes often are suspected in the emergency department (ED), they may be unsuspected in other settings (for example, postoperative delirium tremens in closet alcoholics).
  - Iatrogenic toxicity can occur in patients taking prn (as needed) sedatives, especially the elderly, or be due to unsuspected drug interactions. Antipsychotic medications, for example, may worsen memory in patients with underlying Lewy body disease, a type of progressive dementia.
  - Prescription medicines may be used inappropriately. Prednisone, dexamethasone, and other steroids can cause paradoxical confusion, as can a host of other medications.

- Focal brain lesions
  - Focal brain lesions occasionally can cause acute confusion. Subdural hematomas, strokes, and mass lesions may be found on CT scan and MRI. If the confusion is due to increased intracranial pressure, as in a subdural hematoma, arousal may be most affected and the patient may be sleepy. If due to a stroke, the "confusion" is likely to be misdiagnosed aphasia, unless a huge lesion is present, in which case associated hemiparesis makes the diagnosis obvious.

- Uncommonly, strokes can present as confusional states with highly select lesion loci. Brain tumors often develop slowly, allowing the brain to compensate; therefore, they are somewhat less likely to present as acute confusional states.

- Occasionally, focal lesions can result in confusion. Patients develop an agitated confusion with head lesions affecting the caudate, thalamus, or basal forebrain. Patients may appear agitated with lesions of the Wernicke area or of the mirror-image homologous area of the right hemisphere.

- Infections
  - Urinary tract infections and pneumonias are common infections that cause confusion in debilitated, nursing home, and other elderly patients. If these common infections are not present, patients should be checked for other common metabolic abnormalities, including abnormalities of glucose, sodium, BUN, calcium, magnesium, and phosphorus.

  - The blood oxygen should be checked and the anion gap measured. Once these are sent for investigation, other common conditions should be sought, including cobalamin deficiency, thyroid disease, vasculitis, and latent syphilis. Ammonia should be checked, especially if asterixis is present.

- Neurological diseases
  - Specific neurological diseases besides stroke, tumor, and subdural hematoma need to be considered. Paramount among these are neurological infections, especially those that are treatable. Young patients presenting with high fever and confusion should be evaluated for herpes virus and treated presumptively until the condition is ruled out.

  - Chronic meningitis is not the exclusive domain of the immunosuppressed; in fact, cryptococcal meningitis, tuberculous meningitis, and carcinomatous meningitis may occur even with minimal symptoms, such as mild headache and confusion. Diabetics and elderly patients may have bacterial meningitis with minimal fever. Elderly nursing home residents may have Listeria meningitis that responds to ampicillin rather than third-generation cephalosporins. Patients from areas of endemic tuberculosis may be susceptible to tuberculous meningitis.

- Epilepsy
  - Epilepsy can present as confusion. Patients may have nonconvulsive status epilepticus, a condition that can be easily diagnosed and treated. Two types may occur—absence status may occur in patients who may or may not have had prior absence seizures, and complex partial status epilepticus may occur in patients with or without a history of complex partial seizures. The 2 types are differentiated by EEG. In absence epilepsy, spike-and-wave discharges are seen at a rate of 3 per second. In complex partial status (the more common type), a focal discharging pattern may be seen.
  - In younger patients, the Landau-Kleffner syndrome is a potentially treatable epileptic condition. Landau-Kleffner syndrome involves acquired aphasia with a convulsive disorder in previously "normal" children who acutely or progressively lose language function. Patients typically have a severe comprehension defect, especially involving an auditory agnosia. The patients' seizures usually respond to anticonvulsive therapy, although their language disorder often persists.
- Occasionally, a patient with an underlying developmental disorder persisting into adulthood or even metabolic disease commonly presenting in adulthood may present with confusion. These conditions typically are diagnosed after much labor and contemplation by the treating team. For more information on the many metabolic diseases, the interested reader is referred to textbooks of child neurology, because such illnesses were once not recognized or sufficiently appreciated in the adult patient.
  - These illnesses appear to be particularly prevalent in homeless or institutionalized patients, and tragically, only a few of the diseases are treatable. To cite two examples of many, somewhat arbitrarily, adrenoleukodystrophy and cerebrotendinous xanthomatosis may present in adults. The former condition may be diagnosed by a characteristic pattern of demyelination on MRI. The latter condition ought to be suspected in an individual with an abnormal gait and xanthomas of the Achilles tendons, eyelids, and patellae. It is due to deposition of cholestanol in the central and peripheral nervous systems and can be prevented with appropriate medical treatment.

106

- Inflammatory conditions in the CNS include the rare, but treatable, conditions of CNS vasculitis and Hashimoto encephalopathy. Of note, patients with known lupus often have strokes due to nonbacterial thrombotic endocarditis (NBTE) or CNS dysfunction due to antibodies to neuronal tissues (antineuronal antibodies with ribosomal p protein, with CNS appearing normal on light microscopy) so that the coexistence of lupus and encephalopathy more often than not leads to a diagnosis other than vasculitis.

- Certain patterns of disease that suggest CNS vasculitis occur in conjunction with very specific vasculitides. Their importance is related in part to the specificity of the respective treatments. Polyarteritis nodosa, a disease of small- and medium-sized blood vessels, often affects the heart and kidneys. Neurological disease includes peripheral neuropathies, seizures, visual loss (due to involvement of optic structures), subarachnoid hemorrhage, and stroke. The survival rate is markedly better in patients who receive the therapeutic combination of cyclophosphamide (Cytoxan) and corticosteroids than in those who receive corticosteroids alone or no treatment (5-year survival rates, 18% in untreated patients; 55%, corticosteroids alone; 79%, combined treatment).

- Churg-Strauss syndrome includes asthma, eosinophilia, vasculitic neuropathy and, rarely, CNS disease.

- Wegener granulomatosis, a systemic necrotizing granulomatosis, involves the upper and lower respiratory tracts, glomeruli, peripheral nerves, and cranial nerves. Patients often have circulating antineutrophilic circulating cytoplasmic antibodies. The disease once was considered fatal within 4–6 months in untreated patients and within 11 months in those treated with prednisone. Long-term survival now is routine in patients treated with the combination of prednisone and cyclophosphamide. Trimethoprim-sulfamethoxazole may decrease the relapse rate in some patients.

- Isolated CNS vasculitis can present with headaches, encephalopathy, and multifocal signs. Isolated CNS vasculitis should be diagnosed only according to strict criteria, including recurrent, multifocal vascular disease, exclusion of a systemic inflammatory of infectious process, angiography supportive of the diagnosis, and brain biopsy to exclude infection or neoplasia. Without the presence of these criteria, the diagnosis can be considered to be speculative. Therapy with cyclophosphamide and prednisone may result in a cure in some patients.

- Hashimoto encephalopathy is a condition characterized by severe encephalopathy and high circulating titers of antithyroid antibodies, although the patient may clinically be euthyroid. EEG findings may be moderately abnormal and the patient may respond to steroids.

- Dementia

  - Underlying dementia may well be present but is a diagnosis of exclusion. Dementia, unlike an acute confusional state, is not readily reversible with correction of an underlying toxic, metabolic, or infectious disorder. Like delirium and an acute confusional state, dementia involves abnormal perceptions, attention, and memory. Unlike delirium, however, dementia usually is defined as a more or less permanent state without an aura of ready reversibility based upon treatment of an underlying medical condition.

  - Dementia, once thought to be monolithic and more or less untreatable, often can be further fractionated and diagnosed by clinical examination and laboratory testing. Markers exist for Alzheimer disease and Creutzfeldt-Jakob disease, although the limitations of these markers are not adequately known to make them completely reliable.

  - Visual hallucinations and a paradoxical response to antipsychotic medications make Lewy body disease, rather than Alzheimer disease, the likely diagnosis. Prominent behavioral or language disturbance increases the possibility of Pick or other frontotemporal dementia. The so-called "useless hand" (unilateral), also misreferred to as an "alien" hand, makes the diagnosis of corticobasal ganglionic degeneration more likely.

  - Presence of abnormal eye movements (especially vertical eye movements) may indicate progressive supranuclear palsy, although the physician should not forget to consider thiamine deficiency or Whipple disease in this situation.

  - Again, dementias can present acutely but continue chronically and are diagnoses of exclusion. Diagnosis usually does not require lumbar puncture, except in the case of Whipple disease or if chronic meningitis needs to be excluded.

- Alcohol
  - Confusional states due to alcohol are sufficiently important, complex, and common to merit their own category.
  - The discussion of alcoholic dementia overlaps with that of nutritional dementia, traumatic dementia, epileptic dementia, vascular dementia, and toxic dementia due to illegal drugs, as these conditions tend to exist in the same patients.
  - Alcoholic patients typically are malnourished and require thiamine followed by glucose on arrival to the ED.
  - The CT scans may show atrophy and hemorrhage due to thiamine deficiency, orbitofrontal or temporal contusions that may be signatures of prior trauma, or subdural hematomas. EEG results may be significant for seizure activity.
  - As mentioned above, closet alcoholics can present with delirium tremens several days after admission to the hospital. Various electrolyte imbalances are common.

- Vascular dementia
  - Vascular dementia refers to dementia that is due to strokes. The strokes may be cortical and have localizing features depending upon what part of the cortex is involved.
  - Vascular dementia also refers to dementia due to multiple subcortical strokes, which are due to extensive disease of the smallest caliber blood vessels.
  - This has been known by multiple names, including Binswanger disease, état lacunaire, leukoariosis (referring to the radiographic appearance), and others.
  - Notably, the presence of subcortical strokes, even extensive ones, does not preclude Alzheimer disease.
  - Clinically, patients with Binswanger disease have not only the radiographic characteristics but also distinct presenting features. These may include gait abnormalities and difficulties with memory, such as 3-word recall, and frontal lobe tests, such as the Thurstone or the go, no go paradigm.

- Typically such patients do not have "cognitive features" such as anomia, apraxia, agnosia, and neglect as are seen with cortical lesions.

- Some cases are associated with severe hypertension or elevation of the fibrinogen level.

Further Inpatient Care

Once a diagnosis is made, the patient requires follow-up until the confusional state resolves or a plateau is reached. In general, good follow-up and acting as a general internist are the same thing. The follow-up depends entirely on the diagnosis. Many clinicians underestimate the degree of improvement that is possible in confused patients, even confused elderly patients.

Prognosis

The prognosis of confusional states is highly variable. Patients frequently become much better than the expected recovery predicted by the admitting physicians. The prognosis may depend on general medical care and attention, rather than specific management of the encephalopathy. Many patients with confusional episodes recover completely.

Chapter 17

Dementia with Lewy Bodies (DLB)

Definition

Dementia with Lewy bodies (DLB) is a progressive degenerative disease or syndrome of the brain. It shares symptoms—and sometimes overlaps—with several diseases, especially with two common diseases of older adults, Alzheimer's and Parkinson's.

Persons who develop DLB have behavioral and memory symptoms of dementia like those of Alzheimer's disease and, to varying extents, the physical, motor system symptoms seen in Parkinson's. However, the mental symptoms of a person with DLB might fluctuate frequently, motor symptoms are milder than for Parkinson's disease, and DLB patients usually have vivid visual hallucinations.

Facts

"Dementia with Lewy Bodies" is the preferred term for several disorders or conditions that cause dementia. Dementia is a gradual, progressive decline in mental ability (cognition) that affects memory, thinking processes, behavior and physical activity. In addition to these mental symptoms, persons with DLB experience physical symptoms of parkinsonism, including mild tremor, muscle stiffness and movement problems. Strong visual hallucinations also occur.

"Fact Sheet: Dementia with Lewy Bodies," © 2000 Family Caregiver Alliance; reprinted with permission. For more information from Family Caregiver Alliance, visit www.caregiver.org.

111

DLB is named after smooth round protein lumps, called Lewy bodies, that are found in the nerve cells of affected brains. Lewy bodies are often present in the nuclei (nerve cells) of brains afflicted with a variety of disorders. In DLB, the Lewy bodies are found throughout the outer layer of the brain (the cerebral cortex) and deep inside the midbrain or brainstem. These "abnormal protein structures" were first described in 1912 by Frederich Heinrich Lewy, M. D., a contemporary of Alois Alzheimer who first identified the more common form of dementia that bears his name.

Because Lewy bodies are also often found in the brains of those diagnosed with Alzheimer's, Parkinson's, Down syndrome, and other disorders, researchers agreed in 1995 to use the term "Dementia with Lewy Bodies" to describe both a single disease (sometimes called "pure DLB") and a spectrum of disorders with similar or related pathology.

It is believed that DLB, as a defined disease process, accounts for as many as 20% of the seven million cases of dementia in the United States and for as much as one-third of dementing illness in elderly Americans. This makes DLB the second most common form of dementia after Alzheimer's.

Doctors and other clinical experts sometimes use other terms to describe DLB or variations of Lewy body syndromes, including "Diffuse Lewy Body Disease," "Cortical Lewy Body Disease," "Lewy Body Dementia," or "Lewy Body Variant of Alzheimer's Disease." Although debate about the nature of Lewy body-related disorders continues, most clinicians now follow the terminology and diagnosis recommendations for DLB developed in 1995 by an international consortium.

The cause of DLB is unknown and no specific risk factors are identified. Cases have appeared among families but there does not seem to be a strong tendency for inheriting the disease. Genetic research may reveal more information about causes and risk in the future.

Symptoms

Initial symptoms of DLB usually are similar to those of Alzheimer's or vascular dementia and are cognitive (mental) in nature. Other patients may first show the neuromuscular symptoms of Parkinson's disease. A small number of patients will begin with dementia and parkinsonism symptoms at the same time.

Key symptoms are:

- For most DLB patients, mild problems with recent memory, such as forgetting very recent events.

- Brief episodes of unexplained confusion and other behavioral or cognitive problems. The individual may become disoriented about the time or where he or she is; have trouble with speech, finding words or following a conversation, and experience visuospatial difficulty (such as finding one's way or working a jigsaw puzzle); and problems in thinking such as inattention, mental inflexibility, indecisiveness, lack of judgment, and loss of insight.

- Fluctuation in the occurrence of these cognitive symptoms from moment to moment, hour to hour, day to day, or week to week. For example, the person may converse normally one day and be mute, unable to speak, the next day—or even from one moment to the next. While this is often felt to be an important part of DLB, it may occur in other dementias and is sometimes it is very difficult to determine whether fluctuation truly occurs in a given patient.

- Well-defined, vivid, visual hallucinations. In DLB's early stage, the person may even acknowledge and describe the hallucinations. Other types of hallucinations are less common but sometimes occur. These might be auditory ("hearing" sounds), olfactory ("tasting" something), or tactile ("feeling" something that isn't there).

- Movement (motor function) problems of parkinsonism, sometimes referred to as "extrapyramidal" signs. These symptoms often seem to start spontaneously and may include flexed posture, shuffling gait, reduced arm-swing, limb stiffness, a tendency to fall, bradykinesia (slowness of movement), and tremor.

Movement and motor problems occur in later stages for 70% of persons with DLB. But for 30% of DLB patients, and more commonly those that are older, Parkinson's symptoms occur first, before dementia symptoms. In these individuals cognitive decline tends to start with depression or mild forgetfulness.

Testing and Diagnosis

Dementia with Lewy bodies is difficult to diagnose. Not only does it resemble other dementias, it overlaps with Alzheimer's, Parkinson's, and other disorders, which may be difficult to rule out or exclude. Because no single test exists to diagnose DLB, a variety of medical, neurological, and neuropsychological tests are used to pinpoint it and its possible overlap with other illnesses.

Although Lewy bodies are found in brains of patients with other diseases and because testing will involve several approaches, it is useful to understand what happens to the brain of a person who has DLB. Three significant changes or pathological features are seen in brains afflicted by Dementia with Lewy Bodies:

- The brain's cerebral cortex (the outer layers of the brain) degenerates or shrinks. This can affect reasoning and complex thinking, understanding, personality, movement, speech and language, sensory input, and visual perceptions of space. Degeneration also occurs in the limbic cortex at the center of the brain, which plays a major role in emotions and behavior. Lewy bodies form throughout these degenerating cortical areas.

- Nerve cells die in the midbrain, especially in an area that also degenerates in Parkinson's disease, the substantia nigra, located in the brainstem. These cells are involved in making the neurotransmitter (brain messenger) dopamine. Lewy bodies are found in the nerve cells that remain. The midbrain is involved in memory formation and learning, attention, and psychomotor (muscular movement) skills.

- Lesions called Lewy neurites that affect nerve cell function are found in DLB brains, especially in the hippocampus, an area of the brain essential for forming new memories.

None of the symptoms of dementia with Lewy bodies is specific only to DLB. To address this problem, an international group of researchers and clinicians developed a set of diagnostic criteria in 1995, called the Consensus Guidelines, that can reliably point to DLB:

Must be present:

- Progressive cognitive decline (decrease in thinking ability) that interferes with normal social or occupational activities. Memory problems do not necessarily occur in the early period but will occur as DLB progresses. Attention, language, understanding and reasoning, ability to do arithmetic, logical thinking, and perceptions of space and time will be impaired.

Two of the following are present (one also indicates possibility of DLB):

- Fluctuating cognition: mental problems vary, especially attention and alertness.

- Visual hallucinations: detailed and well-formed visions occur and recur.

- Parkinsonism: motor-related and movement problems appear.

A DLB diagnosis is even more likely if the patient also experiences repeated falls, fainting, brief loss of consciousness, delusions, or is sensitive to neuroleptic drugs that are given to control hallucinations and other psychiatric symptoms. Hearing, smell, or touch hallucinations support the diagnosis of DLB.

Finally, the timing of symptoms is a reliable clue: If both mental and motor symptoms appear within one year of each other, DLB is more likely the cause. Signs of stroke or vascular dementia usually negate the likelihood of DLB.

It is not presently clear how accurate the clinical diagnosis of DLB is. While some reports suggest the diagnosis can be made with good accuracy, other studies show that it is difficult to accurately diagnose DLB. Nevertheless, other testing should be done to exclude other causes or illnesses such as Creutzfeldt Jakob or vascular disease. Brain imaging (CT scan or MR imaging) can detect brain shrinkage and help rule out stroke, fluid on the brain (normal pressure hydrocephalus), or subdural hematoma. Blood and other tests might show vitamin B12 deficiency, thyroid problems, syphilis, or human immunodeficiency virus (HIV). Depression is also a common cause of dementia-like symptoms. Additional tests can include an electroencephalogram (EEG) or a spinal tap. Scans using SPECT and PET (Positron Emission Tomography) technology have shown promise in detecting differences between DLB and Alzheimer's disease.

Alzheimer's and Parkinson's: Differences and Overlap with DLB

DLB's similarity to Alzheimer's and Parkinson's diseases and the fact that Lewy bodies are often found in the brains of patients with these diseases means that clinicians must pay close attention to the factors that distinguish DLB:

- Memory and other cognitive problems occur in both DLB and Alzheimer's. However, in DLB they fluctuate frequently.

- DLB patients experience more depression than do Alzheimer's patients.

- Hallucinations are experienced by Alzheimer's patients in late stages, and by Parkinson's patients who take medications to improve movement and tremor. In DLB, hallucinations occur in early stages, and they are frequent, vivid, and detailed.

- Neuroleptic drugs (sometimes called psychotropic drugs) prescribed to lessen the so-called psychiatric symptoms of dementia, such as hallucinations, agitation, or restlessness will induce Parkinson's in some DLB patients.

- Life expectancy is slightly shorter for DLB than for Alzheimer's patients.

- At autopsy the brains of DLB patients have senile plaques, a hallmark of Alzheimer's. Another Alzheimer's feature, neurofibrillary tangles, are absent or found in fewer numbers and are concentrated in the neocortex. Other Alzheimer's features— regional neuronal loss, spongiform change and synapse loss, neurochemical abnormalities, and neurotransmitter deficits— are also seen. However, DLB-afflicted brains are less damaged than are Alzheimer's brains.

- In DLB movement problems are spontaneous; the symptoms begin suddenly.

- Tremor is less pronounced in DLB than in Parkinson's. Also, DLB patients respond less dramatically to drugs such as Levodopa that are used to treat Parkinson's. Nerve cell loss in the subtantia nigra is not as severe in DLB.

- Both DLB and Parkinson's patients may sometimes experience fainting and wide alterations in blood pressure.

- Some Parkinson's patients develop dementia in later stages. Dementia is usually the presenting symptom in DLB.

- Parkinson's patients lose the neurotransmitter dopamine; Alzheimer's patients lose the neurotransmitter acetylcholine. DLB patients lose both.

- In DLB, Alzheimer-like and Parkinson-like symptoms appear within one year of each other.

Despite these differences, a diagnosis of dementia with Lewy bodies does not preclude a positive diagnosis of Alzheimer's, Parkinson's, or other diseases common in older age.

Duration and Treatment

With an average lifespan after onset of 5 to 7 years, the progress of dementia with Lewy bodies is relentless, resulting in severe dementia and immobility. DLB does not follow a pattern of stages as is seen in some other dementias. A few patients progress very rapidly through the disease. Death usually occurs from pneumonia or other illness. There is no cure nor specific treatment to arrest the course of the disease.

Caution must be used in treating a person who is suspected of having DLB, again pointing to the need for an accurate diagnosis. Medications must be monitored closely for proper balance because some patients—not all—are adversely affected. Neuroleptic (tranquilizing) anti-psychotic drugs such as haloperidol or thioridazine that are often given to Alzheimer's patients to help lessen symptoms such as agitation or hallucinations can cause extreme adverse reactions in many DLB patients and can bring on motor-related symptoms. A patient treated with these drugs could become catatonic, lose cognitive function, and/or develop more muscle rigidity, results that could threaten life. Likewise, levodopa drugs used to treat Parkinson's motor symptoms may increase the hallucinations of DLB patients and aggravate other symptoms. Levodopa is not usually very helpful in treating the motor symptoms of DLB patients.

Some drug therapies are showing promise, however. Cholinesterase inhibitors, such as Tacrine, may be an alternative treatment and have been effective in stopping hallucinations. Some newer antipsychotic drugs (Seroquel, sertindole) may be safe.

DLB patients can live at home with frequent reassessment and careful monitoring and supervision. Caregivers must watch them closely because of the tendency to fall or lose consciousness. Dementia prevents patients from learning new actions that might help them overcome movement problems. They may need more assistance some days than others, and can be reassured by a caregiver's help in turning attention away from hallucinations. Caregivers can turn to a regional Caregiver Resource Center in California for assistance, and to a qualified diagnostic center for initial diagnosis and follow-up. In other states, resources can be found through local and state offices on aging and health.

Credits

LewyNet, The University of Nottingham, Division of Pathology, University Park, Nottingham, England NG7 2RD. Telephone +44 115 9515151. Web site: http://www.ccc.nottingham.ac.uk/~mpzjlowe/lewy/lewyhome.html.

"Dementia with Lewy Bodies: A Distinct Non-Alzheimer Dementia Syndrome?" by Paul G. Ince, Elaine K. Perry, and Chris M. Morris,

Brain Pathology, April, 1998. (Available with extensive bibliographies at LewyNet web site—see above.)

"Similarities to Alzheimer's and Parkinson's Make Lewy Body Dementia Difficult to Recognize and Challenging to Treat," *John Douglas French Center for Alzheimer's Disease Journal*, 1998/1999.

Parkinson's Disease UPDATE, a monthly newsletter, Medical Publishing Company, P. O. Box 450, Huntingdon Valley, PA 19006. Issue #10, 2000.

"Dementia with Lewy Bodies" by Ian G. McKeith, M.D., FRCPsych., *High Notes, News from the John Douglas French Alzheimer's Foundation*, Fall, 1996.

"Consensus guidelines for the clinical and pathological diagnosis of dementia with Lewy bodies (DLB): report of the consortium on DLB International Workshop," by I. G. McKeith, D. Galasko, K. Kosaka, E. K. Perry, et al, 1996. *Neurology*, 47:1113-24.

Dementia with Lewy Bodies, by Robert H. Perry, Ian G. McKeith, and Elaine K. Perry (editors), Forward by Jeffrey L. Cummings, 1996. Cambridge University Press, Cambridge.

Other References

Ala, T. A., Yang, K. H., Sung, J. H., Frey, W. H., 1997. Hallucinations and signs of parkinsonism help distinguish patients with dementia and cortical Lewy bodies from patients with Alzheimer's disease at presentation: a clinicopathological study. *Journal of Neurology*, Neurosurgery and Psychiatry, 62:16-21.

Dickson, D. W., Ruan, D., Crystal, H., Mark, M. H., et al, 1991. Hippocampal degeneration differentiates diffuse Lewy body disease (DLBD) from Alzheimer's disease. *Neurology*, 41:1402-9.

Galasko, D., Katzman, R., Salmon, D. P., Hansen, L., 1996. Clinical features and neuropathological findings in Lewy body dementias. *Brain Cognition*, 31:166-75.

Graham, C., Ballard, C., Saad, K., 1997. Variables which distinguish patients fulfilling clinical criteria for dementia with Lewy bodies from those with dementia, Alzheimer's disease. *International Journal of Geriatric Psychiatry*, 12:314-8.

Hansen, L. A., Samuel, W. 1997. Criteria for Alzheimer's disease and the nosology of dementia with Lewy bodies. *Neurology*, 48:126-32.

Ince, P., Irving, D., MacArther, F., Perry, R.H., 1991. Quantitative neuropathology of the hippocampus: comparison of senile dementia of Alzheimer type, senile dementia of Lewy body type, Parkinson's disease and non-demented elderly control patients. *J Neurol Sci*, 106:142-52.

Ince, P. G., McArthur, F. K., Bjertness, E., Torvik, A., et al, 1995. Neuropathological diagnoses in elderly patients in Oslo: Alzheimer's disease, Lewy body disease and vascular lesions. *Dementia*, 6:162-8.

Klatka, L. A., Louis, E. D., Schiffer, R. B., 1996. Psychiatric features in diffuse Lewy body disease: a clinicopathological study using Alzheimer's disease and Parkinson's disease. *Neurology*, 47:1148-52.

Kosaka, K., Iseki, E., Odawara, T., et al, 1996. Cerebral type of Lewy body disease. *Neuropathology*, 16:32-5.

Louis, E. D., Klatka, L. A., Lui, Y., Fahn, S., 1997. Comparison of extrapyramidal features in 31 pathologically confirmed cases of diffuse Lewy body disease and 34 pathologically confirmed cases of Parkinson's disease. *Neurology*, 48:376-80.

McKeith, I. G., Fairbairn, A., Perry, R. H., Thompson, P., Perry, E. K., 1992. Neuroleptic sensitivity in patients with senile dementia of Lewy body type. *British Medical Journal*, 305:673-8.

Mega, M. S., Masterman, D. L., Benson, D. F., Vinters, H. V., et al, 1996. Dementia with Lewy bodies: reliability and validity of clinical and pathological criteria. *Neurology*, 47:1403-9.

Perry, E. K., Haroutunian, V., Davis, K. L., Levy, R., et al, 1994. Neocortical cholinergic activities differentiate Lewy body dementia from classical Alzheimer's disease. *Neuroreport*, 5:747-9.

Salmon, D. P., Glasko, D., Hansen, L. A., Masliah, E. et al, 1996. Neuropsychological deficits associated with diffuse Lewy body disease. *Brain Cognition*, 31:148-65.

Samuel, W., Alford, M., Hofstter, C. R., Hansen, L., 1997. Dementia with Lewy bodies versus pure Alzheimer's disease: differences in cognition, neuropathology, cholinergic dysfunction, and synaptic density. *Journal of Neuropathology and Experimental Neurology*, 56:499-508.

Chapter 18

Frontotemporal Dementia

Definition

Frontotemporal dementia (FTD) is a degenerative condition of the front (anterior) part of the brain. It differs from other causes of dementia such as Alzheimer's, Pick's, and Creutzfeldt Jakob's diseases. The areas of the brain affected by FTD—the frontal and anterior temporal lobes—control reasoning, personality, movement, speech, social graces, language, and some aspects of memory.

FTD is marked by dramatic changes in personality, behavior, and some thought processes. Changes in personal and social conduct occur in early stages of the disease, including loss of inhibition, apathy, social withdrawal, hyperorality (mouthing of objects), and ritualistic compulsive behaviors. These symptoms may lead to misdiagnosis as a psychological or emotionally-based problem, or, in the elderly, be mistaken for withdrawal or eccentricity. FTD progresses to immobility and loss of speech and expression. Structural changes in the FTD patient's brain can be seen via scans or neuroimaging.

"Fact Sheet: Frontotemporal Dementia," Reviewed by Bruce Miller, M.D., Director, Memory and Aging Center, University of California at San Francisco. Prepared by Family Caregiver Alliance in cooperation with California's Caregiver Resource Centers, a statewide system of resource centers serving families and caregivers of brain-impaired adults. May 2000. Funded by the California Department of Mental Health. © 2000 Family Caregiver Alliance; reprinted with permission. For more information from Family Caregiver Alliance, visit www.caregiver.org.

Facts

As many as 7 million Americans may be afflicted with a form of dementia. Frontotemporal dementia may account for 2–5% or 140,000–350,000 cases of dementia and for as many as 25% of presenile dementias.

FTD occurs predominantly after age 40 and usually before age 65, with equal incidence in men and women. In nearly half of the patients, a family history of dementia exists in a first degree relative (parent or sibling), suggesting a genetic component in these cases. Additionally, a form of dementia found in persons with motor neuron disease (amyotrophic lateral sclerosis, commonly known as, "Lou Gehrig's Disease") may be associated with FTD.

Symptoms

Initial symptoms of FTD are primarily changes in personality and behavior. In addition to the symptoms described below, FTD patients often present two seemingly opposite behavioral profiles in the early and middle stages of the disease. Some individuals are overactive, restless, distractible, and disinhibited. Others are apathetic, inert, aspontaneous, and emotionally blunted. These differences in outward activity disappear in the late stages of the disease.

Major symptoms of FTD are:

- Dramatic change in personal and social conduct. The individual may lack initiative, seem unconcerned, and neglect domestic, financial, and occupational responsibilities.

- Loss of empathy toward others. Patients may show shallow affect (flat facial expression or lack of emotional response). Or they may be inappropriately jocular and sing, dance, clap, or recite phrases repeatedly.

- Rigid and inflexible thinking and impaired judgment.

- Loss of insight into personal and social misconduct, such as small sexual or moral transgressions.

- Stereotyped (repetitive) or compulsive behavior. For example, the person with FTD may become compulsive about rituals of hygiene and dress while at the same time neglecting proper hygiene. They may echo what others say, wander restlessly over a fixed route, or adhere to a fixed daily schedule.

- Hypochondriasis, including bizarre somatic complaints.

- Excessive eating or gluttony, food fads (especially a craving for sweet foods) and even excessive alcohol consumption. (The tendency of FTD patients to consume alcohol often leads to a misdiagnosis of alcohol-related dementia.) The person may refuse to eat, however, due to a behavioral pattern called "negativism" or to inability to use motor skills needed for eating.

- Decreased motor skills in later stages.

- Change in sleep patterns, with prolonged sleepiness shown, especially in those that present more apathetic behaviors.

In late stage FTD symptoms include:

- A gradual reduction in speech, culminating in mutism.

- Hyperoral traits.

- Failure or inability to make motor responses to verbal commands.

- Akinesia (loss of muscle movement) and rigidity with death due to complications of immobility.

Differences Between FTD and Other Dementias

FTD differs markedly in several ways when compared to other dementias, especially Alzheimer's disease:

- FTD is characterized by cerebral atrophy in the frontal and anterior temporal lobes of the brain, while Alzheimer's affects the hippocampal, posterior temporal, and parietal regions. The neurofibrillary tangles, senile plaques, and Lewy bodies present in the brains of Alzheimer's and other dementia patients are absent. (Pick bodies are also usually absent.)

- Alzheimer's patients experience severe memory loss. While FTD patients exhibit memory disturbances, they remain oriented to time and place and recall information about the present and past.

- FTD patients, even in late stages of the disease, retain visuospatial orientation, and they negotiate and locate their surroundings accurately.

- Intellectual failure in FTD is distinctly different from that of Alzheimer's patients. Results of intelligence tests are normal in those with FTD until the point in the disease when disinterest results in lower scores.

• Life expectancy is slightly longer for FTD.

Testing and Diagnosis

FTD can be accurately diagnosed with brain scans or imaging. Computed tomography (CT scan) and magnetic resonance imaging (MRI) reveal cerebral atrophy in the frontotemporal regions. Degeneration of the corpus striatum, thalamus, and other subcortical structures occurs. Functional brain imaging and single photon emission tomography may reveal dysfunction of the frontal lobes, decreased blood flow, and a selective reduced uptake of tracer in the anterior (front) cerebral hemispheres. Electroencephalography (EEG) remains normal, however, even in advanced stages. In autopsies, brain tissue changes include large neuronal cell loss with secondary spongiform change and astrocytic gliosis.

Neuropsychological testing is useful to obtain a clinical assessment of the disease. Tests evaluate conduct, language, visuo-spatial abilities, memory, abstraction, planning and mental control, motor skills, and intelligence. Tests might show:

• An economy of mental effort and unconcern. Responses may be impulsive and tasks readily abandoned, while other patients may be slow, inert, and persistent.

• Conversation is not spontaneous; responses are brief and one does not elaborate. Some patients may make mechanical, repetitive remarks, echo words spoken by others, or repeat responses. Apathetic patients may be hypophonic (have a weak voice) and have an odd or halting speaking pattern. Overactive patients may be the opposite, with unconstrained speech. Failure to respond or inappropriate responses should not be assumed to be incomprehension, but rather a concreteness of thinking or inattention.

• Visuo-spatial skills remain normal except for those compromised by behavioral abnormalities.

• Memory problems do not occur except as a result of ineffective use of memory.

• Thought processes show impaired powers of abstraction, verbal response and design fluency. For example, in card and block sorting or picture arrangement, the FTD patient may abandon tasks, produce items eccentrically, not follow instructions, violate "rules," etc. Comprehension is normal, however.

Duration and Treatment

The length of FTD varies, with some patients declining rapidly over two to three years and others showing only minimal changes over a decade. Studies have shown persons with FTD to live with the disease an average of eight years, with a range from three years to 17 years.

No medications are known currently to treat or prevent FTD. Serotonin-boosting medications may alleviate some behaviors.

Credits

D. Neary, J. S. Snowden and D. M. A. Mann, 1994, "Dementia of Frontal Lobe Type," *Dementia*, Edited by Alistair Burns and Raymond Levy, Chapman & Hall Medical, London, pp. 815-822.

Bruce L. Miller, M.D., "Degenerative Dementia," Family Caregiver Alliance Conference Presentation, 1999.

Gustafson, L., 1987, "Frontal lobe degeneration of non-Alzheimer's type. II. Clinical picture and differential diagnosis." *Arch. Gerontol. Geriatr.* 6(3):209-23.

M. Jackson and J. Lowe, 1996, "The new neuropathology of degenerative frontotemporal dementias." *Acta Neuropathol.* 91(2):127-34.

Other References

Brun, A., 1987, Frontal lobe degeneration of non-Alzheimer type. I. Neuropathology. *Arch. Gerontol. Geriatr.*, 6:193-208.

Brun, A., 1993, Frontal Lobe Dementia of the non-Alzheimer Type Revisited. *Dementia*, 4:126-31.

Brun, A., Englund, B., Gustafson, L., et al, 1994, Clinical and neuropathological criteria for frontotemporal dementia. *J. Neurol. Neurosurg. Psychiatry*, 57:416-418.

Mann, D. M. A., South, P. W., Snowden, J. S. and Neary, D., 1993, Dementia of frontal lobe type: Neuropathology and immunohistochemistry. *J. Neurol. Neurosurg. Psychiatry*, 56:605-14.

Miller, B. L., Cummings, J. L., Villanueva-Meyer, J., *et al*, 1991, Frontal Lobe Degeneration: clinical, neuropsychological and SPECT characteristics. *Neurology*, 41:1374-1382.

Miller, B. L., Chang, L., Mena, I., Boone, K. B., Lesser, I, 1993, Clinical and imaging features of right focal lobe degenerations. *Dementia*, 4:204-213.

Miller, B. L., Darby, A. L., Swartz, J. R., Yener, G. G., Mena, I., 1995, Dietary changes, compulsions and sexual behavior in fronto-temporal degeneration. *Dementia*, 6:195-199.

Neary, D., Snowden, J. S., Shields, R. A., et al, 1987, Single photon emission tomography using 99mTc-HMPAO in the investigation of dementia. *J. Neurol. Neurosurg. Psychiatry*, 50:1101-9.

Neary, D., Snowden, J. S., Northern, B. and Goulding, P. J., 1988, Dementia of frontal lobe type. *J. Neurol. Neurosurg. Psychiatry*, 51:353-61.

Orrell, M. W., Sahakian, B. J. and Bergmann, K., 1989, Self-neglect and frontal lobe dysfunction. *Br. J. Psychiatry*, 155:101-5.

Risberg, J., 1987, Frontal lobe degeneration of non-Alzheimer type. III. Regional blood flow. *Arch. Gerontol. Geriatr.*, 6:225-33

Snowden, J. S., Neary, D., Mann, D. M. A., 1996, Fronto-temporal lobar degeneration: Fronto-temporal dementia, progressive aphasia, semantic dementia. Churchill-Livingstone, New York, pp. 9-41.

Chapter 19

Huntington's Disease

Introduction

Huntington's disease (HD) is a hereditary brain disorder that affects people of all races all over the world. It takes its name from Dr. George Huntington, a Long Island physician who published a description of what he called "hereditary chorea" in 1872. From the Greek word for "dance," chorea refers to the involuntary movements which are among the common symptoms of HD.

Until recently, little was known or published about Huntington's disease. Yet in the last 20 years, much has been learned about the causes and effects of HD and about treatments, therapies and techniques for managing the symptoms of the disease. In 1993, after a ten-year search, scientists found the gene that causes HD, and important advances have flowed from this dramatic discovery. Many scientists are actively engaged in the search for effective treatments to stop or reverse the effects of HD, and eventually to cure it altogether. HD is a degenerative disease whose symptoms are caused by the loss of cells in a part of the brain called the basal ganglia. This damage to cells affects cognitive ability (thinking, judgment, memory), movement, and emotional control. Symptoms appear gradually, usually in mid-life,

Reprinted with permission from *Huntington's Disease*, part of the Family Guide Series of booklets produced by the Huntington's Disease Society of America (HDSA) © 2003 Huntington's Disease Society of America. To obtain a copy of this booklet, or other informational materials, contact HDSA, 158 West 29th Street, 7th Floor, New York, NY 10001-5300, 800-345-HDSA, www.hdsa.org.

between the ages of 30 and 50. However, the disease can strike young children and the elderly.

In most cases, people can maintain their independence for several years after the first symptoms of HD appear. A knowledgeable physician can prescribe treatment to minimize the impact of symptoms. Allied health professionals, such as social workers, occupational and physical therapists, speech-language pathologists (speech therapists), and nutritionists can all play a useful role in maximizing abilities and prolonging independence.

Inheritance

HD is a family disease for two reasons. First, it is passed from one generation to the next by the transmission from parent to child of a "mutated" (altered) gene. Each child of an affected parent has a one in two, or 50 percent, chance of inheriting the gene that causes HD, and is said to be "at risk." People who carry the gene will eventually develop Huntington's unless they die of some other cause before the onset of symptoms.

HD occurs in approximately 1 in 10,000 people in the United States. Currently about 30,000 people in the U.S. have HD and a further 150,000 are at risk.

Males and females have an equal chance of inheriting the gene from an affected parent. Those who do not inherit the gene will not develop the disease, nor will their children; HD does not "skip a generation." Genetic testing is available to determine whether or not a person carries the gene for HD.

The Family

HD is also a family disease because of its impact on every family member. As the disease progresses, the family role of the affected person will gradually change. The spouse or partner will have to assume more and more of the housekeeping, decision-making and parenting duties, which his/her partner may no longer be able to fulfill. In addition the spouse or partner will most likely become the primary care giver.

Children and adolescents must face living with a mother or father who is ill and whose behavior may be erratic. They may even be asked to participate in the parent's care. For parents, telling children about HD can pose difficult questions. Should a child/children be told about HD? If so, at what age? When is a child old enough to cope with the idea of being at risk for HD?

There are no easy answers, particularly since children develop at different rates and each family situation is different. Generally, it is a good idea to be as open as possible without being alarmist, and to convey the facts bit by bit. This way, a child can develop a gradual awareness of HD rather than being suddenly overwhelmed by information.

It is not helpful to treat HD as a shameful family secret, as a child or adolescent will find out about it eventually. Withholding the truth can lead to mistrust and resentment.

Symptoms and Stages of HD

Symptoms

The symptoms of HD vary widely from person to person, even within the same family. For some, involuntary movements may be prominent even in the early stages. For others, these may be less evident and emotional and behavioral symptoms may be more obvious. The following are common features of HD:

Emotional/Behavioral Symptoms. Depression, irritability, anxiety, and apathy are often encountered in HD. Some people can experience depression for a period of months or even years before it is recognized to be an early symptom of Huntington's. Behavioral changes may include aggressive outbursts, impulsiveness, mood swings, and social withdrawal. Often, existing personality traits will be exacerbated by HD, e.g., a person who had a tendency to be irritable. Schizophrenia and other serious psychiatric problems are uncommon in HD but do occur.

Cognitive/Intellectual Symptoms. Slight intellectual changes are often the first signs of cognitive disturbance. These may involve reduced ability to organize routine matters or to cope effectively with new situations. Short-term memory loss may occur while long-term memory generally stays intact. Work tasks become more difficult.

Motor Symptoms. Physical symptoms may initially consist of "nervous" activity, fidgeting, twitching, or excessive restlessness. Handwriting may change and facial grimaces may appear. Day-to-day skills involving coordination and concentration, such as driving, become more difficult.

These initial symptoms will gradually develop into more marked involuntary movements of the head, trunk and limbs—which often lead to problems in walking and balance. Speech and swallowing can become impaired. Movements generally tend to increase during voluntary effort, stress or excitement, and decrease during rest and sleep.

The Stages of HD

Though the pattern and severity of symptoms vary from person to person, the course of HD can be roughly divided into three stages.

Early in the disease, manifestations include subtle changes in coordination, perhaps some involuntary movements, difficulty thinking through problems, and often, a depressed or irritable mood. At this stage, medications are often effective in treating depression and other emotional symptoms. It is a good time to begin planning for the future. Financial plans should be made and legal documents (a Living Will, for example) drawn up. Huntington's Disease Society of America (HDSA) chapter social workers and family service coordinators can help to determine what is needed.

In the middle stage, involuntary movements (chorea) may become more pronounced. A staggering gait can sometimes be mistaken for drunkenness (it can be helpful to carry documentation that clearly refers to a diagnosis of Huntington's disease). Speech and swallowing will begin to be affected. It is important to consult a speech-language pathologist (speech therapist) who will be able to offer suggestions and strategies for improving communication and swallowing abilities. Likewise, occupational and physical therapists can develop programs to help maintain the highest level of functioning and thereby improve the quality of life.

Thinking and reasoning skills will also gradually diminish. At this stage it may become increasingly difficult to hold a job and to carry out household responsibilities. Here again, simple strategies may be employed to help decrease frustration, increase functioning, and prolong independence. For example, disorientation and short-term memory loss can be addressed by labeling drawers, maintaining a daily routine and posting a calendar listing appointments and events.

People with late-stage HD may have severe chorea, but more often have become rigid. Choking on food becomes a major concern, as does weight loss. At this stage people with HD are totally dependent on others for all aspects of care, can no longer walk, and are not able to speak.

Although cognitive abilities are severely impaired, it is important to remember that the person is generally still aware of his/her environment, remains able to comprehend language, and retains an awareness of loved ones and others. He/she may continue to enjoy looking at photographs and hearing stories of family and friends.

People do not die from HD itself but rather from a complication of the disease, such as choking or infection. Death generally occurs about 15 to 20 years after onset.

Diagnosis

A clinical diagnosis of HD can only be accomplished by a comprehensive examination, which generally entails a series of neurological and psychological exams and a detailed family history. MRI (magnetic response imaging) or CT (computerized tomography) scans may be included in the exam but the findings from these procedures are not sufficient to form a diagnosis.

Similarly, a genetic test may be used to help confirm, or rule out, a diagnosis of HD. However, a positive test result (indicating the presence of the HD gene) is not sufficient in and of itself (i.e., without a neurological exam) to confirm a diagnosis of HD.

It is best to see a neurologist who is very familiar with HD, as the symptoms can mimic those of other disorders such as Parkinson's disease or alcoholism. Referrals to knowledgeable professionals can be provided by your local HDSA chapter.

For some, diagnosis of HD can be a relief. It may provide an explanation for why their memory is not quite as sharp as it used to be or why they are feeling irritable or depressed. Others find the news very upsetting.

It is not uncommon for people to be in a state of "denial" when they are first diagnosed with HD. Regardless of their initial reaction, it can help to discuss the situation with others, either in a support group, with an HDSA social worker or with another counselor or therapist.

Juvenile Huntington's Disease

In approximately ten percent of cases, Huntington's disease affects children or adolescents. Children most often inherit the disease from their fathers (adult-onset HD is inherited from both parents with the same frequency). The symptoms of the juvenile form, or Westphal variant, of HD are somewhat different from adult-onset HD.

Initial symptoms usually involve slow, stiff and awkward walking and talking, choking, clumsiness and falling. Later, the child may become slow to respond and performance at school may become erratic. The course of the juvenile variant is generally more rapid than adult-onset

HD. The booklet, "Living with Juvenile Huntington's Disease," and the videotape, "Claudia's Challenge," both provide more information on juvenile HD and are available from HDSA.

Being at Risk for HD

Being at risk for Huntington's disease affects different people in different ways. Some choose not to think or talk about their at-risk status, even to the point of shunning other family members. Others think constantly about being at risk and about the possibility of developing HD. This can have an insidious influence and may lead to behavior, which is impulsive or self-destructive. Still others are able to find a balanced approach to their at-risk status and approach decision-making in this way.

Being at risk for HD influences major life choices such as marriage, family planning and career decisions. It can also have a pervasive influence on everyday activities. An episode of clumsiness, twitching or forgetfulness, such as everyone experiences from time to time, may be seen as a potential symptom of HD and can take on nerve-racking significance.

Many people come to accept the uncertainty of being at risk for HD, especially in the absence of an effective treatment or cure for the disease. Indeed, faced with the choice, most prefer to live with this uncertainty rather than taking a test which could remove hope by confirming that they will develop HD.

For others, genetic testing for HD offers a chance to end the uncertainty and to gain information, which they believe will enable them to make informed choices about the future.

Genetic Testing

Soon after the Huntington's disease gene was found in 1993, a test was developed which enabled people to find out if they were carrying the gene that causes HD. Earlier tests were based on a process of "linkage analysis" which required blood samples from several family members. The new "direct gene test" is much more accurate and requires blood only from the individual taking the test.

The HD gene was found to contain a specific section that was expanded in people with HD. In all people, this stretch of genetic material, or DNA, contains a pattern of so-called "trinucleotide repeats." Nucleotides are the building blocks of DNA and are represented by the letters C, A, G and T. In most people, the repeated pattern, CAG, occurs 30 times or less. In Huntington's disease, it occurs more than 40 times. By analyzing a person's DNA and counting the number of CAG's, it is possible to tell if that person will develop HD. The test cannot predict age of onset.

The decision to undergo genetic testing is an intensely personal one and one that cannot be taken lightly. Everyone has their own circumstances to take into consideration, and there are no "right" or "wrong" answers. Testing should never be forced upon an at-risk individual. Children are generally not able to consider the full implications of testing and may be vulnerable to pressure from others. Therefore, the minimum age requirement is usually 18.

Various resources are available to assist you in making this decision. HDSA chapter social workers and genetic counselors at testing centers can help, and there may be a support group for people at risk for HD in your area.

The Huntington's Disease Society of America recommends that at-risk persons who wish to undergo presymptomatic testing do so at an HD testing center. The testing centers involve teams of professionals who are knowledgeable about HD, and a list of these centers is available from HDSA.

The testing procedure involves sessions with various professionals. It typically includes one session devoted to each of the following: genetic counseling; a neurological exam; a psychological interview; discussion of the results; and follow-up. The genetic test itself is a blood test.

The purpose of the preliminary sessions is to ensure that the person understands the potential implications of his/her genetic status and is prepared to receive the results. The neurologic exam will determine if any early symptoms of HD are present. If the person is found to be symptomatic, he/she will be offered the option of discontinuing the testing procedure.

It is important to note that presymptomatic testing for HD cannot determine when the disease will begin its course or severity. People who test positive for the gene may remain healthy for many years. HD can only be diagnosed by a neurological exam.

For couples planning a family, prenatal testing of a fetus is also an option. A "nondisclosing" variation of the prenatal test can also be done using linkage analysis. Instead of examining the gene, this method of testing compares patterns of chromosomal inheritance in several family members with the chromosomes inherited by the fetus. In this way, the approximate risk that the fetus is carrying the HD gene can be determined without disclosing the genetic status of the at-risk parent.

Treatment

Treatment for HD takes many forms. While current treatments do not alter the course of HD, medications can be effective in treating common symptoms such as depression and anxiety, for example. Involuntary movements can also be lessened by medication. Some drugs have significant side effects, however, so it is important that these be explained by the physician before the treatment begins.

Some doctors may prescribe drug treatment when it is not absolutely necessary. In many cases, people with HD do better when medication is kept to a minimum. Often, drugs that are effective at one stage of the disease may not be effective at another.

For these reasons, it is preferable to locate a neurologist with expertise in HD. Not all neurologists are familiar with the disease. Though a family physician is not likely to have much experience with HD, that physician should remain involved in ongoing care and treatment. The person with HD and family members play a critical role in monitoring and assessing the effectiveness of any care and treatment.

A Physicians Guide to the Management of Huntington's Disease contains useful and detailed information on the treatment of specific symptoms of HD and is available from HDSA.

It is also helpful to consult a physician or occupational therapist and speech-language pathologist (speech therapist) so that strategies that can have a positive and lasting impact on the quality of life can be implemented early.

Nutrition is important in everyone's life, but it takes on added significance in HD. People with HD require an unusually high number of calories to maintain their body weight. Maintaining, or even gaining, weight can help reduce involuntary movements and other symptoms, particularly in the later stages of HD. Nutritional supplements such as Ensure can help, and a nutritionist can offer other valuable suggestions.

Often the best advice and emotional support one gets is from someone who "has been there." The mutual support given and the knowledge shared are the reasons that many find HD support groups to be an important part of their lives. Support groups are located in most states and HDSA can help you locate the one closest to you.

The Search for a Cure

The key to better treatments and an eventual cure for HD is research. There have been several exciting breakthroughs in recent years, notably the HD gene discovery of 1993. Since then, certain brain proteins have been discovered which appear to interact with huntingtin, the protein expressed by the HD gene. Research is under way to determine how these substances combine to cause the symptoms of HD, and to find ways of stopping this interaction as a possible means of treatment.

After the gene discovery, an international coalition of scientists, known as the Huntington Study Group (HSG), was formed to conduct basic and clinical research in a coordinated fashion. HSG sites combine research facilities with teams of doctors with expertise in treating HD. The group has begun to test new drugs which could potentially lead to effective treatments for Huntington's disease.

In 1997, the Huntington's Disease Society of America established the HDSA Coalition for the Cure, a consortium of 14 top laboratories in North America and Europe. Coalition investigators focus on four key areas of study: animal models, cell models, biochemistry and cell biology. Through HDSA funding, semi-annual meetings and the sharing of data and ideas, the Coalition is accelerating the pace of HD research.

Huntington's Disease Society of America

With over 30 chapters throughout the country, the Huntington's Disease Society of America is often the first place people go for information or assistance in coping with the effects of HD. HDSA chapters can provide information about local resources, including knowledgeable physicians and other health professionals, genetic testing centers, support groups, and long-term care facilities. In most cases, a chapter social worker is available for information and support.

HDSA publishes and distributes a wide variety of informational materials, including newsletters, books, booklets, brochures and videotapes covering care, treatment, research, and related topics.

The Society's commitment to research is demonstrated by its continued increases in funding to HDSA research programs each year. In 2003 the Society dedicated over $2.5 million for medical and research initiatives including the HDSA Coalition for the Cure, the HDSA Grants and Fellowships program, and the HDSA Centers of Excellence for Family Services and Research. For more information about how you can help or to find out more about HDSA, please write to Huntington's Disease Society of America, 158 West 29th Street, 7th Floor, New York, NY 10001-5300. Or call us at 800-345-HDSA or visit our national web site at www.hdsa.org. We look forward to hearing from you.

Chapter 20

Mild Cognitive Impairment

What is MCI?

Mild cognitive impairment (MCI) refers to a condition characterized primarily by a memory problem in the presence of otherwise
normal cognitive functioning. MCI is not a form of dementia; however,
people with MCI are at greater risk of eventually developing signs of
Alzheimer's disease (AD), than similarly aged people in the general
population.

What causes MCI, and does it run in families?

As with Alzheimer's disease, the causes of MCI remain unclear. No
genetic link has been found for the condition. Nevertheless, it is possible that, like AD, a genetic component might be a risk factor for
people with MCI to develop AD.

How is MCI diagnosed?

The diagnosis of MCI is usually precipitated by a complaint from
the patient and/or an informant regarding trouble remembering specific incidents that occur on a daily basis. Given this information, the

"Q and A: Mild Cognitive Impairment," by Heather Greene, MA; Joy Taylor,
PhD; and Helen Davies, MS, RNCS, in *Stanford/VA Alzheimer's Research
Center of California Newsletter*, Winter/Spring 2002. © 2002 Stanford/VA
Alzheimer's Center; reprinted with permission.

clinician will most likely obtain pertinent medical history and administer routine paper and pencil tests to get an objective assessment of the patient's memory and cognitive functioning. The following guidelines are typically used by health care professionals in making the diagnosis of MCI:

- Subjective memory complaint corroborated by an informant

- Objective indicators of memory impairment (i.e., testing) in relation to age and education

- Normal general cognitive function

- Intact activities of daily living

- Not demented

Will my memory problems get worse?

Although different theories have been developed to determine which MCI patients are at risk of progressing to AD, so far there are no sure answers. Unfortunately, this means that thousands of people are given a diagnosis with no clear understanding of what it means for the future. Many people get stuck at this stage trying to prove that "they" are wrong and there is no problem, while the family struggles with how to deal with the difficulties they see the patient experiencing.

So what can I do?

Health professionals suggest that first and foremost patients learn to "let go" and accept that there is a problem. The sooner this happens, the easier it will be to cope with the stresses of daily life. In doing so both the patient and family will feel better and can focus on what is under their control. Admit that there are no easy answers and move on with your life. Live each day to the fullest and try not to focus on what may or not happen down the line. This does not mean that you should ignore the problem, but instead that you should make the best of what you have. If you don't let go, the chances for family conflict increase and valuable time can be lost unnecessarily.

In addition, we know that there are certain things that can exacerbate memory problems, including stress. Therefore it is suggested that patients try keeping stress levels down through exercise, good nutrition, support groups, open communication, pleasurable activities and information seeking.

What is the best way for my family and me to communicate about the diagnosis?

Communication is key to healthy relationships so it is important to be open with one another. This can be difficult with a diagnosis as confusing and uncertain as MCI because more often than not, each person has a different idea of what the problem actually is and how it should be dealt with. Identifying problems and acknowledging feelings that emerge, is a good way to begin. Working together can reduce stress and identify new ways of coping. The more open everybody is to addressing the issue, the less chance of conflict and the better life will be.

Final Thoughts

If you or a family member has been diagnosed with MCI, you are not alone. If you are looking for help, you may want to consider joining a support group. To find out about support groups and get further information about MCI and current research, ask your healthcare provider or call the local Alzheimer's Association (800-660-1993). You can also find additional support at these websites: www.alz.org (Alzheimer's Association) and www.caregiver.com (Family Caregiver Alliance).

Although we are hopeful to have more answers in the future, there are many people living with the uncertainty of MCI now. What we recommend: talk to your doctor, join a support group, keep informed, communicate with one another and, most importantly, advocate for yourselves.

Chapter 21

Multi-Infarct Dementia

Serious forgetfulness, mood swings, and other behavioral changes are not a normal part of aging. They may be caused by poor diet, lack of sleep, or too many medicines, for example. Feelings of loneliness, boredom, or depression also can cause forgetfulness. These problems are serious and should be treated. Often they can be reversed.

Sometimes, however, mental changes are caused by diseases that permanently damage brain cells. The term dementia describes a medical condition that is caused by changes in the normal activity of very sensitive brain cells. These changes in the way the brain works can affect memory, speech, and the ability to carry out daily activities.

Alzheimer's disease is the most common cause of dementia in older people. The second most common cause of dementia in older adults is vascular dementia, which affects the blood vessels in the brain.

Alzheimer's disease (AD) affects approximately four million people in the U.S. Abnormal proteins collect in the brain and appear to cause loss of nerve cells in the areas vital to memory and thinking.

Alzheimer's disease develops slowly. At first, people with AD may have trouble remembering recent events, or the names of familiar people or things. Skills are lost continuously and gradually, though some people decline faster than others. As the disease goes on, symptoms become more easily noticed and serious enough to cause people with AD or their family members to seek medical help.

"Multi-Infarct Dementia," Alzheimer's Disease Education and Referral (ADEAR) Center, National Institute on Aging, National Institutes of Health, NIH Pub. No. 02-3433, May 2002.

Multi-infarct dementia is the most common form of vascular dementia, and accounts for 10–20% of all cases of progressive, or gradually worsening, dementia. It usually affects people between the ages of 60–75, and is more likely to occur in men than women.

Multi-infarct dementia is caused by a series of strokes that disrupt blood flow and damage or destroy brain tissue. A stroke occurs when blood cannot get to part of the brain. Strokes can be caused when a blood clot or fatty deposit (called plaque) blocks the vessels that supply blood to the brain. A stroke also can happen when a blood vessel in the brain bursts.

Some of the main causes of strokes are:

• untreated high blood pressure (hypertension)
• diabetes
• high cholesterol
• heart disease

Of these, the most important risk factor for multi-infarct dementia is high blood pressure.

Because strokes occur suddenly, loss of thinking and remembering skills—the symptoms of dementia—also occurs quickly and often in a step-wise pattern. People with multi-infarct dementia may even appear to improve for short periods of time, then decline again after having more strokes.

Symptoms

Sudden onset of any of the following symptoms may be a sign of multi-infarct dementia:

• confusion and problems with recent memory
• wandering or getting lost in familiar places
• moving with rapid, shuffling steps
• loss of bladder or bowel control
• laughing or crying inappropriately
• difficulty following instructions
• problems handling money

Multi-infarct dementia is often the result of a series of small strokes. Some of these small strokes produce no obvious symptoms and are noticed only on brain imaging studies, so they are sometimes called "silent strokes." A person may have several small strokes before noticing serious changes in memory or other signs of multi-infarct dementia.

Transient ischemic attacks, or TIAs, are caused by a temporary blockage of blood flow. Symptoms of TIAs are similar to symptoms of stroke and include mild weakness in an arm or leg, slurred speech, and dizziness. Symptoms generally do not last for more than 20 minutes. A recent history of TIAs greatly increases a person's chance of suffering permanent brain damage from a stroke. Prompt medical attention is required to determine what may be causing the blockage in blood flow and to start proper treatment (such as aspirin or warfarin).

If you believe someone is having a stroke—if a person experiences sudden weakness or numbness on one or both sides of the body, or difficulty speaking, seeing, or walking—call 911 immediately. If the physician believes the symptoms are caused by a blocked blood vessel, treatment with a "clot buster," such as t-PA (tissue plasminogen activator), within three hours can reopen the vessel and may reduce the severity of the stroke.

Diagnosis

People who show signs of dementia and who have a history of strokes should be evaluated for possible multi-infarct dementia. The doctor usually will ask the patient and the family about the person's diet, medications, sleep patterns, personal habits, past strokes, and other risk factors (such as high blood pressure, diabetes, high cholesterol, and heart disease). The doctor also may ask about recent illnesses or stressful events, like the death of someone close or problems at home or work, which may account for the symptoms. To look for signs of stroke, the doctor will check for weakness or numbness in the arms and legs, difficulty with speech, or dizziness. To check for other health problems that could cause symptoms of dementia, the doctor may order office or laboratory tests. These tests may include a blood pressure reading, an electroencephalogram (EEG), a test of thyroid function, or blood tests.

The doctor also may ask for x-rays or special tests such as a computerized tomography (CT) scan or a magnetic resonance imaging (MRI) scan. Both CT scans and MRI scans take pictures of sections of the brain. The pictures are displayed on a computer screen to allow the doctor to see inside the brain and check for signs of stroke,

143

tumors, or other sources of brain injury. Specialists called radiologists and neurologists interpret these scans. In addition, the doctor may send the patient to a psychologist or psychiatrist to assess reasoning, learning ability, memory, and attention span.

Sometimes multi-infarct dementia is difficult to distinguish from AD because their symptoms can be very similar. It is possible for a person to have both diseases, making it hard for the doctor to diagnose either.

Treatment

While no treatment can reverse brain damage that has already been caused by a stroke, treatment to prevent further strokes is very important. For example, high blood pressure, the primary risk factor for multi-infarct dementia, and diabetes are treatable. To prevent more strokes, doctors may prescribe medicines to control high blood pressure, high cholesterol, heart disease, and diabetes. They will counsel patients about good health habits such as exercising, avoiding smoking and drinking alcohol, and eating a low-fat diet.

To reduce symptoms of dementia, doctors may change or stop medications that can cause confusion, such as sedatives, antihistamines, strong painkillers, and other medications. Some patients also may have to be treated for additional medical conditions that can increase confusion, such as heart failure, thyroid disorders, anemia, or infections.

Doctors sometimes prescribe aspirin, warfarin, or other drugs to prevent clots from forming in small blood vessels. Medications also can be prescribed to relieve restlessness or depression or to help patients sleep better.

To improve blood flow or remove blockages in blood vessels, doctors may recommend surgical procedures, such as carotid endarterectomy, angioplasty, or stenting. Studies are under way to see how well these treatments work for patients with multi-infarct dementia. Scientists are also studying drugs that can improve blood flow to the brain, such as anti-platelet and anti-coagulant medications; drugs to treat symptoms of dementia, including Alzheimer's disease medications; as well as drugs to reduce the risk of TIAs and stroke, such as cholesterol-lowering statins and blood pressure medications.

Helping Someone with Multi-Infarct Dementia

Family members and friends can help someone with multi-infarct dementia cope with mental and physical problems. They can encourage individuals to maintain their daily routines and regular social and physical activities. By talking with them about events and daily experiences, family members can help loved ones use their mental abilities as much as possible. Some families find it helpful to use reminders such as lists, alarm clocks, and calendars to help the patient remember important times and dates.

A person with multi-infarct dementia should see their primary care doctor regularly. Health problems such as high blood pressure, diabetes, high cholesterol, and heart disease should be carefully monitored. If a person has additional medical conditions, such as depression, mental health experts may be consulted as well.

Help for home caregivers is available from a variety of sources, including nurses, family doctors, social workers, and physical and occupational therapists. Home health care and respite or neighborhood day care services can provide much-needed relief to care-givers. Support groups offer emotional support for family members caring for a person with dementia. A state or local health department, a local hospital, or the patient's doctor may be able to provide telephone numbers for such services.

Chapter 22

Pick's Disease

What is it?

A progressive dementia occurring in middle life characterized by slowly developing changes in character and social behavior, or impairment of language, due to degeneration of the frontal and temporal lobes of the brain.

Where does the name come from?

Arnold Pick was the doctor who was the first to describe the disease in 1892.

Other names for the disease. Many doctors now prefer to reserve the name "Pick's" for just one of the types of changes in the brain tissue (histology) that may be seen with the disease. You may come across several different names which are explained below: Frontotemporal lobar degeneration, frontotemporal dementia, semantic dementia and primary progressive aphasia.

Frontotemporal lobar degeneration. Many doctors now prefer this name for the disease. Patients who would have previously been told they had Pick's disease may now be told they have frontotemporal

Reprinted with permission from "Pick's Disease (frontotemporal lobar degeneration)," by Dr. Alison Godbolt, Dementia Research Unit, and Penelope Roques, Pick's Disease Support Group (PDSG). © 2003 PDSG. Additional information from PDSG is available online at www.pdsg.org.uk.

lobar degeneration. The name refers to the parts of the brain that are affected: the frontal and temporal lobes (at the front and side of the brain respectively).

Frontotemporal lobar degeneration can present with three different patterns of symptoms: frontotemporal dementia, semantic dementia or primary progressive aphasia. In frontotemporal dementia the frontal lobes (controlling behavior, organization and planning) are affected first, whilst in semantic dementia it is the temporal lobes (controlling language) that are affected first. In primary progressive aphasia, the disease starts in an area at the back of the frontal lobes and front of the temporal lobes.

What are the symptoms?

Frontotemporal dementia. Personality change is an early feature. The person may lose their inhibitions and become extrovert, or alternatively may become apathetic and withdrawn. They may talk to strangers, make inappropriate remarks in public and be rude or impatient. They may become aggressive which may be quite out of character, and may develop fixed routines. Some people begin to hoard things and become obsessive. Behavior may be sexually suggestive, though a loss of interest in sexual acts themselves is also common. Often the person with dementia will be unaware of the problems.

People may also develop a sweet tooth and overeat leading to gain in weight. Excessive alcohol intake may occur. Spending money and losing cash often causes problems. In the later stages people with the illness may compulsively put objects in their mouths.

In the early stages memory is not usually affected. However sometimes difficulties in organization and concentration may lead to an apparent memory problem. People may be very distractible. Later in the disease a more generalized dementia can develop.

Semantic dementia. This begins with loss of knowledge about the world, which often presents as problems with language. Although people can still speak fluently they lose the words for certain items and also lose the knowledge of the meaning of the word. For example, someone may not only forget the word "hippopotamus" when shown a picture, but also loses all the knowledge they once had about this (e.g. that it is an African animal that lives in rivers). However, unlike Alzheimer's disease, memory for day to day events may be good. People may also have difficulty recognizing what things are. At later stages, personality is often affected.

Primary progressive aphasia. People gradually develop difficulties with their speech (aphasia), which becomes slow and laboured and contains errors. This can be an isolated problem, and personality, memory and understanding may be almost normal for a long period. Eventually other areas do become involved and at a late stage a more generalized dementia becomes apparent.

What is the life span of the disease?

This varies quite a lot between individuals. It may last from 2 to more than 10 years, and a long duration of illness is quite common.

Is Pick's disease linked to other diseases?

A small number of people who have motor neuron disease may go on to develop frontotemporal lobar degeneration, with symptoms like those described above. Occasionally, the change in behavior develops before any weakness or wasting, and so before motor neuron disease is diagnosed. This is not common however.

Who can get Pick's disease?

It usually affects men or women in their 40s and 50s. However a few patients are affected as young as in their 20s, and older people do sometimes develop the disease.

What is known about brain changes associated with Pick's disease?

Loss of cells from the frontal and temporal lobes of the brain leads to shrinkage (atrophy) of these areas that may be visible on a brain scan. Brain changes have also been studied in post mortem examinations when the brain can be examined under a microscope ("histology"). Several different types of brain changes can cause the same symptoms. One example is deposition of a protein called tau.

Is it inherited?

In less than a half of cases a person with the disease may have a family history of the disease in one of their parents, brothers, or sisters. In these cases the cause may be genetic. Mutations (faults) in the tau gene on chromosome 17 are the cause in some of these cases. In other families with several members affected and no tau mutation

149

found, it is likely that other yet-to-be-discovered genes cause the disease.

How is it diagnosed?

The diagnosis is based on a clinical assessment and further tests are often suggested to investigate the problems. These may include brain scans (MRI or CT), neuropsychology assessments, blood tests and EEG (electroencephalography). Not all tests are suitable for every person. There is no one test that proves or disproves the diagnosis, but they all provide information that overall aids the doctor in reaching a diagnosis.

Can it be treated?

There is no cure for the disease at present. Sometimes antidepressants or tranquilizers may be suggested to control particular problems. Knowing more about the disease and why the person is behaving as they are can in itself be an effective means of helping people cope with the disease.

Chapter 23

Vascular Dementia

What Is Vascular Dementia?

Dementia is the general term for a gradual progressive decline in a person's memory and other mental abilities. Vascular dementia is the second most common cause of dementia and recently its incidence has been found to be higher than previously expected. The most common type of vascular dementia is multi-infarct dementia (MID) where the brain has been damaged by repeated small strokes. However, vascular dementia can be caused by a number of other conditions including high blood pressure (hypertension), irregular heart rhythms (arrhythmias) and diseases which cause damage to the arteries in the brain. Indeed, any condition which causes the circulation to the brain to be impaired or damaged carries a risk to mental abilities.

Vascular dementia accounts for almost 20% of all cases of dementia, with at least another 20% of people having both Alzheimer's disease and vascular dementia (Brown 1993).[1] It usually affects people between the ages of 60–75 years and is slightly more common in men than women.

Vascular dementia is similar to Alzheimer's disease in that it results in the progressive deterioration of the higher functions of the brain, such as:

Excerpted from "Vascular Dementia," © 2002 Alzheimer Scotland - Action on Dementia; reprinted with permission. For more information from Alzheimer Scotland - Action on Dementia, visit their website at www.alzscot.org.

- memory
- new learning
- recognition
- fine motor movements
- planning

One major difference with vascular dementia is that these changes will generally occur in a stepwise pattern due to the sudden occurrence of strokes.

The person will usually deteriorate at the point that they have a stroke, but they may improve or remain stable for a while before the next stroke occurs, when they will again deteriorate. It is often difficult to decide with certainty whether a person has Alzheimer's disease or vascular dementia and often a patient will have both types of dementia.

Causes of Vascular Dementia

Vascular dementia is due to impaired blood supply to the brain and can be divided into different types depending on the nature of the vascular disease.

- Arteriosclerotic dementia—reduced oxygen supply to the brain (chronic ischemia).

- Vascular dementia following a stroke. Major strokes can be fatal or may lead to physical disability or vascular dementia due to damage to the brain.

- Multi-infarct dementia (MID) which develops gradually following a number of mini-strokes or transient ischemic attacks (TIAs—see below), which the person may not realize they are having. MID affects the cerebral cortex, which is the outer part of the brain.

- Subcortical vascular dementia (Binswanger's disease) which involves vascular damage to the nerve cell fibres of the inner parts of the brain (deep white matter) by affecting the sheath which insulates nerve fibres in the brain (demyelination).

- There is also a vascular dementia which involves both cortical and subcortical damage to the brain.

- There are rarer causes of vascular dementia which may affect some people with auto-immune inflammatory diseases that affect the arteries such as systemic lupus erythematosus (SLE or lupus) and temporal arteritis.

While vascular dementia can be caused in several different ways, the most common cause is a blockage of small blood vessels (arteries) deep within the brain. When any part of the body is deprived of blood which carries oxygen and nutrients it dies and this is called an infarct. When this happens in the brain it is called a stroke. Depending on where the stroke occurs in the brain different functions of the brain will be affected. Each side of the brain controls the movement on the other side of the body, thus strokes on the left side of the brain can cause problems in moving the limbs on the right side of the body and vice versa. Strokes on the left side are also especially associated with problems in language and memory. Strokes on either side can cause problems with recognition of objects and coordination of complex tasks. Strokes in certain areas of the brain can also cause changes in the person's mood and personality.

Transient Ischaemic Attacks (TIAs)

Transient ischemic attacks (TIAs) are temporary interruptions of blood flow to the brain, (a stroke is a permanent cut off of blood to part of the brain). TIA warning signs include:

- numbness, weakness, or paralysis of the face, arm or leg, especially on one side
- sudden blurred, decreased or complete loss of vision in one or both eyes
- difficulty speaking or understanding simple statements
- loss of balance, dizziness or loss of coordination especially when combined with another warning sign
- sudden severe headache in one part of the head.

These warning signs can last for a few hours and never last longer than 24 hours. They should not be ignored, as diagnosis and treatment may well prevent a serious stroke. *Contact a doctor immediately if these symptoms occur.*

Strokes

Strokes occur when brain cells are deprived of their blood supply and then die. They can be caused by damage to the brain or neck arteries. The damage may be a blockage or bleeding into the brain caused by:

- *Thrombosis:* A gradual narrowing and eventual blockage of an artery, usually because of a build-up of cholesterol and fatty deposits. Approximately 60% of strokes are caused by thrombosis.

- *Embolism:* A blockage of a brain or neck artery by a clot, either a blood clot elsewhere in the body (often the heart) which travels to the brain, or a piece of fatty deposit broken away from the lining of the arteries. Approximately 20% of strokes are caused by embolism.

- *Hemorrhage:* A burst in a brain artery causing bleeding in the brain. Approximately 20% of all strokes are caused by hemorrhage.

Symptoms and Diagnosis

Serious forgetfulness, mood swings and other behavioral changes are not a normal part of ageing. They could be caused by poor diet, malfunctioning thyroid, lack of sleep or too many medicines. Feelings of loneliness and boredom or depression can also cause forgetfulness. These conditions can often be helped and medical advice should be sought.

Sometimes, however, mental changes are caused by diseases that permanently damage the brain cells.

Multi-Infarct Dementia

MID is probably the most common type of vascular dementia and is caused by a number of 'mini-strokes'. The person may not be aware of these small strokes and the symptoms may last for only a few hours up to a few days. A person with MID is likely to have better insight into their condition right up until the later stages, as compared with people who have Alzheimer's disease, where insight is lost relatively early. Parts of their personality may also remain relatively intact for longer.

The symptoms can be quite varied as the stroke can occur in any part of the brain and therefore will affect different functions. Not everyone with MID will suffer from all of these symptoms but they may include:

- mild weakness in an arm or leg
- slurred speech

- dizziness

- trouble remembering things especially recent events

- difficulty following a conversation or communicating properly

- confusion

- hallucinations where they see or hear things which are not real, or delusions

- depression with emotional swings when laughter or tears can occur for no reason

- epileptic fits or partial or total paralysis sometimes occur but are rare

- incontinence of bladder and/or bowel.

Subcortical Vascular Dementia

Binswanger's disease was once considered rare, but it is being reassessed and may in fact be relatively common. It is the 'white matter' deep within the brain which is affected and the pattern of symptoms is different from MID.

Symptoms can include:

- slowness and lethargy in thinking and actions

- difficulty walking and may have to walk with legs far apart

- emotional ups and downs

- loss of bladder control early in the course of the disease

- most people with Binswanger's disease have or have had high blood pressure.

Diagnosis and Tests

Anyone who shows signs of dementia and has a history of strokes should have a complete medical examination. An accurate diagnosis is vital in order to treat the person and reduce the risk of further strokes and to slow the progress of vascular dementia. The doctor will ask about the person's diet, medications, sleep patterns, personal habits, history of high blood pressure, diabetes, cholesterol problems and any abnormal heart patterns. Make sure the doctor knows of any other medical problems or recent stressful events in the person's life which might account for the symptoms.

One caregiver found it very difficult to obtain a diagnosis for his partner and it took years to finally discover she had vascular dementia. 'The doctor said it was just old age'. The initial symptoms were difficulty remembering things, finding household tasks more difficult, becoming less sociable.

Ensure the person you are concerned about receives a thorough examination from the doctor and ask for an appointment with a specialist if you are not happy with the diagnosis.

The doctor will look for signs of stroke by checking for weakness or numbness in the arms or legs and for any difficulty with speech. The doctor may also ask for further tests, which could include blood pressure readings, cholesterol levels, an electrocardiograph (ECG), a chest x-ray and blood tests including thyroid function and vitamin levels. Further tests may be required including a CT scan[2] or a magnetic resonance imaging scan (MRI).[3] The different types of scans allow the specialists to examine the brain and reveal any areas damaged by strokes, which would indicate the person may have vascular dementia.

The person may also be sent to a psychologist or psychiatrist to assess reasoning, learning ability, memory and attention span. People with vascular dementia should be offered a skilled multidisciplinary assessment of their condition through referral to a specialist. This service may be part of the general stroke service or the psychogeriatric service. The services might include:

- rehabilitation to restore as much mental or physical ability as possible.

- diagnosis and treatment of any underlying disease such as high blood pressure (hypertension), high cholesterol, or diabetes

- speech and language therapy to help the person make the best use of their remaining abilities

- occupational therapy to help the person cope better and more safely at home.

Course of the Illness

For each type of vascular dementia there will be a different progression of the illness.

Major strokes. For those who have suffered a major stroke the symptoms will be severe and will start from the date of the stroke.

The brain tissue which has been destroyed cannot be repaired and generally the person will not improve, although in some cases the brain manages to adjust and work around the injured area.

Mini-strokes. Mini-strokes which lead to multi-infarct dementia (MID). If someone has MID caused by mini-strokes the symptoms may not be evident at the beginning of the disease, but will gradually become more obvious as more strokes occur. Usually the disease progresses in a step-wise fashion following the strokes. After a stroke the person will deteriorate, with the symptoms becoming more pronounced, and then will often improve and their condition will stabilize until the next stroke, when they will decline again. If no further strokes occur the progression of vascular dementia may stop and in some cases the abilities of the person may improve. Sometimes the steps are so small that the decline appears gradual, which is very similar to the progression of Alzheimer's disease.

Subcortical vascular dementia. Early symptoms are slowness and lethargy, walking difficulties, emotional ups and downs and lack of bladder control. The dementia will gradually progress later.

Prevention and Treatment

Risk Factors

The risk factors for vascular dementia are the same as those associated with strokes; high blood pressure (hypertension), diabetes, high cholesterol level and heart disease. To a large extent these risk factors are controllable and while no treatment can reverse damage that has already been done, treatment to reduce the risk of strokes occurring or additional strokes is possible. Medicines can be used to control blood pressure, high cholesterol, heart disease and diabetes.

Giving up smoking, avoiding an excessive alcohol intake, having a healthy diet and regular exercise will all lessen the risk of having a stroke. Speak to your physician who will be able to help with advice and information.

Drugs

Aspirin and warfarin are widely used to lessen the risk of further strokes by preventing clots from forming in small blood vessels. There are also drugs available to control high blood pressure, diabetes and high cholesterol levels. Drugs to control depression and relieve restlessness and help the person with vascular dementia to sleep better can also be prescribed.

There are several new drugs recently licensed for treating Alzheimer's disease (like donepezil (Aricept) or galantamine (Reminyl). Although these are usually prescribed for someone with Alzheimer's disease they are now being given to people with vascular dementia, as some studies have suggested they may be of some help.

Very rarely surgery may also be a useful option if there is a significant narrowing in the carotid artery, which is the main blood vessel to the brain.

Notes

1. Brown MM (1993) Vascular Dementia. *Alzheimer's Review* 3(2) 57-62.

2. CT scans or CAT scans use x-rays but show more detail and allow a specialist to see inside a brain.

3. MRI scans use radio waves and a strong magnetic field to give a clear and detailed picture of the brain.

Chapter 24

Wernicke-Korsakoff Syndrome (Alcohol-Related Dementia)

Alternative Names

Korsakoff psychosis; Alcoholic encephalopathy; Encephalopathy—alcoholic; Wernicke's disease

Definition

Wernicke-Korsakoff syndrome is a brain disorder involving loss of specific brain functions caused by a thiamine deficiency.

Causes, Incidence, and Risk Factors

The syndrome is actually a spectrum, including two separate sets of symptoms, one of which tends to start when the other subsides. Wernicke's encephalopathy involves damage to multiple nerves in both the central nervous system (brain and spinal cord) and the peripheral nervous system (the rest of the body).

It may also include symptoms caused by alcohol withdrawal. The cause is generally attributed to malnutrition, especially lack of vitamin B_1 (thiamine), which commonly accompanies habitual alcohol use or alcoholism.

Heavy alcohol use interferes with the metabolism of thiamine, so even in the unusual cases where alcoholics are eating a balanced diet while drinking heavily, the metabolic problem persists because most of the thiamine is not absorbed.

Korsakoff syndrome, or Korsakoff psychosis, tends to develop as Wernicke's symptoms diminish. It involves impairment of memory out of proportion to problems with other cognitive functions.

Patients often attempt to hide their poor memory by confabulating. The patient will create detailed, believable stories about experiences or situations to cover gaps in memory. This is not usually a deliberate attempt to deceive because the patient often believes what he is saying to be true. It can occur whether or not the thiamine deficiency was related to alcoholism and with other types of brain damage.

Korsakoff psychosis involves damage to areas of the brain involved with memory.

Symptoms

- Vision changes
  - Double vision
  - Eye movement abnormalities
  - Eyelid drooping
- Loss of muscle coordination
  - Unsteady, uncoordinated walking
- Loss of memory, can be profound
- Inability to form new memories
- Confabulation (making up stories to explain behavior that have little relation to reality)
- Hallucinations

Note: Symptoms that indicate alcohol withdrawal may also be present or may develop.

Signs and Tests

- Examination of the nervous/muscular system may show polyneuropathy (damage to multiple nerve systems).
- Reflexes may be decreased (or of abnormal intensity), or abnormal reflexes may be present.

- Testing of gait and coordination indicates damage to portions of the brain that control muscle coordination.

- Muscles may be weak and may show atrophy (loss of tissue mass).

- Examination of the eyes shows abnormalities of eye movement.

- Blood pressure and body temperature measurement may be low.

- Pulse (heart rate) may be rapid.

The person may appear cachectic (malnourished). A nutritional assessment may confirm malnourished state.

- Serum B_1 levels may be low.

- Pyruvate is elevated.

- Transketolase activity is decreased.

If the history is significant for chronic alcohol abuse, serum or urine alcohol levels may be elevated (see toxicology screen) and liver enzymes may be elevated.

Other chronic conditions that may cause a thiamine deficiency include the following:

- AIDS

- Hyperemesis gravidarum (continuous nausea and vomiting during pregnancy)

- Thyrotoxicosis (very high thyroid hormone levels)

- Cancers that have spread throughout the body

- Long-term dialysis

- Congestive heart failure, when treated with long-term diuretic therapy

- A brain MRI rarely shows changes in the tissue of the brain indicating Wernicke-Korsakoff syndrome.

Treatment

The goals of treatment are to control symptoms as much as possible and to prevent progression of the disorder. Hospitalization is required for initial control of symptoms.

If the person is lethargic, unconscious, or comatose, monitoring and care appropriate to the condition may be required. The airway should be monitored and protected as appropriate.

Thiamine (vitamin B_1) may improve symptoms of confusion or delirium, difficulties with vision and eye movement, and muscle incoordination. Vitamin B_1 may be given by injection into a vein or a muscle, or by mouth.

Thiamine does not generally improve loss of memory and intellect associated with Korsakoff psychosis.

Total abstinence from alcohol is required to prevent progressive loss of brain function and damage to peripheral nerves. A well-balanced, nourishing diet is recommended.

Support Groups

The stress of illness can often be helped by joining a support group where members share common experiences and problems.

Expectations (Prognosis)

Without treatment, Wernicke-Korsakoff syndrome progresses steadily to death. With treatment, symptoms (such as uncoordinated movement and vision difficulties) may be controlled, and progression of the disorder may be slowed or stopped.

Some symptoms—particularly the loss of memory and cognitive skills—may be permanent. There may be a need for custodial care if the loss of cognitive skills is severe.

Other disorders related to the abuse of alcohol may also be present.

Complications

- Permanent loss of memory
- Permanent loss of cognitive skills
- Injury caused by falls
- Difficulty with personal or social interaction
- Alcohol withdrawal state
- Permanent alcoholic neuropathy
- Shortened life span

Wernicke's encephalopathy may be precipitated in at-risk people by carbohydrate loading or glucose infusion. Supplementation with thiamine must precede glucose infusion to prevent this.

Calling Your Health Care Provider

Call your health care provider if symptoms suggesting Wernicke-Korsakoff syndrome occur, or if the condition has been diagnosed and symptoms worsen or reappear.

Also call if new symptoms develop, particularly symptoms of alcohol withdrawal. Alcohol withdrawal can be fatal, so call the local emergency number (such as 911) or go to the emergency room if any severe symptoms occur.

Symptoms of alcohol withdrawal include:

- Delirium or confusion

- Agitation

- Jumpiness or nervousness

- Insomnia

- Hallucinations

- Palpitations

- Heart rate that is faster than normal without an observable cause, such as:
    - Increased activity
    - Pale skin
    - Profuse sweating
    - Muscle tremors
    - Seizures
    - Headache
    - Fever
    - Nausea/vomiting

Prevention

Abstinence or moderate alcohol use and adequate nutrition reduce the risk of developing Wernicke-Korsakoff syndrome. If a heavy drinker is determined not to quit, thiamine supplementation and a good diet may help prevent the development of this condition, but not if damage has already occurred.

Note: The information provided herein should not be used during any medical emergency or for the diagnosis or treatment of any medical condition. A licensed physician should be consulted for diagnosis and treatment of any and all medical conditions. Call 911 for all medical emergencies.

Part Three

Diagnosing and Treating Dementias

Chapter 25

Questions to Ask the Doctor about Mental Changes

Questions to Ask the Doctor

As we age, we experience many physical and mental changes. Many of these changes are just a part of normal aging, but sometimes, they may be an indicator of a more serious condition. One thing that people with memory problems often fear is that they have Alzheimer's disease—one form of dementia. However, there are many health conditions which mimic the symptoms of Alzheimer's disease but are treatable.

The questions below are designed to help you talk with your doctor about all of the possible causes of your memory loss symptoms, especially those which are treatable, before you and your doctor settle on a diagnosis of Alzheimer's disease or dementia.

Possible Medication Interactions

If you take even two medications, you may be experiencing dizziness, memory loss, or other symptoms due to medication interactions.

- Make a list and be sure to tell your physician about all substances you are taking, including:
  - Prescription Medications
  - Vitamins

This chapter includes text from "Questions to Ask the Doctor," and "Working with Your Doctor," both produced by the Administration on Aging (AOA)'s Alzheimer's Program (www.aoa.gov/alz), 2002.

- Herbal supplements
- Over the counter products (such as aspirin and cold medicine)
- Smoking cessation products
- Water and weight loss products
- Topical items (such as arthritis ointment, athlete's foot treatment, etc.)
- Other items

- Be sure to be thorough, because even things that we don't think about (such as arthritis ointment) can contain substances that can cause problems for some people.

- Your doctor may need to work with you over time or may need to change your prescriptions and over the counter products in order to rule out medication interactions. Of course, this may not solve your problem, but it is an important thing to rule out.

Effect of Weight Loss/Gain and Medications

If you have recently gained or lost even 10 pounds, you should ask your doctor to check your medication levels.

- Some medications are prescribed according to our weight and losing or gaining weight may mean that you have too much or too little medication in your body for your size, and you may experience a variety of symptoms that mimic dementia.
- Use the list suggested above and share it with your physician.
- Be sure to alert your doctor to weight changes and have them adjust your medications if necessary.

Symptoms from Dehydration

If you are dehydrated or malnourished, your body may not be processing your medications correctly.

- You probably know that water is an important element in our bodies. Water is also necessary for our body to digest food and to dissolve and metabolize medications properly. However, many of us do not get enough water and dehydration among older adults is common.

- In talking with your doctor about your symptoms, be sure to alert your physician of any bouts of diarrhea, vomiting, and heat exhaustion you have recently experienced.

- Ask your physician to ensure that you are not dehydrated, because if you are, the medications in your system may be more concentrated than appropriate and your body may not be metabolizing your medicines correctly.

- If you are dehydrated, your physician will work with you to ensure proper hydration and that your medication levels are appropriate.

Falls and Concussions

If you have fallen or hit your head recently, you could have a concussion which can result in sudden memory loss, dizziness, etc.

- Although you may not realize it, a recent fall or serious bump on the head may be the cause of your memory problems. Falls among older adults are common and sometimes, people fall and do not know if they hit their head or even if they were unconscious for any period of time.

- Be sure to tell your doctor about any recent falls or serious bumps on your head so that your doctor can rule out concussions and other potential problems that can arise from such events.

- Your doctor may do a series of tests to see if there is anything that needs to be done and if so, he/she will do what is necessary to address the problem.

Depression

Depression is a common problem among older adults and affects as many as one in five older people. The symptoms of depression are remarkably similar to those of dementia.

- Physicians often mistake depression for dementia, so be sure to ask for specific tests to rule out depression. Blood tests and neurological and psychological evaluations are generally necessary to rule out depression.

- Depression can have many different triggers such as loss, significant life changes, and side effects of medications. Your physician should address all possible underlying causes of depression.

- Don't be afraid to ask for a depression screening, as many older people experience the symptoms of depression but are unaware that they have a treatable condition.

- Remember that depression is treatable, so be sure that your physician checks for depression prior to providing a diagnosis of dementia.

Alcohol Use

Consuming too much alcohol, or drinking alcohol while taking certain medications may result in symptoms of memory loss.

- Be sure to tell your physician if you drink alcohol on a regular basis, or if you experienced symptoms after an occasional drink.

- Use the list suggested above to advise your physician of any medications and treatments you use.

- Carefully follow your physician's advice in regards to the use of alcohol.

Questions and Answers about Working with Your Doctor

How does your physician know if it is Alzheimer's disease?

There is no single test that can diagnose Alzheimer's disease. However, trained physicians are 80%-90% accurate. Your physician needs to do a full assessment that includes:

- An accurate medical and psychiatric history
- A neurological/physical exam
- Lab tests to rule out anemia, vitamin deficiencies, and other conditions
- An evaluation of the person's ability to do common daily activities such as managing finances and medications
- A mental status exam to evaluate the person's thinking and memory
- A caregiver interview

Your physician may also request a brain scan, psychological testing, and additional lab work if he/she needs additional information.

How can you help your physician?

You can be prepared for the appointment by bringing a list of medications, a log of symptoms or behavior changes, and a list of questions or concerns. It is also helpful to provide an accurate history of the person's medical conditions and any previous psychiatric treatment.

What can your physician do if the diagnosis is Alzheimer's disease?

Although there is no cure for Alzheimer's disease, there are ways to treat some of the symptoms of the disease. Your physician may suggest:

- Use of medications to treat cognitive decline and memory loss

- Referral to appropriate activities such as exercise, recreation and adult day care services

- Appropriate treatment of medical or psychological conditions that may contribute to cognitive changes or decline

What can be done for behavioral problems?

At times, a person with a dementing illness may display behavior problems such as wandering, paranoia, suspiciousness, combativeness, or resistance to maintaining personal hygiene. These behavioral problems can seem overwhelming to the caregiver. The physician may suggest various strategies to assist in daily caregiving tasks such as:

- Enrollment in the Alzheimer's Association's Safe Return Program, an identification program for memory impaired adults

- Modifying the person's environment in order to reduce confusion caused by over-stimulation such as reducing noise and glare from windows

- Explaining a task before you do it such as saying, "I am going to help you put on your shirt."

- Providing a predictable routine at home with structured times for meals, bathing, exercise, and bedtime

- Providing reassurance to the confused patient without challenging their accusations or misperceptions and by redirecting their attention

If it seems that suggested strategies aren't helpful in managing the person's behavior, the physician may want to use medications to manage symptoms of depression, restlessness, hallucinations, hostility, and agitation. Be prepared to provide the physician with accurate information regarding the behavior problem such as the onset of the behavior, the frequency of the behavior, the time of day the behavior occurs, and the strategies you have tried.

How can your physician help you plan for the future?

The physician may suggest you start planning for health care needs now by completing an advance directive. An advance directive is a legal document that a patient signs while capable of making sound decisions. It directs how healthcare treatment will be made in the event of future incapacity. There are two types of advance directives:

- **Living Will** which conveys the person's desire to die a natural death and not be kept alive by artificial means.

- **Durable Power of Attorney for Health Care and/or Finances** designates an individual who can make health care/ financial decisions on behalf of the impaired person if he or she is not able to give consent.

We hope that this document is helpful in speaking with your doctor about all of the possible causes of your memory problems. After considering the various treatable conditions that often mimic the symptoms of dementia, your physician may determine that a diagnosis of Alzheimer's disease is correct. If you are diagnosed with Alzheimer's disease or another form of dementia, you may wish to contact your state or Area Agency on Aging or the local chapter of the Alzheimer's Association for assistance in coping with Alzheimer's disease.

Chapter 26

Warning Symptoms of Alzheimer's Disease or Dementia

Symptoms of Dementia

Symptoms that signal the onset of dementia are usually subtle and may not be noticeable for a number of years. In fact, earlier signs usually are identified in retrospect, and often by someone other than the patient. Most people think of memory loss as the central symptom in dementia. While most dementias affect memory, some forms of dementia do not initially involve memory loss. Other areas that may be affected include language, perceptual skills, reasoning, and personality. This is especially true in individuals whose symptoms begin before age 65.

Ten Warning Symptoms of Alzheimer's Disease or Dementia

1. **Memory Loss That Affects Job Skills:** It's normal to occasionally forget assignments, colleagues' names, or a business associate's telephone number and remember them later. Those with a dementia, such as Alzheimer's disease, may forget things more often and not remember them later.

This chapter includes "Symptoms of Dementia," "Who Gets Alzheimer's Disease," and "Alzheimer's Disease: Making a Diagnosis," Northwestern University Medical School–Cognitive Neurology and Alzheimer's Disease Center (www.brain.northwestern.edu), © 2002 Northwestern University, updated 2003; reprinted with permission.

2. **Difficulty Performing Familiar Tasks:** Busy people can be so distracted from time to time that they may leave the carrots on the stove and only remember to serve them at the end of the meal. People with Alzheimer's disease could prepare a meal and not only forget to serve it but also forget they made it.

3. **Problems with Language:** Everyone has trouble finding the right word sometimes, but a person with Alzheimer's disease may forget simple words or substitute inappropriate words, making his or her sentence incomprehensible.

4. **Disorientation of Time and Place:** It's normal to forget the day of the week or your destination for a moment. But people with Alzheimer's disease can become lost on their own street, not knowing where they are, how they got there or how to get back home.

5. **Poor or Impaired Judgment:** People can become so immersed in an activity that they temporarily forget the child they're watching. People with Alzheimer's disease could forget entirely the child under their care. They also may dress inappropriately, wearing several shirts or blouses.

6. **Problems with Abstract Thinking:** Balancing a checkbook may be disconcerting when the task is more complicated than usual. Someone with Alzheimer's disease could forget completely what the numbers are and what needs to be done with them.

7. **Misplacing Things:** Anyone can temporarily misplace a wallet or keys. A person with Alzheimer's disease may put things in inappropriate places: an iron in the freezer, or a wristwatch in the sugar bowl.

8. **Changes in Mood or Behavior:** Everyone becomes sad or moody occasionally. Someone with Alzheimer's disease can exhibit rapid mood swings (from calm to tears to anger) for no apparent reason.

9. **Changes in Personality:** People's personalities ordinarily change somewhat with age. But a person with Alzheimer's disease can show drastic personality changes, becoming extremely confused, suspicious, or fearful.

10.   **Loss of Initiative:** It's normal to tire of housework, business activities, or social obligations, but most people regain their initiative. The person with Alzheimer's disease may become very passive and require cues and prompting to become involved.

[These warning signs were taken from publications of the National Alzheimer's Association.]

Who Gets Alzheimer's Disease?

The two main categories of Alzheimer's disease are familial and sporadic. Familial Alzheimer's disease refers to a genetic form of the disease that is transmitted from one generation to the next. Only 5 percent of all cases of Alzheimer's disease have been associated with a genetic component. These individuals come from families in which as many as half of the members develop Alzheimer's disease. Fortunately, this form of the disorder is rare.

The remaining 95 percent of Alzheimer's disease cases are sporadic, or randomly occurring in the population. Particular dietary habits, professional occupations, or personality types do not seem to lead to the development of Alzheimer's disease.

A variety of "risk factors" have been identified in individuals diagnosed with probable AD (PRAD). In fact, it is quite common to pick up a newspaper or to turn on the TV and hear about the newest "risk factor" that has been identified. While some of these factors may turn out to be useful, it is important to remember that much of the research that has been done in this area is retrospective research. This means that the research is conducted by comparing a group of patients diagnosed with PRAD with a group of healthy age-matched adults. These types of analyses provide information about the number of individuals diagnosed with PRAD who have a certain characteristic compared with the healthy individuals. While these results are useful in directing future research studies, they do not provide information about cause and effect. What is needed is a prospective study in which large numbers of individuals are followed from an early age to the age at which PRAD develops.

Alzheimer's Disease: Making a Diagnosis

The absolute diagnosis of Alzheimer's disease can only be made at autopsy. However, physicians at specialized centers can diagnose

Alzheimer's disease with 90 percent certainty based on clinical information. To make the diagnosis the following may need to be conducted:

- A medical history and neurological exam.

- Neuropsychological testing: Neuropsychological testing involves a careful analysis of a person's memory, problem solving, language, attention, and visuospatial ability.

- Basic blood tests: Blood tests may be used to help exclude other causes of memory difficulties. For example, a person with a thyroid disorder or a vitamin deficiency may have problems with his or her memory.

- Brain scans: A brain scan such as an MRI or a CT scan may need to be done in certain patients to detect brain tumors or strokes. These disorders may cause memory problems.

Chapter 27

Dementia Screening Tests

What is a screening test?

A screening test is a preliminary procedure administered to distinguish individuals who may need further evaluation for a disorder from those who are less likely to need additional testing. Familiar examples of screening tests include Pap smears, mammograms, and kits for collecting small stool samples to be examined for hidden blood. Most such tests are administered under the supervision of a health care professional who orders the test, communicates the result, and discusses appropriate next steps.

What screening tests are marketed directly to consumers?

Test developers, health care facilities, and other sources are marketing a growing number of screening tests directly to consumers. Some of these tests are offered on a "self-referred" basis—individuals taking the test do not need a physician's order for it, and the testing facility reports the results directly to the examinee. Self-referred testing is a controversial practice. It is lucrative for facilities administering these tests because consumers must pay for them directly.

"Facts: About Dementia Screening Tests Marketed to Consumers" is reprinted with permission of the Alzheimer's Association. For additional information, call the Alzheimer's Association national toll-free number, 800-272-3900, or visit their website at www.alz.org. © 2002 Alzheimer's Association. All rights reserved.

Insurance plans generally do not pay for self-referred procedures, so facilities offering them can set their own price and require payment in advance.

What consumer screening tests are marketed for dementia?

The Alzheimer's Association has received numerous questions about two dementia screening tests recently marketed directly to consumers. One is the Early Alert Alzheimer's Home Screening Test, available in pharmacies and from a website. The other is the Minnesota Cognitive Acuity Screen (MCAS), sold by telephone and through a website.

The Alzheimer's Association believes that no single dementia screening procedure is a meaningful substitute for established diagnostic criteria for Alzheimer's disease administered by a skilled physician. Although these screening tests do not claim to offer a definitive diagnosis, any test that may plant the idea of a serious illness in a test-taker's mind has the potential to cause great psychological distress. The whole process of assessment, diagnosis, and diagnostic disclosure should be carried out within the context of an ongoing relationship with responsible health care professionals. Here are some relevant facts about each of the tests currently generating frequent questions:

Facts about the Early Alert Alzheimer's Home Screening Test:

- This test, marketed by FMG Innovations, Inc., sells for around $15–$20 in pharmacies and on the Internet.

- It is packaged in a small box that contains an instruction sheet, a pencil, and a booklet with 12 "scratch and sniff" odor strips. Examinees are instructed to scratch each strip to release the smell, then circle one of four words that best describe the odor. Choices include "cinnamon," "dog," "soap," "garlic," "motor oil," fruit and floral fragrances, and a variety of other scents.

- Correct answers are provided in an answer key at the back of the booklet. Examinees with four or more incorrect choices are advised to consult their physician.

- The instruction sheet states, "Smell loss is among the first signs of Alzheimer's disease. Experts recommend screening for smell loss once a year after the age of 65." It is true that there are legitimate scientific investigations exploring a possible link between smell loss and Alzheimer's disease, but the relationship has not been confirmed or quantified. No currently accepted diagnostic criteria for Alzheimer's include evaluation of smell, and there is no recommendation for annual smell testing from any recognized authority involved in establishing clinical guidelines.

- Many factors other than Alzheimer's disease can impair smell, including current smoking or past smoking, certain drugs, a wide variety of medical conditions, and individual differences in sensitivity to odors.

- Medical and diagnostic equipment, including products marketed directly to consumers, is regulated by the Center for Devices and Radiologic Health (CDRH) of the U.S. Food and Drug Administration (FDA). According to a CDRH spokesperson, the Early Alert smell test has not been cleared or approved for marketing.

Facts about the Minnesota Cognitive Acuity Screen (MCAS):

- The MCAS is sold by telephone and over the Internet for $95 by Nation's CareLink, a care management firm specializing in geriatric assessments.

- The test consists of a 15-minute question-and-answer telephone interview administered by a registered nurse who asks testtakers such questions as their name, address, and birthday, what day it is, and how they would handle an emergency such as a fire in their home. Examinees are also asked to repeat a six-digit number, to remember 10 words, and to tap on the telephone when instructed. Nurses score each examinee, and those whose scores fall below certain levels are considered to need monitoring or to have "failed" the test.

- The test's developers recommend annual testing. This recommendation does not reflect a policy established by any recognized clinical guideline.

- The chief use of the MCAS has been for commercial rather than clinical purposes—the test was developed by Nation's CareLink as a risk management tool to help insurers avoid issuing long-term care policies to individuals judged likely to develop dementia.

- The MCAS website describes the test as "98.1 percent effective in identifying cognitive function." In support of this statement,

MCAS cites an article published by the test's developers in the October 2000 edition of the journal *Neuropsychiatry, Neuropsychology, and Behavioral Neurology*. The abstract of this article on PubMed, the on-line literature database for the U.S. National Library of Medicine, concludes with the developer's own statement that "The Minnesota Cognitive Acuity Screen (MCAS) should undergo further study in unselected elderly populations to better understand its value as a screening tool." The PubMed database contains no additional articles about the test.

Chapter 28

How Is Alzheimer's Disease Diagnosed?

Ruling out Other Causes Memory of Loss or Dementia

A definitive test to diagnose Alzheimer's disease, even in patients showing signs of dementia, has not yet been devised, so the first step is to rule out other conditions that might be causing memory loss or dementia. There are a number of causes for dementia in the elderly:

- Alzheimer's disease.
- Vascular dementia (abnormalities in the vessels that carry blood to the brain).
- Lewy bodies variant (LBV), also called dementia with Lewy bodies.
- Parkinson's disease.

Experts currently believe that 60% of cases of dementia are due to Alzheimer's, 15% to vascular injuries, and the rest are a mixture of the two or caused by other factors. As yet, it is very difficult to differentiate among these dementias. Other diseases, many common in the elderly, can also cause symptoms that resemble Alzheimer's disease.

Vascular Dementia. Vascular dementia is primarily caused by either multi-infarct dementia (multiple small strokes) or Binswanger's disease (which affects tiny arteries in the midbrain). One major analysis suggests that patients with vascular dementia have better long term verbal memory than Alzheimer's patients, but poorer executive function (less ability to integrate and organize).

Lewy Bodies Variant. Lewy bodies are abnormalities found in the brains of patients with both Parkinson's disease and Alzheimer's. They can also be present in the absence of either disease; in such cases, the condition is called Lewy bodies variant (LBV). In all cases, the presence of Lewy bodies is highly associated with dementia. LBV was defined in 1997 and some experts believe it may be responsible for about 20% of people who have been diagnosed with Alzheimer's. They can be difficult to distinguish. Compared to AD patients, those with LBV may be more likely to have hallucinations and delusions early on, to walk with a stoop (similar to Parkinson's disease), to have more fluctuating attention problems, and to perform better than AD patients on verbal recall but less well organizing objects.

Parkinson's Disease. Dementia is about six times more common in the elderly Parkinson patient than in the average older adult. It is most likely to occur in older patients who have had major depression. Unlike in Alzheimer's, language is not usually affected in Parkinson's related dementia. Visual hallucinations occur in about a third of people on long-term medications.

Other Conditions that Cause Similar Symptoms. Some elderly people have a condition called mild cognitive impairment, which involves more severe memory loss than normal but no other symptoms of Alzheimer's. A number of conditions, including many medications, can produce symptoms similar to Alzheimer's:

- Severe depression.
- Drug abuse.
- Thyroid disease.
- Severe vitamin B_{12} deficiency.
- Blood clots.
- Hydrocephalus (excessive accumulation of spinal fluid in the brain).
- Syphilis.
- Huntington's disease.

- Creutzfeldt-Jakob disease.
- Brain tumors.

It is important that the physician recognize any treatable conditions that might be causing symptoms or worsening existing dementia caused by Alzheimer's or vascular abnormalities.

Psychological Testing. A number of psychological tests are used or being developed to assess difficulties in attention, perception, and memory and problem-solving, social, and language skills.

- Two commonly used tests that are very useful in identifying individuals who may be at risk for Alzheimer's are the Mini-Mental State Exam (MMSE) and the Mattis Dementia Rating Scale. One study suggests that missing recall items on the MMSE in combination with a cluster of other symptoms is a very reliable way of identifying Alzheimer's at an early stage. The symptoms include difficulty in calculation, repetition, getting lost while driving, forgetting relatives' names, and poor judgment.

- A clock drawing test is also a good test for AD. The patient is given a piece of paper with a circle on it and is first asked to write the numbers in the face of a clock and then to show "10 minutes after 11." The score is based on spacing between the numbers and the positions of the hands. In the study, scoring eight or less identified 71% of Alzheimer's patients and correctly ruled out 82% of subjects without the disease.

Electroencephalography

Electroencephalography (EEG) traces brain-wave activity; in some Alzheimer's patients this test reveals "slow waves." Although other diseases may evidence similar abnormalities, EEG data helps distinguish a potential Alzheimer's patient from a severely depressed person, whose brain waves are normal.

Imaging Tests

Imaging tests include computerized tomography (CT) and magnetic resonance imaging (MRI and the more advanced techniques single photon emission computed tomography (SPECT), and positron-emission tomographic (PET). The are sometimes used to rule out other disorders such as multi-infarct dementia, stroke, blood clots, tumors, or hydrocephalus. Eventually imaging techniques, particularly PET or SPECT, may be able to specifically detect AD in early stages, but at this time attempts to accurately identify AD changes in the brain are limited to trials.

Investigative Tests

Blood Tests. High blood levels of a substance called p97 may prove to help detect the presence of Alzheimer's, but more research is needed. Other blood tests may rule out metabolic abnormalities.

Cerebrospinal Fluid Test. A screening test the detects high levels of beta-amyloid proteins in the cerebrospinal fluid is expected to be approved in Europe. The manufacturers are hoping to eventually develop a blood test that can give similar results.

Odor Test. Investigators are also using the impairment of smell in AD to develop tests that require patients to distinguish between odors.

Determining Severity after a Diagnosis Has Been Made

Once a diagnosis has been made, some experts observe that certain factors at the time of diagnosis indicate a higher risk for a more rapid decline:

- Older age.
- Being male.
- The presence of high blood pressure.
- Signs of loss of motor control and coordination.
- Tremor.
- Social withdrawal.
- Loss of appetite and severe weight loss.
- Accompanying sensory problems, such as hearing loss and a decline in reading ability.
- General physical debility.

Chapter 29

Verbal Memory and Odor Identification Testing May Help Identify Early Alzheimer's Disease

Verbal Memory Test Best Indicator of Who Will Have Alzheimer's Disease, New Study Says

Early Detection of Alzheimer's Could Lessen the Impact

Incidence of Alzheimer's Disease is expected to increase as the population of elderly grows. Early diagnosis and treatment will be the key to lessening the disease's worst effects, but, how to spot the disease before its symptoms become serious (and harm is already done) is a challenge for health professionals. A new study by psychologists Konstantine K. Zakzanis, Ph.D., and Mark Boulos, B.Sc., of the University of Toronto has determined that the best predictor of future Alzheimer's type dementia is a verbal memory test.

In a meta-analysis of 31 studies amounting to 1,144 Alzheimer's patients and 6,046 healthy controls, Zakzanis and Boulos looked at both neuropsychological and neuroimaging tests to determine their ability to detect preclinical dementia and/or Alzheimer's disease. They also paired a genetic susceptibility (presence of the apoE gene) to dementia/Alzheimer's with results on both neuropsychological and neuroanatomic tests again attempting to identify which types of tests

This chapter includes text from "Verbal Memory Test Best Indicator of Who Will Have Alzheimer's Disease, New Study Says," © 2002 American Psychological Association, reprinted with permission; and, "Odor Identification Test May Help Predict Alzheimer's Disease," Alzheimer's Disease Education and Referral (ADEAR) Center, National Institute on Aging, 2002.

would prove most accurate in identifying preclinical disease in patients with the apoE gene.

Specifically, their findings support the use of the California Verbal Learning Test (long delay recall and percent recall) as the best predictor of Alzheimer's type dementia, with executive function type measures also being predictive but less so than both the long and short delay memory tests.

Changes in the hippocampus were the best volumetric or neuroimaging measure but in general volumetric measures were less sensitive to preclinical stages of the dementia than were the neuropsychological tests.

Ironically, while memory assessments were also more predictive of preclinical Alzheimer's than neuroimaging tests for people with the apoE gene, the most predictive test for such persons still appears to be an odor identification test.

In presenting their findings, the authors note that decline in memory, especially in verbal episodic memory, can be observed in normal elderly people as well as in elderly with mild cognitive impairments and that most of those people will not become future victims of Alzheimer's. How can we tell the difference between those elderly with normal memory impairments and those with preclinical Alzheimer's? The answer, according to the researchers, lies in the magnitude of the memory deficit. Because their study was a meta-analysis of effect sizes, the results allowed them to compare the size of the difference between normal older adults with normal memory decline and older adults with actual dementia.

Odor Identification Test May Help Predict Alzheimer's Disease

A simple odor identification test might help doctors more accurately predict which individuals with mild cognitive impairment will go on to develop Alzheimer's disease, according to research funded by the National Institute on Aging and the National Institute of Mental Health, two components of the National Institutes of Health in Bethesda, Maryland.

In the study, D. P. Devanand, M.D., and colleagues at Columbia Presbyterian Medical Center in New York asked 90 men and women who had minor memory problems and other mild cognitive impairments to participate in a 15 to 20 minute "scratch and sniff" test. The participants, whose mean age was 67, were exposed to 40 distinct smells such as menthol, peanuts, and soap. Each odor was embedded in a microcapsule on a separate page. After scratching open the capsule and smelling its contents, each participant was asked to identify the odor from four alternatives listed for each capsule. The study is reported in the September 2002 issue of the *American Journal of Psychiatry*.

None of the 30 individuals who scored well on the test developed Alzheimer's disease during the follow-up period, which averaged 20 months. But the researchers found 19 of 47 people with mild cognitive impairment who had difficulty identifying these smells or odors went on to develop Alzheimer's disease during the follow-up period. Of those 19, 16 reported that they had a good sense of smell at the time of the test, yet scored poorly on it. This finding suggests that the inability to recognize smells, when combined with a lack of awareness that olfactory senses are impaired, might be used as a predictor of impending Alzheimer's disease. Thirteen of the 90 participants in this study had not completed follow-up at the time of publication.

Chapter 30

What Treatments Are Available for Alzheimer's Disease?

Although Alzheimer's disease is currently incurable, it can be treated with medications, at least in its earlier stages. Many of the medications that have been developed and that show some promise act to increase the amount of acetylcholine in the brain. Acetylcholine is the chemical messenger that sends messages from one neuron (brain cell) to another. Other medications being tested for the prevention and treatment of Alzheimer's disease include anti-inflammatory drugs, estrogen, and antioxidants. Behavioral programs are also an important part of any treatment plan for the person with Alzheimer's disease.

Cholinergic Medications

Levels of acetylcholine, the main chemical messenger in the brain, are lowered in Alzheimer's disease. Medications that serve to increase its levels can improve behavior and thinking in patients with Alzheimer's disease. Some of the medications in this category include:

- Tacrine was the first drug in this class to be approved for use. It improves thinking to a mild degree, but it has drawbacks. It must be taken four times per day, and it has been shown to be

---

"What Treatments Are Available for Alzheimer's Disease," Alzheimer's Information Center, © 2001 American Federation for Aging Research. Reprinted with permission from the American Federation for Aging Research. For further information, please visit www.infoaging.org.

toxic to the liver in many people. It can also cause nausea and diarrhea.

- Donepezil has similar benefits to tacrine, but it is less toxic to the liver. It is given only once a day, and it may be slightly more effective than tacrine.

- Rivastigmine was recently approved for the treatment of mild to moderate symptoms of Alzheimer's disease. In preliminary trials, rivastigmine was associated with greater improvement in performance tests than any other drug in its class.

- Galantamine (also called galanthamine) has been recently approved by the Food and Drug Administration after a number of studies showed that it offered benefit to persons with Alzheimer's disease.

- Metrifonate is another once-a-day drug that has shown promise in clinical trials.

- Physostigmine also confers some cognitive benefits, but can cause severe gastrointestinal side effects.

- Acetylcarnitine mimics the effects of acetylcholine and has shown promise in clinical trials in treating the dementia of Alzheimer's disease.

Anti-Inflammatory Drugs

In the 1980s, it was observed that the incidence of Alzheimer's disease was lower in those older people who regularly took a certain class of pain relievers called nonsteroidal anti-inflammatory drugs (NSAIDs). Some of these are commonly used for minor pain, and several, including ibuprofen (for example, Advil®), acetaminophen (for example, Tylenol®) and naproxen, are available over the counter. Two large studies, one based in Rotterdam, The Netherlands, and one in Baltimore, confirmed that regular use of NSAIDs, particularly ibuprofen, did indeed decrease the risk of developing Alzheimer's disease. However, aspirin was of no benefit and neither was acetaminophen. One significant problem with regular use of NSAIDs is that they can cause serious problems, such as gastrointestinal bleeding and kidney damage.

COX-2 inhibitors are a new class of anti-inflammatory medications that function like NSAIDs, but are protective of the stomach and far less likely to cause bleeding. One clinical trial that looked at the use of COX-2 inhibitors in slowing Alzheimer's disease symptoms found no benefit. This might be due to the fact that COX-2, the enzyme inhibited by these drugs, is itself protective of brain cells, and inhibiting it may remove that protection.

CT scans and MRIs of the brain can be done if signs and symptoms point to the possibility of a brain tumor, stroke, bleeding around the brain, or a condition called normal pressure hydrocephalus (an excess of brain fluids).

A special blood test can be ordered to look for the presence of apolipoprotein E4, the gene that increases the risk of Alzheimer's disease, but the absence of the gene does not exclude Alzheimer's.

Antioxidants

Antioxidants are substances that combat the effects of oxidative damage in our bodies. Oxidative damage to proteins and DNA occurs when our cells utilize oxygen to produce energy. Toxic byproducts of that process are called reactive oxygen species, a kind of free radical. Natural substances in the body (antioxidants) act to scavenge these dangerous molecules and render them less harmful, but this protection fails over time. Oxidative damage has been implicated as a possible cause or contributor to the damage in Alzheimer's disease.

While many antioxidants occur naturally in our bodies, we take others in through foods (or supplements). Those studied for their effects on Alzheimer's disease include:

- Vitamin E was found in at least one study to slow the progression of dementia, but it can cause bleeding in people who take blood-thinning medications like warfarin. One study compared the effects of vitamin E to selegiline (a psychiatric drug in the category monoamine oxidase inhibitors, which can have a number of adverse effects) or placebo. Both vitamin E and selegiline delayed the progression of Alzheimer's disease equally, but the combination of the two was actually worse than either alone. Because the side effects of selegiline can be high, vitamin E, if approved by your doctor, at 1,000 units per day, would be the safer choice.

- Gingko biloba is an herb that may increase blood flow to the brain. Some studies have suggested benefit in Alzheimer's disease, but these studies were conducted in Europe, where the content and dosage of herbal supplements is much more consistently regulated than in the United States. Gingko biloba can also increase the risk of bleeding and should not be taken without first checking with your doctor.

Behavioral Programs

Simple steps can be taken that can reduce the confusion felt by persons with Alzheimer's disease and decrease the agitation that such confusion can produce. Large calendars and digital clocks and familiar objects in a simple, uncluttered environment are useful. Exercise, occupational therapy, group therapy, music, and family activities are often helpful too.

As the disease progresses, the person with Alzheimer's disease can become progressively more agitated. Simple distractions, touching, and talking can often calm them. Home movies and videos can be soothing as well.

In later stages of the disease, the caregivers must assume full responsibility for all aspects of daily living. Alzheimer's patients need help with dressing, bathing, and eating. They must be prevented from driving. As the disease progresses, wandering can become a serious problem. Door locks and alarms may be needed; identification bracelets, such as those issued by the Alzheimer's Association (http://www.alz.org), are recommended.

End-of-Life Care

In the later stages of the disease, Alzheimer's patients become totally incontinent (cannot control their urine or bowels). They become bedridden, with the risk of pressure sores and pain from muscle contractures. They lose the ability to swallow and can neither eat nor drink. Though many spouses and children strive for years to keep their loved ones with Alzheimer's disease at home, most patients come to require around the clock nursing care. Families must make critical decisions about end-of-life care (feeding tubes, respirator use). Ideally, the patient, the family, and the physician have come to these decisions well in advance and are all in agreement.

Caregivers and family members of persons with Alzheimer's can be devastated by the slow deterioration and loss of their loved ones. No one can provide care for a person with Alzheimer's without help. Doctors, nurses, hospital social service departments, local elderly service administrations, local support groups, and the Internet can provide referrals for assistance to caregivers.

Chapter 31

Alzheimer's Disease Medications

Four prescription drugs currently are approved by the U.S. Food and Drug Administration to treat the symptoms of mild to moderate Alzheimer's disease (AD). These medications are called "cholinesterase inhibitors." Scientists do not yet fully understand how these medications work to treat AD, but current research suggests that each acts to prevent the breakdown of acetylcholine, a brain chemical believed to be important for memory and thinking. These medications can help delay or prevent symptoms from becoming worse for a limited time and may help control some behavioral symptoms. Treating the symptoms of AD can provide patients with comfort, dignity, and independence for a longer period of time and can encourage and assist their caregivers as well.

None of these medications stops the disease itself. As AD progresses, the brain produces less and less acetylcholine, and the medications may eventually lose their effect. No published study directly compares these drugs. Because all four work in a similar way, it is not expected that switching from one of these drugs to another will produce significantly different results. However, an AD patient may respond better to one drug than another.

Some additional differences among these medications are summarized in Table 31.1. The medications (listed from most recent to last as approved by the FDA) are:

"Alzheimer's Disease Medications Fact Sheet," Alzheimer's Disease Education and Referral Center (ADEAR), National Institute on Aging, May 2002.

- Reminyl®
- Exelon®
- Aricept®
- Cognex® (Note: Cognex is still available but is not actively marketed by the manufacturer.)

Table 31.1. Medications Summary (continued on next page)

Note: The brief summary provided below does not include all information important for patient use and should not be used as a substitute for professional medical advice. Consult the prescribing doctor and read the package insert before using these or any other medications or supplements. Drugs are listed from most recent to last, as approved by the FDA.

Drug Name	Manufacturer's Recommended Dosage	Common Side Effects	Possible Drug Interactions
Reminyl® (galantamine) Prevents the breakdown of acetylcholine and stimulates nicotinic receptors to release more acetylcholine in the brain.	4 mg, twice a day (8 mg/day) Increase by 8 mg/day after 4 weeks to 8 mg, twice a day (16 mg/day). After another 4 weeks, increase to 12 mg, twice a day (24 mg/day), if well tolerated.	Nausea, vomiting, diarrhea, weight loss	Some antidepressants such as paroxetine, amitriptyline, fluoxetine, fluvoxamine, and other drugs with anticholinergic action may cause retention of excess Reminyl in the body, leading to complications; NSAIDs should be used with caution in combination with this medication.*
Exelon® (rivastigmine) Prevents the breakdown of acetylcholine and butyrylcholine (a brain chemical similar to acetylcholine) in the brain.	1.5 mg, twice a day (3 mg/day) Increase by 3 mg/day every 2 weeks to 6 mg, twice a day (12 mg/day). Continue up to 6 mg, twice a day (12 mg/day), if well tolerated.	Nausea, vomiting, weight loss, upset stomach, muscle weakness	None observed in laboratory studies, NSAIDs should be used with caution in combination with this medication.*

Benefits reported for these medications tend to occur at higher doses. However, the higher the dose, the more likely are side effects. Doctors usually start patients at low doses, and gradually increase the dosage based on how well a patient tolerates the drug. Patients may be drug-sensitive in other ways, and they should be monitored for unusual symptoms when a drug is started. Report any unusual symptoms to the prescribing doctor right away.

It is important to follow the doctor's instructions when taking any medication, including vitamins and herbal supplements. Also, let the doctor know before adding or changing any medications.

Table 31.1. Medications Summary (continued from previous page)

Drug Name	Manufacturer's Recommended Dosage	Common Side Effects	Possible Drug Interactions
Aricept® (donepezil) Prevents the breakdown of acetylcholine in the brain.	5 mg, once a day Increase after 4–6 weeks to 10 mg, once a day.	Nausea, diarrhea, vomiting	None observed in laboratory studies, but NSAIDs should be used with caution in combination with this medication.*
Cognex® (tacrine) Prevents the breakdown of acetylcholine in the body, not specific to the brain.	10 mg, four times a day (40 mg/day) Increase by 40 mg/day every 4 weeks to 40 mg, four times a day (160 mg/day), if liver enzyme functions remain normal.	Nausea, diarrhea, possible liver damage	NSAIDs should be used with caution in combination with this medication.*

Note: Cognex is still available but no longer actively marketed by the manufacturer.

* Use of cholinesterase inhibitors can increase risk of stomach ulcers, and because prolonged use of non-steroidal anti-inflammatory drugs (NSAIDs) such as aspirin or ibuprofen can also cause stomach ulcers, NSAIDs should be used with caution in combination with these medications.

Chapter 32

Complementary Health Approaches for Alzheimer's Disease

How can overall health and well-being be maintained in a person suffering from Alzheimer's disease?

It's important for the person with Alzheimer's to be under the continual supervision of a qualified medical doctor in order to stay in the best overall health possible. Poor overall health is associated with greater symptoms of Alzheimer's, so maintaining healthy habits may reduce symptoms. Attention must be paid to proper exercise, diet, and to any new or long-standing health problems. Hearing and vision should also be evaluated regularly, and treated appropriately if faltering. Ongoing consultation with a primary physician may be supplemented with visits to specialists or other health professionals as necessary to address specific needs.

Co-existing medical conditions should be identified and properly managed, as they may negatively impact Alzheimer's behaviors. For example, frequent urinary tract infections may increase wandering, and depression disrupts sleep and deepens social withdrawal.

Do people with Alzheimer's need to follow a special diet?

People with Alzheimer's should eat well-balanced, nutrient-rich meals, but a special diet is usually not necessary. However, even

"Treatment of Alzheimer's Disease: Diet, Exercise, and Complementary Health," © 2002 Fisher Center for Alzheimer's Research Foundation; reprinted with permission. Additional information from the Fisher Center for Alzheimer's Research Foundation, as well as a searchable database of resources listed by zip code, is available online at www.alzinfo.org.

healthy older people experience changes in eating habits as they age: Food may not smell or taste the same, it may become more difficult to chew and digest food, and our cells may not be able to utilize the energy from food as efficiently. These problems may be more pronounced in people with Alzheimer's, and may be compounded by other challenges posed by the disease. In addition, Alzheimer's may cause appetite control systems in the brain to malfunction as nerve cells in those areas deteriorate, resulting in extreme eating behaviors (overeating or not eating at all).

In early stages of the disease, people with Alzheimer's may have difficulty preparing meals. They may forget they have food in the oven, or cook something and forget to eat it. Step-by-step written or verbal instructions clearly delineating what to do to prepare and eat meals may be beneficial in such cases.

Food preparation problems may progress to difficulty eating. Nerve cell death eventually steals the ability to recognize thirst or hunger. At the same time, depth perception may be compromised due to changes in the visual and "mapping" areas of the brain, making the process of eating more frustrating. The person may no longer know how to use a knife or fork, and may lose interest in food altogether.

Severe eating problems put the person with Alzheimer's at risk for weight loss, dehydration, and malnutrition. See your doctor if you notice significant weight loss or changes in eating behavior. Ask about ways to increase your loved one's food intake and find out if nutritional supplementation might be warranted. Keep in mind that supplements should be used with caution and only under a doctor's supervision, as they may interact with prescription medications.

Is it important for a person who has Alzheimer's to exercise?

Maintaining a reasonable level of exercise is important for many reasons, both for overall health and to address issues specific to Alzheimer's. Exercise can improve mobility and help one maintain independence. In normal people, moderately strenuous exercise has been shown to improve cognitive functioning.

In people with Alzheimer's, studies show that light exercise and walking appear to reduce wandering, aggression and agitation. Incorporating exercise into daily routines and scheduled activities can also be beneficial in alleviating problem behaviors. The type of exercise should be individualized to the person's abilities. Talk with your doctor about what is right.

What kinds of complementary health approaches might benefit a person with Alzheimer's?

Health treatments for people with Alzheimer's disease can also employ so-called "complementary" health approaches. These may include herbal remedies, acupuncture, and massage. This area of treatment is presently the subject of a great deal of research, with far more proposed. It's important to understand that complementary or alternative health approaches, including vitamins and herbal supplements, are not subject to the same kind of critical government review for safety and efficacy that new drugs are, so one must be cautious when considering such approaches. While there are a growing number of legitimate researchers investigating these approaches, there is also a great deal of misinformation in the public domain, and unsubstantiated claims are rampant. Ask your doctor to help you understand the benefits and risks of such approaches, and do not take herbal or vitamin supplements without first discussing it with your doctor, since many of these pills can interact negatively with prescription or nonprescription medications.

Gingko biloba, an herbal supplement with antioxidant properties, has been the subject of much hype regarding it's supposed effects on cognition and memory. Some studies have shown that some people with dementia (of unspecified types) may benefit from gingko biloba supplements, but rigorous evidence of the herb's effectiveness is so far lacking. More studies are ongoing, including ones that are investigating whether gingko biloba can help improve symptoms of mild cognitive impairment. Like other herbal supplements, gingko biloba can have side effects and may interact with prescription medications, so it should only be taken under a doctor's supervision.

Acupuncture, a core component of traditional Chinese medicine that has been used for thousands of years to treat all manner of health complaints, has recently been investigated for its use in Alzheimer's disease. Scientists at two medical institutions, the Wellesley College Center for Research on Women in Wellesley, Mass. and the University of Hong Kong, reported the promising findings of two small studies at a recent medical meeting for Alzheimer's researchers.

In the Wellesley study, 11 people with dementia (10 with Alzheimer's, one with vascular dementia, a related condition) were treated with acupuncture twice a week for three months. Tests completed before and after the study measured cognitive function and mood in the study subjects, and an analysis showed that the treatments significantly reduced depression and anxiety. The Hong Kong study, in which eight patients with Alzheimer's were treated for a total of 30 days each, demonstrated significant improvements in cognition, verbal skills, motor coordination and in an overall measure of the severity of Alzheimer's symptoms. Additional studies are ongoing to repeat the results and further explore the effectiveness of acupuncture for treating mood and behavioral disturbances associated with Alzheimer's disease.

Massage can be therapeutic for a number of health conditions, and a great deal of research has documented its benefits in general health. Fewer studies have investigated its usefulness in Alzheimer's, but there is some evidence that massage therapy may reduce behaviors such as wandering, aggression and agitation.

Part Four

Coping with Alzheimer's Disease: Information for the Newly Diagnosed

Chapter 33

I Have Alzheimer's Disease

A diagnosis of Alzheimer's disease may be the last thing you wanted to hear. But the first thing you should know is that you are not alone.

In this chapter, you will find tips and resources to increase your comfort, allow you to remain active, and help you cope. But more important, we hope you will find the inspiration to make your years ahead the best that they can be.

Taking Care of Yourself

If you have Alzheimer's disease, it's important to understand that your life is not over. Living with Alzheimer's means dealing with some life changes sooner than you had anticipated. You can live a meaningful and productive life by taking care of your physical and emotional health, by engaging in activities you enjoy, and by spending time with family and friends. This chapter has suggestions for how you can take care of yourself.

Caring for Your Physical Health

Caring for your physical health can improve the quality of your life for years to come.

"I Have Alzheimer's," is reprinted with permission of the Alzheimer's Association. For additional information, call the Alzheimer's Association national toll-free number, 800-272-3900, or visit their website www.alz.org. © 2002 Alzheimer's Association. All rights reserved.

- Get regular checkups.
- Take your medication.
- Eat healthy foods.
- Exercise every day.
- Rest when you are tired.
- Drink less alcohol.

Coping with Your Feelings

After receiving a diagnosis, you may experience a range of emotions, including:

- denial about having dementia
- fear of losing people important to you
- loneliness because no one seems to understand what you are going through
- frustration with not making yourself understood
- loss of the way you used to see yourself
- depression or anger about the way your life is changing.

The feelings you may be experiencing are normal. But it is important to find ways to deal with those feelings. The following suggestions may help you take care of your emotional needs:

- Write in a journal about your experiences and feelings.
- Join a support group.
- Talk to your physician, who can determine if there is an appropriate treatment.
- See a counselor.
- Talk to a clergy member or other person who can help with your spiritual needs.
- Share your feelings with your friends and family.
- Do the activities you enjoy as long as you are able.

For more information about support groups, check with your local Alzheimer's Association chapter.

Helping Your Family and Friends

When you learn that you have a diagnosis of Alzheimer's disease, you may hesitate to tell others. You may be coming to terms with the diagnosis yourself or fear that others may feel uncomfortable around you. It is true that your relationship with family and friends will change. But it is important to talk to the people in your life about Alzheimer's disease and about the changes you will all experience together.

Talking about Your Diagnosis

Talking about your diagnosis is important for helping people understand Alzheimer's disease and learning about how they can continue to be a part of your life. The following suggestions may be helpful:

- Explain that Alzheimer's disease is not a normal part of aging but a disease of the brain that results in impaired memory, thinking, and behavior.

- Share educational information on Alzheimer's disease or invite family and friends to attend Alzheimer education programs.

- Be honest about how you feel about your diagnosis and allow other family members to do the same.

- Assure friends that although the disease will change your life, you want to continue enjoying their company.

- Let family and friends know when and how you may need their help and support.

If you have Alzheimer's disease, you will find that eventually there will be many changes in your relationships with family members and friends. Planning for these changes and talking about them honestly will help everyone.

Working with Your Spouse

Most people with Alzheimer's disease continue to live at home even as the disease progresses. As a result, your spouse may have to manage the household and your care. He or she may feel a sense of loss because of the changes the disease brings to your relationship. The following suggestions may benefit your relationship.

- Continue to participate in as many activities as you can.

- Modify activities to your changing abilities.

- Talk with your spouse about how he or she can assist you.

- Work together to gather information about caregiver services and their costs, such as housekeeping and respite care, and start a file you can consult when they are needed.

- Seek professional counseling to discuss new factors in your relationship and changes in sexual relations.

- Continue to find ways in which you and your spouse can fulfill the need for intimacy.

- Encourage your spouse to attend a support group for caregivers.

Helping Children and Teens

Children often experience a wide range of emotions when a parent or grandparent has Alzheimer's disease. Younger children may be fearful that they will get the disease or that they did something to cause it. Teenagers may become resentful if they must take on more responsibilities or feel embarrassed that their parent or grandparent is "different." College-bound children may be reluctant to leave home.

- Reassure young children that they cannot "catch" the disease from you.

- Be straightforward about personality and behavior changes. For example, you may forget things, such as their names, and say and do things that may embarrass them. Assure them that this is not their fault or intentional but a result of the disease.

- Find out what their emotional needs are and find ways to support them, such as meeting with a counselor who specializes in children who have a loved one diagnosed with Alzheimer's.

- School social workers and teachers can be notified about what the children may be experiencing and be given information about the disease.

- Encourage children and teens to attend support group meetings and include them in counseling sessions.

- Record your thoughts, feelings, and wisdom to "be with them" as they experience important events in their lives (graduations, dating, marriage, births, and deaths).

Coping with Changes in Daily Life

Alzheimer's disease will bring significant changes in your day-to-day experiences. Things you once did easily will become increasingly difficult. The following suggestions may help you cope with changes in your daily life and plan for changes that will occur in the future.

Doing Difficult Tasks

You may find familiar activities such as balancing your checkbook, preparing a meal, or doing household chores more difficult. Try the following tips:

- Do difficult tasks during the times of the day when you normally feel best.

- Give yourself time to accomplish a task, and don't let others rush you.

- Take a break if something is too difficult.

- Arrange for others to help you with tasks that are too difficult.

Communicating with Others

You may begin to experience difficulty understanding what people are saying or finding the right words to express your thoughts. The following tips are important in communicating:

- Take your time.

- Ask the person to repeat a statement, speak slowly, or write down words if you do not understand.

- Find a quiet place if there is too much distracting noise.

Driving

- Understand that at some point it may no longer be safe for you to drive. Discuss with your family and physician about how and when you will make decisions about driving.

- Make plans for other transportation options, such as family members, friends, or community services.

- Contact your local chapter of the Alzheimer's Association to learn what local transportation services are available.

Dealing with Memory Changes

- Post a schedule of the things you do every day, such as meal times, regular exercise, a medication schedule, and bed time.

- Have someone call to remind you of meal times, appointments, or your medication schedule.

- Keep a book containing important notes, such as phone numbers, people's names, any thoughts or ideas you want to hold on to, appointments, your address, and directions to your home.

- Post important phone numbers in large print next to the phone.

- Have someone help you label and store medications in a pill organizer.

- Mark off days on a calendar to keep track of time.

- Label photos with the names of those you see most often.

- Label cupboards and drawers with words or pictures that describe their contents.

- Have someone help you organize closets and drawers to make it easier to find what you need.

- Post reminders to turn off appliances and lock doors.

Living Alone

Many individuals manage on their own during the earliest stages of Alzheimer's disease, with support and assistance from others. The following suggestions may help if you live by yourself.

- Arrange for someone to help you with housekeeping, meals, transportation, and other daily chores. To get information about assistance available in your community, talk to your local chapter of the Alzheimer's Association or your physician.

- Make arrangements for direct deposit of checks, such as your retirement pension or Social Security benefits.

- Make arrangements for help in paying bills. You can give a trusted individual the legal authority to handle money matters.

- Plan for home-delivered meals if they are available in your community.

- Leave a set of house keys with a neighbor you trust.

- Make arrangements for someone to regularly check your smoke alarm.

- Have family, friends, or a community service program call or visit daily.

  - Keep a list of questions and concerns to discuss with them during your time together.

  - Keep a list of things for them to check out around the house, such as electrical appliances, mail, and food items.

Making Job Decisions

If you are still working when you are diagnosed with Alzheimer's disease, you will need to make decisions about eventual changes in work life. The following suggestions may help you make decisions and discuss options with your employer.

- Talk to your employer about your diagnosis. You may want to provide educational materials and bring someone with you to help explain your situation.

- Discuss with your employer the possibility of switching to a position that better matches your abilities and strengths or of reducing your work hours.

- Continue to work as long as you and your physician feel you are able.

- Decide with your employer who else will need to know about your diagnosis, such as co-workers and clients with whom you work.

- Tell co-workers that you may become frustrated with yourself, or frustrating to them, when you have trouble recalling information or finding the right words.

- Use reminders, memos, and a calendar to help you perform your job effectively.

- Research early-retirement options.

- Educate yourself and family about employee benefits that may be available to you. Find out how to make benefit claims.

- When you stop working, find an activity to take the place of your job. Consider volunteer work or a new hobby.

Planning for the Future

After a diagnosis of Alzheimer's, you may worry about the impact the disease will have on you and your family. Planning ahead is one way to deal with those fears. By participating in decisions now, you can determine the kind of life you want for the years ahead. In this section, you will find information and tips to help you begin planning.

Choosing Health Care Providers and Facilities

You may be able to live independently and safely for some time on your own or with the help of a family member or hired caregiver. As Alzheimer's advances, there may come a time when your day-to-day care will require the skills of a full-time health care staff.

To make sure that your needs and preferences for care are understood, talk about the options available to you with a family member or trusted friend. The sooner you do this, the more likely you are to find those options with services you prefer.

Care services tend to fall into three categories: respite care, residential care, and hospice care. The cost for each type of care differs by service and community. Financial assistance may be available through state or federal programs (for example, Medicaid or the Veterans Administration).

Selecting a Care Provider

There are important questions to ask when deciding on care providers.

Questions to ask in-home caregivers:

- What is your training and experience in working with people with dementia?
- What times are you available?
- Who would substitute if you can't come?
- Whom can I talk to at the agency if I have a concern?

Concerns when choosing a residential care facility:

- Observe how the environment promotes independence of the residents, provides safety and security, and reflects your own preferences for comfort.

- Ask the care provider if the staff is continually trained on dementia care issues, what kind of programs are offered for people with Alzheimer's, and how they address an increasing need for care.

- Ask the provider if residents and family members can participate in creating and reviewing care and service plans.

- Spend time in a variety of facilities observing what goes on and how people are treated. Talk with residents and visitors about their opinions of the facility and staff. See if the residents look happy, comfortable, relaxed, and involved in activities.

- Talk with staff working directly with residents to see if they are competent and content in their jobs. Also, meet with the administrator and directors of nursing and social services.

- Visit a facility more than once before making a decision.

Respite Care

Respite care provides your caregiver temporary relief from tasks associated with caregiving. You benefit from opportunities to socialize with others and live in the community longer. Respite care is mainly offered through community organizations or residential facilities. The most common respite care programs are in-home care and adult day services.

In-home services offer a range of options, including companion services, personal care, household assistance, and skilled care services to meet specific needs. In-home helpers can be employed privately, through an agency, or as part of a government program.

Adult day services provide you with opportunities to interact with others, usually in a community center or facility. Staff lead various activities such as music programs and support groups. Transportation and meals are often provided.

Residential Care Facilities

The following are types of facilities that may meet your needs, depending on the level of care you require:

- Retirement housing generally provides each resident with an apartment or room that includes cooking facilities. This type of housing usually does not have round-the-clock staff on-site. Staff members may have little or no knowledge about dementia.

This setting may be appropriate for persons in the early stage of Alzheimer's who can still care for themselves independently and live alone safely.

- Assisted living facilities (or board and care homes) bridge the gap between living independently and living in a nursing home. Facilities typically offer a combination of housing and meals; supportive, personalized assistance; and health care services.

- Skilled nursing facilities (also known as nursing homes) may be the best choice when a person needs round-the-clock care or on-going medical treatment. Most nursing homes have services and staff to address issues such as nutrition, care planning, recreation, spirituality, and medical care. Many facilities have special care units designed to meet the unique needs of people with dementia.

- Continuum care retirement communities (CCRC) provide all of the different types of options described above. In these facilities, a person may receive all of the different levels of care on one campus but may need to be moved between buildings to receive different services.

Hospice Care

Hospice programs provide care to persons in the late stages of Alzheimer's disease. Hospice emphasizes a philosophy of comfort and care at the end of life without using drastic lifesaving measures. This service is available through local hospice organizations and some home care agencies, hospitals, and nursing homes.

Financial Matters

You may be worried about the cost of your future care and if you will have enough money to cover these costs. Discussing your immediate and future financial needs and goals will help protect you, the people who depend on you financially, and the people who will care for you. Work with a financial adviser and trusted family member or friend to determine the following:

- potential care expenses, such as follow-up physician visits, prescription medications, care services, and housing

- current sources of income, such as insurance, personal savings, investments, and employee or retirement benefits

- other financial resources available through government assistance or community based organizations.

Health Care Insurance

Health care insurance may include private and retiree insurance and Medicare.

- **Medicare.** Medicare is a federal health insurance program generally for people age 65 or older who are receiving Social Security retirement benefits. Medicare covers inpatient hospital care and a portion of the doctor's fees and other medical expenses. There are specific eligibility requirements in order for a person to receive assistance from this program. Medicare covers some, but not all, of the services a person with Alzheimer's disease may require. Applications for Medicare may be sent to a local Social Security office.

- **Medigap.** Medicare coverage can be supplemented with Medigap, a private insurance that covers copayments and deductibles required by Medicare. The more expensive policies may cover prescription drugs. To find Medigap information on Medicare's website, go to: http://www.medicare.gov/MGcompare/home.asp

- **Medicare HMO (Medicare Managed Care).** A Medicare HMO offers some additional benefits and less paperwork in exchange for restrictions on choices of hospitals, doctors, and other professionals. Most Medicare HMOs cover nursing home and home health care for limited periods only under special circumstances. For more information, visit Medicare's website: http://www.medicare.gov/.

- **Medicaid.** Because Medicaid is a federal program typically administered by each state's welfare agency, eligibility and benefits vary from state to state. The program is typically administered by a state welfare agency. Medicaid covers all or a portion of nursing home costs. A person with Alzheimer's can qualify for long-term care only if he or she has minimal income and cash assets. For more information, visit the Centers for Medicare and Medicaid Services website: http://cms.hhs.gov.

Personal Resources

Retirement benefits that provide critical financial resources include retirement plans, individual retirement accounts (IRAs), annuities, and Social Security.

Investment assets (stocks and bonds, savings accounts, real estate, etc.) and personal property (jewelry and artwork) can be sources of income. Money from the sale of a home can be invested, or a reverse mortgage can be taken out on a home.

Social Security Disability

This is a program to assist wage earners under 65 who can no longer work because they are disabled. To apply, you must have worked a minimum of five nonconsecutive years in the past ten years and establish disability status. You do this by submitting physician statements and other documentation to your local Social Security office. For more information, visit the Social Security Administration's Web site: http://www.ssa.gov/.

Supplemental Security Income

This program guarantees a minimum monthly income to persons who are age 65 or over, disabled, or blind and have limited income and assets. It is important to apply soon after a diagnosis is made because payments ordinarily begin with the date of application or eligibility.

Legal Issues

It is important to obtain legal advice and services from an attorney. You may want to hire an attorney who practices elder law, a specialized area of law focusing on issues that typically affect older adults. Bring a family member with you when you see your attorney.

Free legal advice may be available in your community. Contact your local Legal Aid Society, Area Agency on Aging, or nonprofit legal assistance organizations. Your local chapter of the Alzheimer's Association may be able to provide referrals for legal advice and services.

Advance Directives

Legal documents called advance directives enable you to document your preferences regarding treatment and care, including end-of-life wishes. Talk with your family and your doctor about your preferences for end-of-life care. If you do not decide on your care now, your family may have to later. With advance directives, your family will know your preferences.

Two common forms of advance directives are a living will and a durable power of attorney for health care.

- A living will states your choices for future medical care decisions, including the use of artificial life support systems. You have the legal right to limit or forgo medical or life-sustaining treatment, including the use of mechanical ventilators, cardio-pulmonary resuscitation, antibiotics, feeding tubes, and artificial hydration.

- A durable power of attorney for health care allows you to appoint an agent (usually a trusted family member) to make all decisions regarding health care. These decision may be about health care providers, medical treatment, and end-of-life decisions. The term durable means that this agent can act on your behalf after you are unable to make decisions yourself.

Other Legal Documents

- A durable power of attorney gives you an opportunity to authorize an agent (usually a trusted family member or friend) to make legal and financial decisions for you when you no longer can make them on your own. The term durable means that this agent can act on your behalf after you are unable to make decisions yourself.

- Living trusts allow you to create a trust and to appoint someone else as trustee (usually a trusted individual or bank) to carefully invest and manage your assets.

- A will is a document you create that names an executor (the person who will manage your estate) and beneficiaries (those who will receive the estate at the time of your death).

Once you have filled out these documents, make sure that you, your caregiver or a trusted family member, your attorney, and your doctor all have a copy.

215

Chapter 34

Tips for Living with Alzheimer's Disease

A person in the early stages of Alzheimer's disease will notice many changes. It's getting to be more difficult to remember things, make decisions, and find your way around. It's frustrating a good deal of the time, but there are good days and bad days. Here are some things you can do to make things just a little better and to make things feel a bit more "normal" again.

How can I cope with my memory problems?

- Always keep a book with you to record important information, phone numbers, names, ideas you have, appointments, your address, and directions to your home.

- Place notes around the house when you need to remember things.

- Label cupboards and drawers with words or pictures that describe their contents.

- Place important phone numbers in large print next to the phone.

"Living With Alzheimer's Disease: Tips for the Newly Diagnosed," © 2003 The Cleveland Clinic Foundation, 9500 Euclid Avenue, Cleveland, OH 44195, 800-223-2273 ext. 48950, www.clevelandclinic.org. Additional information is available from the Cleveland Clinic Health Information Center, 216-444-3771, or www.clevelandclinic.org/health.

- Ask a friend or family member to call and remind you of important things you need to remember, such as meal times, medication times and appointments.

- Use a calendar to keep track of time and to remember important dates.

- Use photos of people you see often, labeled with their names.

- Answering machines can help keep track of phone messages.

What's the best way to plan the day?

- Find things to do that you enjoy and are able to do safely on your own.

- It will be easier to accomplish tasks during the times of the day when you feel best.

- Allow yourself the time to do the things you need to do, and don't feel rushed or let other people rush you.

- If something gets too difficult, take a break.

- Ask for help if you need it.

How can I avoid getting lost?

- Ask someone to go with you when you go out.

- Ask for help if you need it, and explain that you have a memory problem.

What will make communicating easier?

- Always take your time and don't feel rushed.

- If you need to, ask the person you're speaking with to repeat what he or she is saying, or to speak slowly if you do not understand.

- Avoid distracting noises and find a quiet place to talk.

Can I continue to drive?

- If you tend to get lost or confused easily, consider alternative modes of transportation.

- Drive only in areas that are familiar to you.

- Contact your local chapter of the Alzheimer's Association to learn what transportation services are available in your area.

- The Department of Motor Vehicles will assess your driving skills if you're not sure whether you should drive. Some hospitals and senior centers also may offer driving assessments.

- You should know that at some point, it no longer will be safe for you to drive. Have someone else drive you where you need to go.

How do I take care of myself at home?

- Your doctor or a local Alzheimer's organization can tell you how to get help with things such as shopping, housekeeping, meals (including home-delivered meals) and transportation.

- Ask a neighbor you trust to keep a set of your house keys.

- Ask a friend or family member to help you to organize your closets and drawers to make it easier for you to find things.

- Keep a list of important and emergency numbers by the phone.

- Have family, friends or a community service program call or visit daily to ensure that everything is all right.

How do I manage my responsibilities?

- Ask a family member to check things around the house, such as electrical appliances, mail and perishable food items.

- Arrange for direct deposit of checks, such as your retirement pension or Social Security benefits.

- Inform your bank if you have difficulty keeping track of your accounts and record keeping. They may provide special services for people who have Alzheimer's disease.

- Ask someone to check your smoke alarm regularly.

It is important to realize that at some point, it will become too difficult or dangerous for you to live by yourself. However, in the earliest stages of the disease, many people do manage on their own, with support and help from friends, family and services, and with simple adjustments and safety practices in place.

Chapter 35

Keeping Alzheimer's Disease at Bay

Doctors are paying closer attention to the early stages of Alzheimer's disease, when there's a greater chance of enabling patients to lead normal lives longer.

The results so far are encouraging, thanks to improved diagnostic techniques and drugs that can slow the degenerative brain disease in its initial phases.

Putting the spotlight on early Alzheimer's is changing "the predominant image of someone with Alzheimer's as not very capable, not very aware, not very able to do things for themselves," says Robyn Yale, a clinical social worker in San Francisco who pioneered early-stage Alzheimer's patient support groups.

Early Warning Signs

People with early-stage Alzheimer's often have difficulty with:

- recalling recent events;
- making decisions and judgments;
- managing routine chores;
- expressing thoughts and feelings;

Reprinted with permission from "Keeping Alzheimer's at Bay," and "Seven Ways for Alzheimer's Patients to Stay Active," © 2002 Peggy Eastman. Peggy Eastman is a freelance writer in the Washington, DC area. These articles originally appeared in the March 2002 issue of the *AARP Bulletin*.

- processing what others say; and

- handling complex tasks such as balancing a checkbook.

In fact, patients in the early throes of the disease can do many things for themselves, Yale says.

Leslie Dennis, 66, of Chicago is one of them. He was diagnosed with the disease more than two years ago, but that hasn't stopped him from volunteering at a local botanical garden and traveling with his wife, Barbara.

"We don't want to be marginalized, [Alzheimer's] or not," says Dennis. After the initial shock of his diagnosis, he says he realized that "life can be beautiful for quite a while."

Neither the cause nor a cure has been found for Alzheimer's, a form of dementia in which memory, language ability and rational thinking decline over time, interfering with the individual's social relationships and ability to function.

People with early Alzheimer's are often able to function well for months and even years longer than those diagnosed in later stages of the disease.

Helping Alzheimer's patients stay active longer has obvious benefits for them, but it can also reduce medical costs as well as the burdens placed on nursing facilities and caregivers.

Experts say that without a cure, an estimated 14 million Americans will have Alzheimer's by 2050, up from 4 million now. The Alzheimer's Association reports that the United States spent more than $50 billion in 2000 on taxpayer-funded Medicare and Medicaid services for people with the disease.

The Pluses of Early Diagnosis

New ways of detecting Alzheimer's are among the biggest breakthroughs, since treatment is most effective early on. Until recently scientists thought the only way to be sure of a diagnosis was by examining brain tissue—after the patient had died.

Doctors today believe they can pinpoint early Alzheimer's with standard tests, such as the widely used Mini-Mental State Examination, to evaluate memory and reasoning abilities.

Researchers are also experimenting with imaging scans that can show changes in the brain that are symptomatic of Alzheimer's.

"Early diagnosis is quite critical," says V. Paul Bertrand, MD, an Illinois neurologist and caregiver for his mother, who has Alzheimer's. Brain cells, he says, are more sensitive to cholinergic drugs in early, mild cases.

Drugs like donepezil (Aricept) boost a chemical in the brain that affects coherent thinking but wanes in Alzheimer's patients. A recent study shows that donepezil delayed the average time between diagnosis and entering a nursing home by 21 months.

The National Institute on Aging is conducting a study on donepezil and vitamin E to learn if they can prevent a condition called mild cognitive impairment from progressing to Alzheimer's.

The primary symptom of mild cognitive impairment is persistent trouble recalling information and events. The condition is more severe than occasionally misplacing keys or forgetting someone's name—but it doesn't encompass the disorientation, confusion and language loss of Alzheimer's.

Scientists estimate more than 80 percent of people with mild cognitive impairment will develop Alzheimer's within 10 years.

Detecting Alzheimer's in the initial stages has other advantages. By understanding lapses in the individual's thinking and behavior, families can take steps to keep the individual safe and functioning as long as possible, says Steven T. DeKosky, MD, director of the Alzheimer's Disease Research Center at the University of Pittsburgh.

Social worker Yale points out that people in the beginning phases of Alzheimer's are often able to participate in decisions about what kind of treatment they want, where they want to live when they need more care and how they want financial and legal issues and medical decisions handled if they become incapacitated.

Staying Engaged

People with early-stage Alzheimer's need more opportunities—from outings and art projects to volunteering and support groups—to stay involved, says Sam Fazio, director of education services for the Alzheimer's Association.

Yale agrees. "Life doesn't end with the diagnosis," she says. "It's something to be faced, just like anything else in life. This is a trauma, but there's a lot to celebrate in the present."

She says people with early Alzheimer's are able to enjoy time with their children and grandchildren, volunteer, exercise, help fellow patients—in other words, they can be engaged in life.

Help at the Start

Sympathetic caregivers can make a big difference for a person with early Alzheimer's. "A lot of things can be done by the caregiver to make things easier," says Bertrand.

Things like laying out clothes to simplify the ritual of what to put on in the morning or keeping a list of channels next to the TV.

Alice Nap, a sales consultant in Joliet, Ill., can tell when her husband—who has early-stage Alzheimer's—is becoming frustrated in an activity. "He wants to do a big project, then he says, 'Maybe I'll start with a small project,' and he doesn't get that done," she explains. The problem for him is following the logical sequence of steps—a sequence in which she can assist.

Barbara Dennis noticed that her husband could no longer write or work on a computer screen; nor could he interpret road signs when he was driving (he decided to stop driving on his own). Barbara could not reverse those losses, but she does support his love of travel by helping him handle trip logistics.

Support groups for people with early-stage Alzheimer's can be very helpful, experts, patients and caregivers agree.

"The disease itself kind of pulls people away from their social life," says Patricia Hunter, family services director for the Western and Central Washington Alzheimer's Association chapter in Seattle.

The support group can become not only a source for socializing but also for information. "What helps people is answering their questions," says Hunter. "We've had couples who've been together for 50 or 60 years. They're used to making decisions together." Finding out what to expect as the disease worsens helps couples prepare in advance.

A support group can also help people deal with issues such as deciding when to stop driving or paying the bills. It can help patients and their families prepare psychologically for the inevitable decline ahead, to deal with anger, depression, anxiety and feelings of isolation and being misunderstood.

Leslie Dennis belongs to a support group, where, he says, "we laugh at our disease and dementia, often with dark humor."

He suggests joining a group of not more than 15 people that meets as long as it's needed. Groups typically are set up to run for eight weeks, but he says "that doesn't do anything. People need to interact with each other and get to know each other."

Robyn Yale says professionals and patients are always on the lookout for ways to keep people with early-stage Alzheimer's engaged in life.

Leslie Dennis has his own ideas. "Simply put, get up and do what you can, or you will fade, fairly quickly."

By doing so, he says, "you remain someone."

Seven Ways for Alzheimer's Patients to Stay Active

Some steps that patients can take to stay active:

- Focus on remaining abilities and develop strategies for dealing with declining ones, such as using reminder notes for appointments;

- Establish a daily routine that provides structure, consistency, mental stimulation and exercise;

- Spend more time with children and grandchildren;

- Establish a relationship with a doctor who answers questions and discusses treatment options clearly and thoroughly;

- Put legal, medical and financial affairs in order;

- Tell trusted friends about the diagnosis, and enjoy low-key social gatherings with them;

- Join a support group.

Where to Get More Information

The Alzheimer's Association. Call 800-272-3900, or go to http://www.alz.org/ for information and referrals to support groups.

Alzheimer's Disease Education and Referral Center (ADEAR), a service of the National Institute on Aging. Call 800-438-4380 or visit their website at www.alzheimers.org.

Eldercare Locator. Call 800-677-1116 to find information on services and programs in your area.

Chapter 36

Early-Stage Alzheimer's Disease: What to Expect

Overview

A diagnosis of Alzheimer's disease (AD) can be difficult to accept. As you read through this chapter, we encourage you to keep an open mind and remember that you are not alone. Organizations that provide assistance and support to people with AD and their families are located in communities all across the nation.

Facts

Alzheimer's disease is a slowly progressing disease that results in the loss of nerve cells in the brain, eventually leading to impairment in memory, judgment and decision-making, orientation to physical surroundings, concentration, and language. Though the loss of nerve cells is irreversible, medications are available that may slow the disease's progress.

AD can affect your ability to perform day-to-day tasks and can lead to changes in behavior and mood. While symptoms often interfere with social, family, and work activities, many AD patients and caregivers have learned a variety of strategies that have helped them maintain an active and productive life. This chapter offers information about this medical condition as well as practical tips for coping with its effects.

"Fact Sheet: Early-Stage Alzheimer's Disease," © 2002 Family Caregiver Alliance; reprinted with permission. For more information from Family Caregiver Alliance, visit www.caregiver.org.

Stages

AD affects people in different ways. The progress of the disease and its symptoms may differ from person to person. However, the general course of the disease is often divided into stages (early, middle and late) based upon memory, thinking, and your ability to care for yourself. Long-term memory (for example, events from childhood and early adulthood) is not affected in the early stages of AD.

Early Diagnosis and Intervention

Although scientists have not found a cure for AD, certain important actions and resources can be helpful to you and your family. The first step is to get a full medical examination to rule out potentially reversible causes of memory loss (e.g., depression, reaction to medication, etc.). In addition, early diagnosis and intervention allow you to:

- Improve your understanding and the understanding—of those around you—about the changes that are taking place.

- Increase your knowledge of AD.

- Access community resources that help AD patients and caregivers.

- Take advantage of medications. Several prescription drugs may delay, for a time, the worsening of symptoms in people with AD.

- Make plans for the future (e.g., financial and health care planning).

- Increase your awareness of local and national research projects and clinical trials of new medications.

- Increase your awareness of safety issues and health.

Early-Stage Symptoms

The following is a list of skills and tasks that may become increasingly difficult for you. The list is intended to help you identify potential difficulties in order to help you plan for future changes and continue living your life to the fullest.

- *Memory for recent events.* Examples: remembering appointments, details of a recent conversation, and names.

- *Carrying out tasks with multiple steps.* Examples: managing money and balancing your checkbook, taking medications as prescribed, shopping, and cooking.

- *Decision-making and problem-solving.* Example: making quick decisions in response to an emergency, such as responding to a flood or fire in your home.

- *Spatial ability and orientation.* Examples: following a map or following directions, judging the distance of objects while driving, and feeling lost in familiar environments.

- *Language.* Examples: finding the right word, writing letters, understanding what you have read or what others have said.

- *Behavior and/or mood.* Examples: loss of interest in new projects, withdrawing in social situations, feelings of anxiety and depression. Keep in mind that anxiety and depression are often treatable, so speak with your physician if these feelings arise.

Transitions

It may be necessary to change your daily routine in the early stages of AD. Although a time may come when you must rely more on others for assistance with some tasks, you will want to stay involved in making decisions that affect your life. The following tasks may require adjustments in your lifestyle:

Driving: Some states have laws requiring physicians to report individuals with a diagnosis of AD to the Department of Motor Vehicles. The intent is to ensure that you and those around you are safe. If you continue driving, ongoing evaluation of your driving abilities and ongoing consultation with your physician are critical. It is also wise to pay attention to the suggestions of those close to you; they may recognize changes in your driving ability before the changes become apparent to you.

In-home responsibilities: Household management may become increasingly difficult for you. Tasks such as cooking and taking medications may pose safety risks.

You may, for example, forget to turn off the stove or forget to take a dose of medication. However, it may be possible to continue to participate in household activities with a minimal amount of assistance from another person. Some individuals may choose to have family or friends assist in certain areas; others may choose to hire help from outside the home. It may be necessary to consider moving to another living situation in order to simplify your lifestyle or to be in closer proximity to family or friends. You may want to start discussing these options with those who are close to you.

Financial responsibilities: Balancing a checkbook, dealing with insurance, and paying bills may become frustrating and overwhelming. Having a trusted family member or friend to help with these tasks is extremely important. A Power of Attorney should be established so that this trusted person can act on your behalf during times when you cannot.

Be sure to include this person in the process very early so that he or she has time to learn what needs to be done. Like driving, managing our own finances is a sign of independence. It can be difficult to allow someone else to do these things for you, but there is no shame in admitting you may need help. The people who are close to you may recognize your need for help before you do.

Treatment

Presently, researchers cannot definitively say what causes AD, and there currently is no cure. However, considerable progress has been made in the field of AD research in recent years resulting in the development of several medications for AD.

The ideal medication for AD would either prevent or cure it, have no side effects, be inexpensive, and be readily available. Researchers have not yet discovered this ideal treatment. It is possible, however, to improve memory and slow the progression of AD with medications. As of the beginning of 2002, four drugs had been approved by the FDA. Tacrine (Cognex), approved in 1993, has many side effects, including potential liver damage, and has proved disappointing with regard to improving memory. For these reasons it is seldom prescribed. Three newer drugs, donepezil (Aricept), rivastigmine (Exelon) and galantamine (Reminyl), have been more beneficial in improving memory with fewer side effects. Unfortunately these drugs are not effective for everyone and their effectiveness is limited to the early and middle stages of AD. Talk to your physician about whether or not one of these medications may be appropriate for you.

New medications are constantly being tested. If you are interested in participating in clinical trials, you should discuss this with both your physician and the people close to you. Information on clinical drug trials and other research is available from the Alzheimer's Disease Education and Referral Center (ADEAR). Many universities and medical schools conduct research projects as well. Your physician may know of research studies seeking participation from people with AD.

It is currently possible to reduce the emotional and behavioral symptoms sometimes associated with AD. For example, a doctor may prescribe drugs to reduce depression, anxiety, and sleep problems. Exercise, diet, education programs, and support groups also help address some problems caused by AD.

Ways of Coping

- Educate yourself about the disease and resources in the community.

- Discuss with family members or other trusted persons your preferences about decisions affecting your life.

- Continue to explore ways to fulfill your needs for intimacy and closeness. The desire for close relationships with others continues throughout the disease.

- Be patient with yourself.

- Exercise can contribute to good physical health and coordination, and can reduce stress. See your physician for an exercise program that will best fit your needs.

- Find productive ways to release anger and frustration—talk with a close friend, a counselor, or join a support group especially for people with AD.

- Use visible and/or accessible reminders—write notes to yourself, leave messages on your answering machine, or set the alarm on a watch as a reminder about an upcoming appointment.

- Engage yourself in meaningful activities—documenting your life story by creating a scrap book, tape recording your autobiography, or keeping a journal can be wonderful ways to reflect upon your life and share yourself with those close to you. Your children and grandchildren will treasure these keepsakes.

- Keep your mind active—do puzzles, write, etc.

- Know that you are not only a "person with AD"—focus on the many and varied personal attributes that you have, such as integrity, kindness, humor.

- Become an advocate for yourself and other individuals with AD. Write letters and make phone calls to local and state represen-tatives, assist community agencies in training staff and profes-sionals about AD, or become involved in a research program.

- Establish a "Power of Attorney for Healthcare" and "Power of At-torney for Finances." These documents will help your loved ones provide you with the type of care you want and need in the future.

- Continue social activities—get together with friends and family as much as possible.

- Maintain an open mind and positive attitude—focus on your present abilities and avoid excessive worry about what might happen in the future. Know that there are many ways to live an active and productive life.

Community Resources

Alzheimer's and senior service organizations: *The Eldercare Locator*, (800) 677-1116, is a free service which will put you in touch with a local Area Agency on Aging or other local sources of help. You can also call the *Alzheimer's Association* at (800) 272-3900 to re-ceive contact information for the appropriate state or regional chap-ter. *Family Caregiver Alliance's National Center on Caregiving* offers help in locating services as well—call (800) 445-8106 or e-mail info@caregiver.org. If either you or your caregiver resides in Califor-nia, you will find help through your local Caregiver Resource Center by calling (800) 445-8106.

Support groups and counseling services: Support groups for those with early Alzheimer's disease can be primarily discussion-oriented or can offer a variety of creative activities including planned outings. Caregiver support groups and education programs are also available in the community for those family members or friends who are assisting you in some way.

Volunteer programs: Volunteer opportunities for persons with AD are now available in some areas. You may enjoy the chance to con-tribute your time and talent to your local community.

Artistic programs: Expressing yourself through work in clay, paint, or photography, for example, may be beneficial to you and can provide you opportunities for self-expression.

Structured day programs: Adult day programs include activities such as art, music, gardening, exercise, discussion groups, and assistance with physical health needs.

Professional assistance: Take advantage of health care professionals who assist with maintaining your physical strength and coordination, such as occupational therapists and physical therapists.

Legal and financial assistance: Again, forming a "Durable Power of Attorney for Health Care" and a "Durable Power of Attorney for Finances" are essential first steps. Call the Eldercare Locator at (800) 677-1116 to find an Area Agency on Aging that provides free and low-cost legal services for seniors in your community.

Care management: A care manager experienced in the field of AD can provide education, assistance with transitions, emotional support, and guidance in locating and coordinating community resources.

Credits

Alzheimer's Disease Educations and Referral Center, (2001). *Progress Report on Alzheimer's Disease: Taking the Next Steps*. Alzheimer's Disease Education and Referral Center (NIH Publication No. 00-4859), Silver Spring, MD.

American Medical Association, (1999). *Diagnosis, Management and Treatment of Dementia: A Practical Guide for Primary Care Physicians*. American Medical Association, Program on Aging and Community Health, Chicago, IL.

Doody, R. S. et al., (2001). Practice Parameter: Management of Dementia (an Evidence-Based Review) Report of the Quality Standards Subcommittee of the American Academy of Neurology. *Neurology*, v. 56, pp. 1154-1166.

Petersen, R. C. et al., (2001). Practice Parameter: Early Detection of Dementia: Mild Cognitive Impairment (an Evidence-Based Review), Report of the Quality Standards Subcommittee of the American Academy of Neurology. *Neurology*, v. 56, pp. 1133-1142.

Zarud, E., (2001). New Treatments of Alzheimer Disease: A Review. *Drug Benefit Trends*, v. 13, no. 7, pp. 27-40.

Resources

Reading

Alzheimer's Early Stages: First Steps in Caring and Treatment, Daniel Kuhn (1999). Hunter House Publishers, P.O. Box 2914, Alameda, CA 94501-0914, (800) 266-5592.

Alzheimer's: The Answers You Need, Helen Davies and Michael Jensen, (1998), Elder Books, P.O. Box 490, Forest Knolls, CA 94933, (800) 909-COPE.

Early Alzheimer's: An International Newsletter on Dementia, Alzheimer's Association of Santa Barbara, 2024 De la Vina Street, Santa Barbara, CA 93105, (800) 563-0020.

Perspectives: A Newsletter for Individuals with Alzheimer's Disease, Alzheimer's Disease Research Center, University of California, San Diego, 9500 Gilman Drive—0948, La Jolla, CA 92093-0948, (858) 622-5800.

Speaking Our Minds: Personal Reflections from Individuals with Alzheimer's, Lisa Snyder, (1999), W.H. Freeman and Company, 41 Madison Ave., New York, NY 10010, (888) 330-8477.

For More Information

Family Caregiver Alliance
690 Market Street, Suite 600
San Francisco, CA 94104
(415) 434-3388
(800) 445-8106
www.caregiver.org
info@caregiver.org

Family Caregiver Alliance (FCA) seeks to improve the quality of life for caregivers through education, services, research and advocacy.

FCA's National Center on Caregiving offers information on current social, public policy and caregiving issues and provides assistance in the development of public and private programs for caregivers.

Chapter 37

Nutrition for Alzheimer's Disease

While no special diet is required for people with Alzheimer's disease—unless they have another condition, such as diabetes, that requires diet monitoring—eating a well-balanced, nutritious diet is extremely beneficial. With the proper diet, your body will work more efficiently, you'll have more energy and your medications will work properly. This chapter addresses the basics of good nutrition. Please consult your physician before making any dietary changes.

The Basics

- Eat a variety of foods from each food category.

- Maintain your weight through a proper balance of exercise and food.

- Choose foods low in saturated fat and cholesterol.

This chapter begins with "Nutrition for Alzheimer's Disease," reprinted with permission from The Cleveland Clinic Foundation, © 2003 The Cleveland Clinic Foundation, 9500 Euclid Avenue, Cleveland, OH 44195, 800-222-2273 ext 48950, www.clevelandclinic.org. Additional information is available from the Cleveland Clinic Health Information Center, 216-444-3771, or www.clevelandclinic.org/health. The section "Can Diet Prevent Alzheimer's Disease?" is from "Alzheimer's Disease and Diet," by Patrick Bird, Ph.D., Dean of the College of Human Health and Performance, University of Florida, Gainesville, FL. © 2000 University of Florida Health and Human Performance. Reprinted with permission.

- Try to limit sugars.

- Moderate your use of salt.

- Drink eight 8 oz. glasses of water per day.

- You may drink alcoholic beverages in moderation (consult your physician).

Medications

Ask your doctor about possible food interactions with the medicines you may be taking.

Preventing Constipation

- Eat foods high in fiber. Good sources of fiber are fruits, vegetables, and whole grains. Fiber and water help the colon pass stool. Most of the fiber in fruits is found in the skins. Fruits with seeds you can eat, like strawberries, have the most fiber.

- Eat bran cereal or add bran cereal to other foods, like soup and yogurt. Bran is a great source of fiber.

- Drink eight 8 oz. cups of water and other fluids a day.

- Exercise.

- Move your bowels when you feel the urge.

Tips to Relieve Constipation

- Drink two to four extra glasses of water a day.

- Add fruits and vegetables to your diet.

- Eat prunes and/or bran cereal.

- If needed, use a very mild stool softener or laxative. Do not use mineral oil or any other laxatives for more than two weeks without calling your health care provider.

Dining Environment

- Minimize distractions in the area where you eat.

- Stay focused on the tasks of eating and drinking.

- Do not talk with food in your mouth.

Amount and Rate

- Eat slowly.

- Cut your food into small pieces and chew it thoroughly.

- Do not try to eat more than ½ teaspoon of your food at a time.

Thirst/Dry Mouth

Often thirst diminishes with age. In addition, some medicines may dehydrate the body.

- Drink 8 or more cups of liquid each day, 10 or more cups if you are feverish.

- Dunk or moisten breads, toast, cookies, or crackers in milk, hot chocolate, or coffee to soften them.

- Take a drink after each bite of food to moisten your mouth and to help you swallow.

- Add sauces to foods to make them softer and moister. Try gravy, broth, sauce, or melted butter.

- Eat sour candy or fruit ice to help increase saliva and moisten your mouth.

- Don't use a commercial mouthwash. Commercial mouthwashes often contain alcohol that can dry your mouth. Ask your doctor or dentist about alternative mouthwash products.

- Ask your doctor about artificial saliva products. These products are available by prescription.

Maintaining Your Weight

Malnutrition and weight maintenance is often an issue for those with Alzheimer's disease.

- Eat smaller meals more frequently. Eating five to six times a day may be more easily tolerated than eating the same amount of food in three meals.

- Take a daily vitamin/mineral supplement.

- Liquid diet supplements may be helpful.

Can Diet Prevent Alzheimer's Disease?

There are hints, unfortunately only hints, in the scientific literature that diet may provide some protection against this devastating disease.

Fats and Cholesterol. In China, for instance, where people eat low-fat diets, the risk of developing Alzheimer's is 1% at age 65, compared to 5% in the U.S. Also, a Netherlands' study recently reported a connection between dementia and diets high in total fat, saturated fat, trans-fats, and cholesterol. On the other hand, omega-3 fatty acids may, according to some research, offer protection against mental decline in old age. Omega-3 fatty acids are a type of fat essential for the development of the nervous system and are found in some fish, mainly salmon, halibut, swordfish, and tuna.

Vitamin E. This antioxidant may slow mental decline by helping to prevent nerve cell damage caused by cell-destroying free radicals. A study published last year in the *New England Journal of Medicine* reported that moderate-stage Alzheimer patients who consumed vary large amounts of vitamin E supplements (2,000 I.U. per day) or took selegiline (a drug prescribed for Parkinson's disease) showed a significant decrease in the advancement of the disease, compared to those who took a placebo. The Alzheimer's Association says that this is an encouraging study, but it is not enough evidence to recommend vitamin E (or selegiline) to treat or prevent Alzheimer's. Also, the vitamin E dosage in this study is very high. The typical recommendation is 200 to 400 I.U. per day.

Good food sources of vitamin E are vegetable oils, whole grains, wheat germ, some nuts and seeds, green leafy vegetables, sweet potatoes, and avocados. Vitamin E supplements, if taken, should be used in moderation.

Vitamin B$_{12}$ and Folic Acid. Data from the Nuns Study, an investigation where 700 nuns are undergoing annual tests and donating their brains for research after they die, suggests that vitamin B$_{12}$ and folic acid (a member of the vitamin B group) deficiencies may contribute to cognitive decline and the onset of Alzheimer's by elevating blood levels of homocysteine. Homocysteine is an amino acid (one of the chemical compounds that forms proteins) that we produce mainly from eating animal products. Normally homocystine is converted into other non-damaging amino acids. But in some people, this conversion is sluggish and results in the accumulation of homocysteine in the blood. In addition to the homocysteine/Alzheimer's link, high blood concentrations of this amino acid are related to cardiovascular disease.

B_{12} is found in all foods of animal origin, and normally we get all of this vitamin we need from animal products in our diet. Still, a significant number of people over age 60 do not absorb enough B_{12} from the food they eat, because of age related changes in their digestive tracts. A way that often works is to take a multivitamin supplement that contains B_{12} or eat B_{12}-fortified cereals. Folic acid is also widely distributed in our food. Good sources are liver and kidney, beats, celery, chickpeas, eggs, fish, green leafy vegetables, nuts, oranges, soybeans, whole wheat products, beets, peas, and tomatoes.

Ginkgo Biloba. There are studies linking ginkgo to improved memory and mental function, especially in the elderly. In addition, some very preliminary evidence suggests that this herbal supplement may benefit Alzheimer's suffers as well. A recent study reported in the *Journal of the American Medical Association* concluded that ginkgo may stabilize, and, in some cases, improve cognitive performance (memory, learning, reading) in Alzheimer sufferers. However, the Alzheimer's Association stresses that it is premature to recommend ginkgo as a specific treatment for the disease. Moreover, there are potential down sides here. Ginkgo may reduce the ability of blood to clot. This could be a problem, especially when the herb is used with anticoagulants such as aspirin.

Aluminum. An enduring Alzheimer's myth is that aluminum in cans, pots, and pans may cause the disease. Most researchers believe that there is not enough evidence to consider aluminum to be either a risk factor for Alzheimer's or a cause of any other form of dementia. The seed for the myth lies in the fact that aluminum is known to be toxic to brain cells, and there seem to be higher concentrations of this metal in the brains of Alzheimer patients.

End Note. One in 10 people over 65 and nearly half of those over 85 have Alzheimer's. The resulting national economic impact—including costs for diagnosis, treatment, and care—of this disease is more than $100 billion each year, according to the Alzheimer's Association. There is currently no medical treatment to cure it or stop its progression, although drugs are available that may temporally relieve some symptoms. Still, as the above suggests, generally healthful eating may provide some protection from Alzheimer's. But a lot more scientific work has to be done to firmly establish any relationship between diet and this disease. If you are concerned about your diet and vitamin intake, nutritionists often recommend a daily multivitamin for a little insurance. And talk to your doctor. For more information about Alzheimer's disease visit the Alzheimer's Association's website: www.alz.org.

Chapter 38

Counseling and Alzheimer's Disease

Alzheimer's disease, as with many chronic illnesses, will affect you both physically and mentally. It is important to realize that you are not alone, and that if you feel you need help coping, you should consider seeking counseling.

The decision to seek counseling is an important step. Too often, people don't get help because they feel guilt, shame or embarrassment. By deciding to get help, you have made a choice to feel better and to improve your life. Counseling services should be chosen with care to meet your needs. Working with a trained mental health care provider, you can develop the right treatment plan.

Where do I start?

First, you will receive an "assessment," a review of your mental health. The assessment is done by a person trained in mental health care. These specialists include family therapists, social workers, psychologists, psychiatrists and other professionals. (Your health care provider can refer you to a mental health care professional.)

The assessment is used to diagnose the problem and determine the best treatment. You will be asked to describe why you want counseling,

---

any symptoms you have (emotional, mental and physical) and your medical history. You may be given a question-and-answer survey.

What happens after the assessment?

Once you complete the assessment, a treatment plan can be chosen. At this time, you and your counselor can discuss:

- The best type of counseling

- The best setting for counseling (counselor's office, outpatient clinic, hospital, residential treatment center)

- Who will be included in your treatment (you alone, family members, others with similar problems)

- How often you should go to counseling

- How long counseling may last

- Any medications that may be needed

What are the types of counseling?

The following list briefly describes common types of counseling. These can be used together or alone, depending on the treatment plan.

Crisis intervention counseling: In cases of emergency (such as initial despair over diagnosis), the counselor will help you get through the crisis and refer you to further counseling or medical care, if needed. These services are provided by community health agencies, helplines and hotlines.

Individual counseling: The person meets one-on-one with the counselor. Counseling often takes place in the privacy of the counselor's office. This type of counseling works well when problems come mainly from you, and your thinking patterns and behaviors. Also, some problems are very personal and difficult to confront with others present. If you are experiencing depression, anxiety or grief in dealing with your Alzheimer's this may be appropriate.

Family therapy: A diagnosis of Alzheimer's disease can affect the entire family. If you are the primary provider in the home, there can be financial strain. If you are a homemaker, there may need to be adjustments in the distribution of chores. These everyday strains combined with the emotional effects of dealing with a chronic illness have an enormous impact on the family dynamic. Family therapy can help family members resolve issues among each other. It also can help them adopt ways to help another family member cope better. Family members can learn how actions and ways of communicating can worsen problems. With help, new and improved ways of communicating can be explored and practiced.

Group therapy: In group therapy, people join in a group and discuss their problems together. The session is guided by a counselor. Members in the group often share the same problem, but not always. The group session provides a place where people can confide with others who understand their struggles. They also can learn how they see themselves and how they are seen by others. Members gain strength in knowing that they are not alone with their problems. Group therapy is useful for a variety of problems.

Long-term, residential treatment: The person receiving therapy lives at a treatment center. The length of stay can vary, depending on the treatment program and progress of therapy. A program can last more than a year or just a week or two. Settings include hospitals, home-like structures and clinics. The person focuses mainly on his or her problem and on getting well. Other activities, such as work, school, family and hobbies, take a backseat to treatment. In most programs, the person receives counseling daily and participates in regular group therapy. Additional counseling after residential treatment has been ended may be needed.

Self-help and support groups: These include a network of people with similar problems. These groups usually meet regularly without a therapist or counselor. There are self-help groups for those coping with Alzheimer's disease.

Chapter 39

Depression Is Treatable

Introduction

Everyone gets the blues now and then. It's part of life. But if you feel little joy or pleasure after visiting with friends or seeing a good movie, you may have a more serious problem. Being depressed for a while, without letup, can change the way a person thinks or feels. Doctors call this "clinical depression."

Being "down in the dumps" over a period of time is not a normal part of growing old. But it is a common problem, and medical help may be needed. For most people, depression will get better with treatment. "Talk" therapies, medicine, or other methods of treatment can ease the pain of depression. You do not need to suffer.

There are many reasons why depression in older people is often missed or untreated. As a person ages, the signs of depression are much more likely to be seen as crankiness or grumpiness. Depression can also be tricky to recognize. Confusion or attention problems caused by depression can sometimes look like Alzheimer's disease or other brain disorders. Mood changes and signs of depression can be caused by medicines older people may take for arthritis, high blood pressure, or heart disease. It can be hard for a doctor to diagnose depression, but the good news is that people who are depressed often feel better with the right treatment.

"Depression: Don't Let the Blues Hang Around," *Age Page*, Alzheimer's Disease Education and Referral (ADEAR) Center, National Institute on Aging, January 2002.

What Causes Depression?

There is no one cause of depression. For some people, a single event can bring on the illness. Depression often strikes people who felt fine but who suddenly find they are struggling with a death in the family or a serious illness. For some people, differences in brain chemistry can affect mood and cause depression. Sometimes those under a lot of stress, like caregivers, can feel depressed. Others become depressed for no clear reason.

People with serious illnesses, such as cancer, diabetes, heart disease, stroke, or Parkinson's disease, sometimes become depressed. They are worried about how this illness will change their lives. They might be tired and not able to deal with something that makes them sad. Treatment for depression helps them manage symptoms of the disease, thus improving their quality of life.

Genetics, too, can play a role. Studies show that depression may run in families. Children of depressed parents may be at a higher risk.

What to Look For

How do you know when you need help? After all, as you age, you may have to face problems that could cause anyone to feel "depressed." Perhaps you are dealing with the death of a loved one or friend. Maybe you are having a tough time getting used to retirement. Possibly, you have a chronic illness. But, after a period of grieving or feeling troubled, most older people do get back to their daily lives. However, if you are suffering from clinical depression and don't get help, you might not feel better for weeks, months, or even years.

Here is a list of the most common signs of depression. If these last for more than two weeks, see a doctor.

- An "empty" feeling, ongoing sadness, and anxiety.
- Tiredness, lack of energy.
- Loss of interest or pleasure in everyday activities, including sex.
- Sleep problems, including trouble getting to sleep, very early morning waking, and sleeping too much.
- Eating more or less then usual.
- Crying too often or too much.
- Aches and pains that won't go away when treated.

- A hard time focusing, remembering, or making decisions.

- Feeling guilty, helpless, or worthless or hopeless.

- Being irritable.

- Thoughts of death or suicide; a suicide attempt.

If you are a family member, friend, or healthcare provider of an older person, watch for clues. Sometimes depression can hide behind a smiling face. A depressed person who lives alone may briefly feel better when someone stops by to say hello or during a visit to the doctor. The symptoms may seem to go away. But, when someone is very depressed, the signs come right back.

Don't ignore the warning signs. If left untreated, serious depression can lead to suicide. Listen carefully if someone of any age complains about being depressed or says people don't care. That person may really be asking for help.

Getting Help

The first step to getting help is to accept that you or your family member needs help. Perhaps you are one of those people who are uncomfortable with the subject of mental illness. Or you might feel that asking for help is a sign of weakness. You might be like many other older people, their relatives, or friends; they believe that a depressed person can quickly "snap out of it" or that some people are too old to be helped. They are wrong. A healthcare provider can help you.

Once you decide to get medical advice, start with the family doctor. The doctor should check to see if your depression could be caused by a health problem or a medicine you are taking. After a complete exam, your doctor may suggest you talk to a mental health specialist, such as a social worker, mental health counselor, psychologist, or psychiatrist. The special nature of depression in older people has led to a different medical specialty—geriatric psychiatry.

Don't avoid getting help because you are afraid of how much treatment might cost. Often, only short-term psychotherapy (talk therapy) is needed. It is often covered by insurance. Also, some community mental health centers may offer treatment based on a person's ability to pay.

Be aware that some family doctors may not understand about aging and depression. They may not be interested in these complaints. Or, they may not know what to do. If your doctor is unable or unwilling to take seriously your concerns about depression, you may want to talk to another healthcare provider who can help.

Are you the relative or friend of a depressed older person who won't go to a doctor for treatment? Explain how treatment may help the person feel better. In some cases, when a depressed person can't or won't go to the doctor's office, the doctor or mental health specialist can start by making a phone call. The telephone can't take the place of the personal contact needed for a complete medical checkup, but it can break the ice. Sometimes the doctor might make a home visit.

Treating Depression

Your doctor or mental health specialist can treat your depression successfully. Different therapies seem to work in different people. For instance, support groups can provide new coping skills or social support if you are dealing with a major life change. A doctor might suggest that you use a local senior center, volunteer service, or nutrition program.

Several kinds of "talk" therapies are useful as well. One method might help give you a more positive outlook on life. Always thinking about the sad things in your life or what you have lost might have led to your depression. Another method works to improve your relationships with others to give you more hope about your future.

Don't forget to let family and friends help you. Getting better takes time, but with support from others and treatment you will get a little better each day.

Antidepressant drugs can also help. These medications can improve your mood, sleep, appetite, and concentration. There are several types of antidepressants available. Some of these can take up to 12 weeks before you are aware of real progress. Your doctor may want you to continue the medication for six months or more after your symptoms disappear.

Some antidepressants can cause unwanted side effects, although new medicines have fewer side effects. Any antidepressant should be used with great care to avoid this problem. Remember:

- The doctor needs to know about all prescribed and over-the-counter medications, vitamins, or herbal supplements you are taking.

- The doctor should be aware of any physical problems you have.

- Be sure to take antidepressants in the proper dose and on the right schedule.

Electroconvulsive therapy (ECT) can also help. It is most often recommended when medications can't be tolerated or when a quick response is needed. ECT, which works quickly in most people, is given as a series of treatments over a few weeks. Like other antidepressant therapies, follow-up treatment with medication or occasional (called maintenance) ECT is often needed to help prevent a return of depression.

Help from Family and Friends

If you are a family member or friend of someone who seems depressed, try to get the person to a healthcare provider for diagnosis and treatment. Then help you relative or friend to stay with the treatment plan. If needed, make an appointments for the person or go along to the doctor, mental health specialist, or support group.

Be patient and understanding. Get your relative or friend to go on outings with you or to go back to an activity that he or she once enjoyed. Encourage the person to be active and busy, but not to take on too much at one time.

Preventing Depression

What can be done to lower the risk of depression? How can people cope? There are a few practical steps you can take. Try to prepare for major changes in life, such as retirement or moving from your home of many years. One way to do this is to keep and maintain friendships over the years. Try to find someone you feel you can talk to. Friends can help ease the loneliness if you lose your spouse. You can also develop a hobby. Hobbies can help keep your mind and body active. Stay in touch with your family. Let them help you when you feel weighed down or very sad. If you are faced with a lot to do, try to break it up into smaller jobs that are more easily finished.

Being physically fit and eating a balanced diet may help avoid illnesses that can bring on disability or depression. Follow the doctor's directions on using medicines to lower the risk of developing depression as a side effect of a drug.

Resources

Many groups offer more information on depression and older people. The following list can help you get started:

American Association for Geriatric Psychiatry
7910 Woodmont Ave., Suite 1050
Bethesda, MD 20814-3004
Phone: 301-654-7850
Fax: 301-654-4137
Website: www.aagponline.org
E-mail: main@aagponline.org

American Psychological Assn.
750 First Street, NE
Washington, DC 20002-4242
Toll-Free: 800-374-2721
Phone: 202-336-5500
Website: www.apa.org
E-mail: webmaster@apa.org

Depression and Bipolar Support Alliance
730 N. Franklin Street, Suite 501
Chicago, IL 60610-7224
Toll-Free: 800-826-3632
Phone: 312-642-0049
Fax: 312-642-7243
Website: www.dbsalliance.org

National Alliance for the Mentally Ill
Colonial Place Three
2107 Wilson Blvd.., Suite 300
Arlington, VA 22201
Phone: 800-950-NAMI (6264)
Website: www.nami.org

National Institute of Mental Health (NIMH)
6001 Executive Boulevard
Room 8184, MSC 9663
Bethesda, MD 20892-9663
Toll-free: 800-421-4211
Phone: 301-443-4513

NIMH, continued
Fax: 301-443-4279
TTY: 301-443-8431
Website: www.nimh.nih.gov
E-mail: nimhinfo@nih.gov

National Mental Health Assn.
2001 N. Beauregard St., 12th Floor
Alexandria, VA 22311
Toll-Free: 800-969-NMHA (6642)
(Mental Health Resource Center)
Phone: 703-684-7722
Fax: 703-684-5968
TTY: 800-433-5959
Website: www.nmha.org

For information about depression in people suffering from Alzheimer's disease and their caregivers:

Alzheimer's Disease Education and Referral (ADEAR) Center
P.O. Box 8250
Silver Spring, MD 20907-8250
Toll-free: 800-438-4380
Phone: 301-495-3311
Fax: 301-495-3334
Website: www.alzheimers.org
E-mail: adear@alzheimers.org

For more information about health and aging, contact:

National Institute on Aging
P.O. Box 8057
Gaithersburg, MD 20898-8057
Toll-Free: 800-222-2225
TTY: 800-222-4225
Phone: 301-496-1752
Website: www.nia.nih.gov

Chapter 40

Should I Stop Driving?

Almost any adult with a driver's license can remember that first trip alone in the family car, feeling completely free and independent. Those same emotions complicate the decision faced daily by many older Americans. They must decide whether to keep driving or give up their car.

Maybe driving is not fun any more. Some people may not drive at night because they have trouble seeing. Others might avoid driving on interstate highways. For many older drivers, these are the first signs that driving is becoming a problem.

But, driving is necessary for many. Gone are the days when most could walk a few blocks to the grocer or doctor. Getting around is a problem for the millions of older people who live in the suburbs or rural areas. In cities there are plenty of taxis and public transportation like buses and subways. However, buses and subways may be hard for someone suffering from arthritis or using a cane. Taxis may seem to cost too much.

In 1983 one out of every 15 licensed drivers in America was over the age of 70. By 1995 this had risen to one out of every 11 drivers. By 2020 one out of every five Americans will be over 65 years of age, and most of them will probably be licensed to drive.

As a group, older drivers are some of the country's safest drivers. Fewer speed or drive after drinking alcohol than at any other age.

From "Older Drivers," *AgePage*, National Institute on Aging (NIA), revised 2002.

However, compared to young and middle-age adults, people over 70 are more likely to be involved in a crash while driving and more likely to die in that crash. There are many reasons for this—some can be changed, but others cannot.

How Does Age Affect Driving?

As we grow older, we do not turn into bad drivers. Some of us stay good drivers. Others simply have changes in their ability to handle a car safely. These include:

- Changes in our bodies
- Changes in the way we think
- Health problems
- Medications

Changes in Your Body

As you age, your joints may stiffen, and muscles weaken. Turning your head to look back or steering and braking the car may become hard to do. Movements are slower and may not be as accurate. Your senses of smell, hearing, sight, touch, and taste might grow weaker.

Vision, being able to see, is a vital part of driving, but age brings changes in the lens of the eye. Eyes need more light in order to see and are more sensitive to glare. Your ability to see things on the edge of the viewing area, peripheral vision, narrows. Vision problems include cataracts, macular degeneration, and glaucoma.

- In cataracts the lens of the eye becomes cloudy, causing problems with the ability to see.

- Macular degeneration is a breakdown of material inside the eye that leads to a loss of vision in the central part of the viewing area.

- The rise in pressure inside the eye that develops in glaucoma may limit the ability to see things on the edge of the viewing area.

Changes in the Way You Think

You probably know your body may change with age. You may not be aware of changes in the way your mind works as you age. Some of you find your reflexes are slower. Or, you may have trouble keeping your attention fixed on one situation. You may have a hard time doing two things at once—something you have to do to drive safely. When you drive, you have to take in new information from many sources and then react. Some of you react more slowly when you find yourself in a new situation.

These are all normal changes in how your brain works as you age. There are, however, two forms of mental problems that can also affect your ability to drive.

- Depression, being "down in the dumps" for a long time, may happen to many older people, but it is not normal. It can, and should, be treated. The attention and sleep problems depressed people of any age sometimes suffer can interfere with safe driving. So can the medicine sometimes used to treat depression.

- Dementia causes serious memory, personality, and behavioral problems that the person can not recognize. Someone with dementia may at first remember how to operate an automobile and how to travel to familiar places. However, at some point as the disease progresses, their driving abilities do become impaired. Unfortunately, people with dementia often cannot recognize when they should no longer drive.

Health Problems

Other illnesses common among older people can affect your ability to drive safely. For example, having arthritis, Parkinson's disease, or stroke, makes it harder to handle a car safely. Sleep problems or fainting make you less alert at an age when you may already have a hard time focusing your attention. If you have an automatic defibrillator or pacemaker, your doctor might suggest that you stop driving. There is a chance that the device might cause an irregular heartbeat or dizziness while driving. Diabetes may cause nerve damage in your hands, legs, or eyes. The eye damage in diabetes is known as diabetic retinopathy. If you also have trouble controlling your blood sugar level and might be in danger of losing consciousness, you should think about giving up your license.

Medications

Older Americans take more prescription medicines than any other age group. They often have one or more long-term illnesses such as arthritis, diabetes, high blood pressure, and heart disease and may

253

be taking several different drugs. Their bodies may be more sensitive to the effects of medicine on their central nervous systems. The older body may not use up a drug as quickly as a younger body does, so the drug can be active in them for a longer time. Sometimes a combination of medicines increases the effects of each drug on the body.

Several types of medication can make driving harder because they affect the central nervous system. Drugs that might interfere with your driving include sleep aids, medicine to treat depression, antihistamines for allergies and colds, strong pain-killers, and diabetes medications. If you are taking one or more of them, talk to your doctor. Perhaps he or she could change your prescription, or help you decide if the medicine is affecting your driving.

Can I Be a Better Driver?

Perhaps you already know some driving situations that are hard—night, highways, rush hour, and bad weather. You might avoid these types of driving and limit your trips to shopping and visits to the doctor. This lowers your chance of having an accident.

While driving, older drivers are most at risk while yielding right of way, turning, especially left turns, lane changing, passing, and using expressway ramps. Pay extra attention at those times. If there is not a left-turn light, look for alternate routes that do provide such lights.

Most of the advice for older drivers is helpful for all drivers. Plan your trips ahead of time. Stick to streets you know. Don't drive under stress. Keep distractions such as the fan, radio, or talking, to a minimum. Leave a big space between your car and the one in front of you. Don't drive when you are tired.

Think about taking a driving refresher class. Some car insurance companies reduce your payment if you pass such a class. The AARP (American Association of Retired Persons) sponsors the "55 ALIVE/ Driver Safety Program." Call 888-227-7669 (888-AARP NOW) for details about courses in your area. The AAA (American Automobile Association) has a similar class called "Safe Driving for Mature Operators." Contact your local AAA's office for class information. These are 8-hour classroom courses that talk about the aging process and help drivers adjust. You might also check with a local private driving school. Ask if they have an instructor who teaches older drivers. You might want to take such a review every few years.

Certain features on your car can make driving easier. Power steering, power brakes, automatic transmission, and larger mirrors are all helpful. Keeping the headlights on at all times and having a light-colored car helps other drivers see you. Hand controls for the accelerator and brakes might be of use to someone with leg problems. Keep the headlights clean and aligned, and check the windshield wiper blades often. A rear-window defroster is a good way to keep that window clear at all times.

Air bags have saved many lives. Advanced age is not a reason for disconnecting an air bag. However, the National Highway Traffic Safety Administration suggests that air bags may not be as effective in preventing serious injury or death in people over 70 years of age as they are in younger people. Older people are more likely to be injured in a traffic accident. Their bones and blood vessels may be rigid. They might break easily. If the accident is minor, emergency personnel may not realize the possibility of internal bleeding in time. People of any age should push their seats as far back as possible from the air bags in both the steering wheel and the passenger side. Of course, everyone in the car should always wear their seat belts.

Should I Stop Driving?

What if you are doing all you can to be a safe driver and still wonder if you should stop driving. This is a difficult decision. There are questions to ask yourself. Do other drivers often honk at you? Have you had some accidents, even "fender benders"? Are you getting lost, even on well-known roads? Do cars or pedestrians seem to appear out of nowhere? Have family, friends, or your doctor said they were worried about your driving? Do you drive less because you are not as confident about your ability as you once were? If you answered yes to any of these, you probably should think seriously about whether or not you are still a safe driver.

There are resources that may help you make this decision. Single copies of the AARP guide, "The Older Driver Skill Assessment and Resource Guide: Creating Mobility Choices," are available free by writing AARP Fulfillment, 601 E Street, NW, Washington, DC 20049, and asking for publication D14957. The AAA Foundation for Traffic Safety has several free books, including "Drivers 55-Plus: Test Your Own Performance," that may be viewed and ordered on their Web site. The Hartford company offers "At The Crossroads: A Guide to Alzheimer's Disease, Dementia & Driving." See the resources at the end of this chapter for the telephone numbers and addresses.

There are currently no upper age limits for driving. Because people age at different rates, it is not possible to choose one age as the limit.

Setting an age limit would leave some drivers on the road too long, while others would be stopped too soon. Heredity, general health, your way of life, and surroundings all influence how you age.

The hard question is whether older drivers should be tested differently and more often. A second question is what would those tests be. The usual road and written tests do not look at the problem areas for older drivers. The useful-field-of-view test is being studied as one possibility. This looks at the amount of viewing area in which someone can absorb information from two different sources and how quickly they respond to it. This area becomes smaller as we age. The smaller the area, the more likely one is to crash. Fortunately, this is a problem that can be improved by training. A doctor who could then certify the driver to the Department of Motor Vehicles would best perform this test.

The Mini Mental Status Exam is also a possible test used to decide if a person is no longer able to drive. This test looks at your ability to perform certain mental tasks. These tasks test those mental skills involved in driving, although they might seem different. You might be asked to copy a particular design or to count backwards from 100 by sevens. Like the useful-field-of-view test, this is not now used for testing drivers.

The aim of these tests is not to get every older driver off the road. Instead, if problem drivers can be identified, some of them could then receive training to improve their driving skills. Unfortunately, others cannot be helped by training and will have to stop driving.

How Will I Get Around?

When planning for retirement, you should think about how you'd get around if you were no longer able to drive. Some communities provide low-cost bus or taxi service for older people. Some offer carpools or transportation on request. Religious groups sometimes have volunteers who take seniors where they need to go.

If such services are not available in your community, taxis may seem too expensive to use often. Remember that you won't have a car to maintain any longer. In fact, the AAA estimates that the cost of owning and running the average car is over $6,500 a year. By giving up your car, you might have as much as $125 a week that could be used for taxis, public transportation, or buying gas for friends and relatives who can drive you places.

You can contact your local Agency on Aging to learn about transportation services available in your area.

Resources

These organizations have information for older drivers.

AAA Foundation for Traffic Safety

607 14th Street, NW, Suite 201
Washington, DC 20005
Phone: 202-638-5944
Fax: 202-638-5943
Website: www.aaafoundation.org

Administration on Aging

One Massachusetts Avenue
Washington, DC 20201
Phone: 202-619-0724
Fax: 202-401-7620
Website: www.aoa.gov
E-mail: AoAInfo@aoa.gov

American Association of Retired Persons (AARP)

601 E Street, NW
Washington, DC 20049
Toll-free: 800-424-3410 (members only)
Phone: 202-434-2277
Website: www.aarp.org

American Automobile Assn.

1000 AAA Drive
Heathrow, FL 32746
Phone: 407-444-7000
Website: www.aaa.com

"At The Crossroads: A Guide to Alzheimer's Disease, Dementia, and Driving"

Available from:
The Hartford
200 Executive Boulevard
Southington, CT 06489
Phone: 860-547-5000
Website: www.thehartford.com/alzheimers

Eldercare Locator

Toll-Free: 800-677-1116
Website: www.eldercare.gov

National Institute on Aging (NIA)

P.O. Box 8057
Gaithersburg, MD 20898-8057
Toll-Free: 800-222-2225 (NIA Information Center)
TTY: 800-222-4225
Phone: 301-496-1752
Website: www.nia.nih.gov

Chapter 41

Planning Ahead for Long-Term Care

Planning for Long-Term Care

Most older people are independent. But later in life—especially in the 80s and 90s—you or someone you know may begin to need help with everyday activities like shopping, cooking, walking, or bathing. For many people, regular or "long-term" care may mean a little help from family and friends or regular visits by a home health aide. For others who are frail or suffering from dementia, long-term care may involve moving to a place where professional care is available 24 hours a day.

The good news is that families have more choices in long-term care than ever before. Today, services can provide the needed help while letting you stay active and connected with family, friends, and neighbors. These services include home health care, adult day care, and transportation services for frail seniors as well as foster care, assisted living and retirement communities, and traditional nursing homes.

Planning Ahead

The key to successful long-term care is planning. You or your family may need to make a decision in a hurry, often after an unexpected

This chapter includes text from "Planning for Long-Term Care," *AgePage*, National Institute on Aging (NIA), 1996, and "Getting Your Affairs in Order," *AgePage*, NIA, 1998. Despite the dates of these documents, the guidelines provided are still helpful. Updated information about Alzheimer's disease resources can be found in the end section of this *Sourcebook*.

emergency like a broken hip. Be prepared by getting information ahead of time. That way, you will know what's available and affordable before there is a crisis. To start:

- If you are having trouble with things like bathing, managing finances, or driving, talk with your doctor and other health care professionals about your need for help. A special type of social worker, called a geriatric case manager, can help you and your family through this complex time by developing a long-term care plan and locating appropriate services. Geriatric case managers can be particularly helpful when family members live a long distance apart.

- If you are helping a family member or friend, talk about the best way to meet his or her needs. If you need help for yourself, talk with your family. For instance, if you are having trouble making your meals, do you want meals delivered by a local program or would you like family and friends to help? Would you let a paid aide in your home? If you don't drive, would you like a friend or bus service to take you to the doctor or other appointments?

- Learn about the types of services and care in your community. Doctors, social workers, and others who see you for regular care may have suggestions. The Area Agency on Aging and local and state offices of aging or social services can give you lists of adult day care centers, meal programs, companion programs, transportation services, or places providing more care.

- Find out how you may—or may not—be covered by insurance. The Federal Medicare program and private "Medigap" insurance only offer short-term home health and nursing home benefits. Contact your state-run Medicaid program about long-term nursing home coverage for people with limited means. Also, your state's insurance commission can tell you more about private long-term care policies and offer tips on how to buy this complicated insurance. These agencies are listed in your telephone book, under "Government."

Be aware that figuring out care for the long term isn't easy. Needs may change over time. What worked 6 months ago may no longer apply. Insurance coverage is often very limited and families may have problems paying for services. In addition, rules about programs and benefits change, and it's hard to know from one year to the next what may be available.

A Need for More Care

At some point, support from family, friends, or local meal or transportation programs may not be enough. If you need a lot of help with everyday activities, you may need to move to a place where care is available around-the-clock. There are two types of residential care:

• Assisted living arrangements are available in large apartment or hotel-like buildings or can be set up as "board and care" homes for a small number of people. They offer different levels of care, but often include meals, recreation, security, and help with bathing, dressing, medication, and housekeeping.

• Skilled nursing facilities—"nursing homes"—provide 24-hour services and supervision. They provide medical care and rehabilitation for residents, who are mostly very frail or suffer from the later stages of dementia.

Sometimes, health care providers offer different levels of care at one site. These "continuing care communities" often locate an assisted living facility next to a nursing home so that people can move from one type of care to another if necessary. Several offer programs for couples, trying to meet needs when one spouse is doing well but the other has become disabled.

Finding the Right Place

To find the residential program that's best for you:

• **Ask Questions:** Find out about specific facilities in your area. Doctors, friends and relatives, local hospital discharge planners and social workers, and religious organizations can help. Your state's Office of the Long-Term Care Ombudsman has information about specific nursing homes and can let you know whether there have been problems at a particular home. Other types of residential arrangements, like "board and care" homes, do not follow the same Federal, state, or local licensing requirements or regulations as nursing homes. Talk to people in your community or local social service agencies to find out which facilities seem to be well run.

• **Call:** Contact the places that interest you. Ask basic questions about vacancies, number of residents, costs and method of payment, and participation in Medicare and Medicaid. Also think

261

about what's important to you, such as transportation, meals, housekeeping, activities, special units for Alzheimer's disease, or medication policies.

- **Visit:** When you find a place that seems right, go talk to the staff, residents, and, if possible, family members of residents. Set up an appointment, but also go unannounced and at different times of the day. See if the staff treats residents with respect and tries to meet the needs of each person. Check if the building is clean and safe. Are residents restrained in any way? Are social activities and exercise programs offered—and enjoyed? Do residents have personal privacy? Is the facility secure for people and their belongings? Eat a meal there to see if you like the food.

- **Understand:** Once you have made a choice, be sure you understand the facility's contract and financial agreement. It's a good idea to have a lawyer look them over before you sign.

A Smooth Transition

Moving from home to a long-term care facility or nursing home is a big change. It affects the whole family. Some facilities or community groups have a social worker who can help you prepare for the change. Allow some time to adjust after the move has taken place.

Regular visits by family and friends are important. They can be reassuring and comforting. Visits are necessary, too, for keeping an eye on the care that is being given.

Getting Your Affairs in Order

Plan for the Future

We all need to prepare for the uncertainties of the future. Making decisions and arrangements before they are needed simplifies caring for an older person or planning for your own old age. Complete personal and financial records will have most of the details you need to plan for any changes that might come up in the years ahead—such as retirement, a move, or a death in the family.

The first step is to assemble as much information as possible about you and your income and savings. A trusted family member or friend should know where you keep all these records and documents, including your will. It is not necessary to tell them what's in your will, but they should know where you keep it. If you don't have a relative or friend you trust, ask a lawyer to help. One day, you might need help managing your money or be unable to make important decisions. Helping you is much simpler for the person who steps in if all your papers are already in order.

Everyone's life history is different. So are their income, savings, debts, and investments. Still, some general suggestions may help you begin to organize your important papers. You might wish to set up a file, assemble everything in a desk or dresser drawer, or just list the information and the location of documents in a notebook. Review these records regularly to make sure they are up-to-date.

Personal Records

Personal records are facts, dates, names, and documents that are part of your history. A personal records file should include the following information:

- Full legal name

- Social Security number

- Legal residence

- Date and place of birth

- Names and addresses of spouse and children (or location of death certificate if any are deceased)

- Location of "living will" or other advance directive if one exists

- Location of birth certificate and certificates of marriage, divorce, and citizenship

- List of employers and dates of employment

- Education and military records

- Religious affiliation, name of church or synagogue, and names of clergy

- Memberships in organizations and awards received

- Names and addresses of close friends, relatives, doctors, and lawyers or financial advisors

- Requests, preferences, or prearrangements for burial.

Financial Records

A financial records file is a place to list information about insurance policies, bank accounts, deeds, investments, and other valuables. Here are some suggestions:

- Sources of income and assets (pension funds, IRA's, 401K's, interest income, etc.)
- Social Security and Medicare information
- Investment income (stocks, bonds, property, and any brokers' names and addresses)
- Insurance information (life, health, and property) with policy numbers and agents' names
- Bank account numbers (checking, savings, and credit union)
- Location of safe deposit boxes
- Copy of most recent income tax return
- Liabilities—what is owed to whom and when payments are due
- Mortgages and debts—how and when paid
- Location of deed of trust and car title
- Credit card and charge account names and numbers
- Property taxes
- Location of all personal items such as jewelry or family treasures.

Sometimes the person helping you may have questions about a bill or a health insurance claim. They may need to talk directly with the people involved. The law does not allow this without your consent. You might consider giving permission to Medicare, a credit card company, or your bank, for example, to discuss your affairs with this person. Sometimes this can be done over the telephone. Sometimes the company has a form for you to sign and return.

Legal Documents

When people think of legal documents associated with aging, they probably think of a will. A will is your chance to say who should receive the things you own. Another way to do that is a trust. Sometimes, before death, older people need other legal documents. Perhaps, someone has to take over an older person's affairs. A standard power of attorney or a durable power of attorney can give one person the right to handle personal or financial matters for another. A standard power of attorney is not useful, however, if the person being cared for cannot make their own decisions. A durable power of attorney may be a better choice because it is effective even if a person becomes unable to make decisions for himself.

Another type of document, an advance directive, describes in writing what your wishes about health care are in case you become terminally ill. Advance directives such as a living will or durable power of attorney for health care can help avoid family conflict. They make it easier for family members facing hard health care decisions on a relative's behalf. For example, your aunt may not wish to have her life extended by being placed on a ventilator or breathing machine, or your brother may want to be an organ donor. An advance directive can provide for this. They are recognized in most, but not all, states.

Because state laws vary, check with your area office on aging, a lawyer, or financial planner. They will have information on wills, trusts, estates, inheritance taxes, insurance, Medicare, and Medicaid.

Chapter 42

Advanced Directives

Advanced Directives and Do Not Resuscitate Orders

What is an advance directive?

An advance directive tells your doctor what kind of care you would like to have if you become unable to make medical decisions (if you are in a coma, for example). If you are admitted to the hospital, the hospital staff will probably talk to you about advance directives.

A good advance directive describes the kind of treatment you would want depending on how sick you are. For example, the directives would describe what kind of care you want if you have an illness that you are unlikely to recover from, or if you are permanently unconscious. Advance directives usually tell your doctor that you don't want certain kinds of treatment. However, they can also say that you want a certain treatment no matter how ill you are.

Advance directives can take many forms. Laws about advance directives are different in each state. You should be aware of the laws in your state.

What is a living will?

A living will is one type of advance directive. It only comes into effect when you are terminally ill. Being terminally ill generally means that you have less than six months to live. In a living will, you can describe the kind of treatment you want in certain situations. A living will doesn't let you select someone to make decisions for you.

What is a durable power of attorney for health care?

A durable power of attorney (DPA) for health care is another kind of advance directive. A DPA states whom you have chosen to make health care decisions for you. It becomes active any time you are unconscious or unable to make medical decisions. A DPA is generally more useful than a living will. But a DPA may not be a good choice if you don't have another person you trust to make these decisions for you.

Living wills and DPAs are legal in most states. Even if they aren't officially recognized by the law in your state, they can still guide your loved ones and doctor if you are unable to make decisions about your medical care. Ask your doctor, lawyer or state representative about the law in your state.

What is a do not resuscitate order?

A do not resuscitate (DNR) order is another kind of advance directive. A DNR is a request not to have cardiopulmonary resuscitation (CPR) if your heart stops or if you stop breathing. (Unless given other instructions, hospital staff will try to help all patients whose heart has stopped or who have stopped breathing.) You can use an advance directive form or tell your doctor that you don't want to be resuscitated. In this case, a DNR order is put in your medical chart by your doctor. DNR orders are accepted by doctors and hospitals in all states.

Most patients who die in a hospital have had a DNR order written for them. Patients who are not likely to benefit from CPR include people who have cancer that has spread, people whose kidneys don't work well, people who need a lot of help with daily activities, or people who have severe infections such as pneumonia that require hospitalization. If you already have one or more of these conditions, you should discuss your wishes about CPR with your doctor, either in the doctor's office or when you go to the hospital. It's best to do this early, before you are very sick and are considered unable to make your own decisions.

Should I have an advance directive?

Most advance directives are written by older or seriously ill people. For example, someone with terminal cancer might write that she does not want to be put on a respirator if she stops breathing. This action can reduce her suffering, increase her peace of mind and increase her control over her death. However, even if you are in good health, you might want to consider writing an advance directive. An accident or serious illness can happen suddenly, and if you already have a signed advance directive, your wishes are more likely to be followed.

How can I write an advance directive?

You can write an advance directive in several ways:

- Use a form provided by your doctor.
- Write your wishes down by yourself.
- Call your state senator or state representative to get a form.
- Call a lawyer.
- Use a computer software package for legal documents.

Advance directives and living wills do not have to be complicated legal documents. They can be short, simple statements about what you want done or not done if you can't speak for yourself. Remember, anything you write by yourself or with a computer software package should follow your state laws. You may also want to have what you have written reviewed by your doctor or a lawyer to make sure your directives are understood exactly as you intended. When you are satisfied with your directives, the orders should be notarized if possible, and copies should be given to your family and your doctor.

Can I change my advance directive?

You may change or cancel your advance directive at any time, as long as you are considered of sound mind to do so. Being of sound mind means that you are still able to think rationally and communicate your wishes in a clear manner. Again, your changes must be made, signed and notarized according to the laws in your state. Make sure that your doctor and any family members who knew about your directives are also aware that you have changed them.

If you do not have time to put your changes in writing, you can make them known while you are in the hospital. Tell your doctor and any family or friends present exactly what you want to happen. Usually, wishes that are made in person will be followed in place of the ones made earlier in writing. Be sure your instructions are clearly understood by everyone you have told.

Chapter 43

Financial Strategies for Elder Care

There are now, more than ever before, innovative financial strategies available to free up assets of older adults that have not traditionally been liquid. These assets can be utilized to pay for the services older adults both need and desire, providing the independence of choice and the ability to enhance quality of life in their later years. Americans are growing older in record numbers and people are living longer than ever before. This has created more elder care alternatives, many of them home based, but the payment for services has shifted from the government to the individual. The challenge for older adults and their caregivers is how do we finance the services we need and want to maintain our quality of life as we grow older. Almost without question an older adult prefers to stay in their home and when that is not a viable choice, they choose a community based housing or health care alternative other than nursing home care. Too often the outcome is determined by affordability, limiting choice. The big question is how do we pay for it? Today, not only do we have more choices in elder care services, but we have new and innovative alternatives to finance those services.

"Innovative Financial Strategies for Elder Care: How to Pay the Bills and Maintain Independence," reprinted with permission of AgeNet, Inc., providing a comprehensive offering of elder care products, services, and information through its Solutions for Better Aging program, (888) 405-4242 and at www.caregivers.com © 2001 AgeNet, Inc.

New Life for Reverse Mortgages

For many older adults the single largest asset they have is their home. An alternative that has existed for a number of years and is being used more frequently by older adults is a reverse mortgage. A reverse mortgage is a special type of home loan that lets a homeowner convert equity into cash, converting a non-liquid asset for immediate use. The equity can be paid in a lump sum or monthly payments and there are no restrictions on how the proceeds can be used. Unlike a traditional mortgage or home equity loan, repayment is not required until the homeowner no longer uses the home as their primary residence. Under the terms of a reverse mortgage you will be able to live in your home as long as you wish as long as you keep current on the taxes and insurance. The primary requirements are the homeowner must be at least 62 years of age and have a significant amount of equity in the home. Increased utilization of reverse mortgages for eldercare financing is, in part, due to the government guarantee programs through HUD and FHA, making the loans more accessible to more older adults. This is an excellent strategy for making use of a substantial asset that is otherwise non-liquid. Loan proceeds might be utilized for home renovation to install special bathroom features or to pay for the services of a home health aid to come in three times a week and provide the additional support needed for a person to continue living in their own home. For some people a reverse mortgage can be a financial alternative that sustains their ability to continue living in their home.

Cash Now from Your Life Insurance

A financial strategy every older adult should consider is "Senior Life Insurance Settlements." This alternative is new within the last few years and simply put, it enables an individual to sell their life insurance to a third party in exchange for a reduced amount of the face value. The amount you receive depends on your age, health, death benefit, and the number of years your policy has been in force (e.g., You'll probably receive more of the policies face value the older you are.). This works well for any person that has a life insurance policy and could enhance the quality of their life by accessing a significant portion of that asset while they are still alive. An example is an older adult who would like to move to an assisted living facility but finds the monthly fees more than they can manage. The financial benefits of liquidating their life insurance policy might be the difference between being able to afford their choice of long-term care options. Any person age 64 and older is eligible. All types of life insurance policies qualify; including group policies issued through an employer or an association as well as term, whole life, universal, federal employee and converted veterans. Look for an arrangement where there is no fee to the policy holder. An additional benefit is that the proceeds from a settlement are not taxed federally.

Transfer Risk of Nursing Home Care to Protect Assets

A third strategy that warrants attention is long-term care insurance. While the cost for this type of insurance is substantial, there are a number of situations when a long-term care insurance policy is a prudent way to mitigate or transfer the financial risk of nursing home care. This alternative provides several distinct benefits. Policies are available that pay a daily rate for nursing home, assisted living, or home care which preserves the freedom of choice for the policy holder while providing financial protection from the high cost of long-term care. For an individual or couple with a significant net worth, long-term care insurance is a viable financial strategy to preserve and protect your assets. In many instances, a qualified long-term care policy may be tax deductible helping to defray the costs of the premiums. As with any type of insurance you are protecting against a future risk. According to the National Association of Insurance Commissioners, one person in three who turned 65 in 1990 will stay one year in a nursing home and one person in ten will stay five years or more. The risk is much higher for women than men. Every individual needs to assess the risks to determine if it is more beneficial to self-insure or transfer the risk to an insurance policy. While long-term care insurance is not for everyone it can be utilized effectively to preserve choice and protect assets and at the very least should be explored to see if it is right for you. The premium costs have a direct relationship to your age at the time you take out a policy, so the sooner you investigate the better off you will be.

273

Part Five

Coping with
Alzheimer's Disease:
Information for Caregivers

Chapter 44

Talking to Your Care Recipient's Doctor

An aging parent deserves the best possible health care—but if the communication between the patient and the doctor isn't good—the health care actually delivered can be less than satisfactory. Caregivers may be tempted to bypass the patient and speak to the doctor directly, but leaving the patient out of the loop is a mistake. For one thing, patient confidentiality considerations may prevent a physician from being candid when a (competent) patient is not present. For another, direct communication is always best. The effort to improve communication between a patient and the attending physician is a process in which the patient should be intimately involved. Caregivers need to learn how to facilitate the process—not take it over. Depending on circumstances, your older relative may need help learning how to communicate with their doctor and how to partner with their caregivers to get the best care. If it's handled properly, doctors will welcome the participation of caregivers—since such participation will give them greater assurance that what they recommend will be carried through.

How can you assess when it might be a good idea to insert yourself in the process? And as a concerned caregiver—how exactly do you do that? Let's take one step at a time.

"Talking to Dad's Doc," by Rod Clark, reprinted with permission of AgeNet, Inc., providing a comprehensive offering of elder care products, services, and information through its Solutions for Better Aging program, (888) 405-4242 and at www.caregivers.com © 2001 AgeNet, Inc.

Communicating with the Patient

"I think the first thing to realize is that the relationship between the caregiver and the older patient needs to be a good one," says Linda Walker, a nurse practitioner with Meriter Health Services, Inc., who works closely with many geriatric patients. "Often, people don't want to see neglect occur, but the caregiver has to realize there may be a limit to how much they will be able to enter the process. As we age, there is often a feeling that we are gradually losing control over our lives. If we are not careful, a well-intentioned offer of help may be perceived as an intrusion." In discussing these things with an older adult it is important not to seem challenging or threatening, Walker explains. Sometimes a patient can see health care as one more thing that they are losing control over. To counter this, it is vital to encourage the patient to take an active role in their health care—and offer your services as a partner in the process.

Open a Dialog about the Doctor/Patient Relationship

The first thing you need to do is open up a personal, candid dialog with the patient about their health, and the quality of health care they are receiving. In the early stages of the conversation it is critical to establish trust. Use tact and diplomacy, and be sensitive to the issue of control. Remember that there may be some delicate areas (sex, incontinence, etc.) that the patient may not be comfortable talking about. Nevertheless it's important to discuss them. Sometimes, when an older adult is silent—health care needs are not met.

Things to Ask about

Part of the challenge you will face lies in the fact that the way doctors and patients relate to each other has changed a great deal since the years when your older relative first established such relationships. In the past patients tended to defer to the doctor and place the responsibility for their health care totally in the hands of their physician, but in today's health care systems—optimum health care is best delivered is a result of an interactive partnership.

Linda Walker recommends asking a series of simple questions along the following lines:

- How are you feeling?

- How was your last visit to the doctor? (Who, when and where.)

- How do you feel about the care you are getting from the doctor?
- What is your relationship with the doctor like?
- Does the physician make you feel rushed? Uncomfortable?
- Do you feel that there is enough time to address your concerns?

As you talk to your relative about the patient/doctor relationship, there are questions you should be asking yourself:

- Does the patient have good opportunities to discuss health issues?
- Is there a real partnership between the patient and the doctor?
- An adversarial relationship?
- What is the doctor's agenda?
- Does it match that of the patient?
- Can they trust their physician? And do they?

At some point during your discussion of health and care, try to secure an agreement from the patient to allow you to accompany them on a visit to the doctor.

Preparing for a Visit

Here are three vital things to prepare when planning a visit to the doctor:

Key questions. In today's managed care systems, time is often at a premium. To fully leverage the physician's time and expertise, it is smart to prepare a list of questions in advance that the patient needs answered.

Medical history. Bring along a medical history that is as detailed as possible. Try and make sure that it is as complete as possible. Are there significant time gaps in the record? Are records from all the relevant doctors and health professionals included? Make sure to make notes about allergies or any special conditions.

Medications. The medications area is very important says Ms. Walker, "Sometimes a patient is seeing several doctors in a variety of clinical settings. Communication between these parties is not always perfect and one doctor may not know every drug or medication that has been prescribed by another. What I recommend is that people bring along all meds in use—including prescriptions and over the counter medications. Just empty the drawer into a bag and bring it all to the appointment."

Going Along on a Doctor Visit

When you accompany the patient to the doctor, make sure that you encourage the highest level of communication possible between doctor and patient. Direct your gaze to the patient when the doctor asks a question to give them the opportunity to answer it first. This will encourage the physician to focus on communicating on a primary level with the patient. Make sure that you get answers to the key questions you developed with the patient earlier, but also make sure that the following matters are discussed.

Diagnoses. Find out what the diagnoses of the patient's conditions are and how the doctor arrived at them.

Tests. If any tests need to be conducted find out what they are, what the reasons for conducting them are, and what they involve.

Treatments. Find out what treatments are proposed or ongoing. What are the impacts and hoped for results? What are the alternatives? Is surgery the only option? What about other treatments? Physical therapy? Explore the options.

New medications. Or alternative remedies (medications, prescription or otherwise are not always the only answer). Ask about side effects, availability of less expensive generics, what risks exist for those that use the medications, what kinds of interactions may be dangerous.

Advanced directives. Are advanced directives in place? Whatever may happen in the future, it may be useful to know the patient's wishes now. How does the patient feel about long term nutritional support? What are the plans for follow-up care?

Need for a specialist? Does the patient's condition call for a specialist? What does the physician think? Does she/he have any recommendations?

Additional meetings. Would it help to have a meeting with other family members as well? If needs aren't being met and the family is part of the caregiving equation, it might be useful, under some circumstances, to bring them into the loop.

Basic communication. Remember, in this era of managed care, the time of medical professionals is often at a premium, so it's important to leverage it. Have vital questions been answered? If relevant, have you described the role of family and friends in the patient's care? Does the patient have the doctor's phone number in wallet or purse? What is the name and number of the nurse that can be called with questions or concerns in the event of a problem?

Consider Psychological Factors

Care is not just about taking stock of physical health, but of psychological and spiritual health as well—and these factors may interfere with a patient's ability to communicate with medical personnel and manage their own care. In considering these broader issues of well being, it is important to look for indications of depression, irrational episodes, and memory loss.

Practitioner Linda Walker suggests that you watch for subtle changes in the patient: weight loss, decline in personal care, or disengagement from social situations. Sometimes, she says, older patients display what we call "failure to thrive." All these may be signs that a patient's ability to monitor their own care is eroding, and that you may need to intercede at a more serious level. "What is perhaps most critical," says Ms. Walker, " is that whatever the circumstances, the patient should be treated with dignity and respect. They should be allowed and encouraged to participate in their health care and health care decisions as much as possible."

Chapter 45

Helping a Person with Dementia Maintain Skills

A person with dementia is a unique individual. As a caregiver, you will want to do everything you can to preserve their dignity and confidence. Each person experiences dementia in their own way but, using encouragement, a reassuring routine and common-sense measures, you can help them to continue to make the best use of their skills and abilities as their condition changes.

Introduction

Try to encourage the person with dementia to do whatever they can for themselves and only offer as much help as is necessary. If they are struggling with a task, avoid the temptation to take over completely, even though it may seem easier and quicker. If you take over, the person is likely to lose confidence and cope less well.

- If you do need to offer assistance, try to do things with the person rather than for them. The person will then be more likely to feel involved.

- Always try to focus on what the person can do rather than what they cannot do.

- Remember that they will have a short attention span and will be finding it hard to remember because of the dementia.

"Maintaining Skills," © 2000 Alzheimer's Society (UK); reprinted with permission. Additional information is available from the Alzheimer's Society at www.alzheimers.org.uk.

- Try to be patient and allow plenty of time. If you feel yourself becoming irritated, take time out. Make sure that the person is safe, then go into another room for a few minutes to give yourself some space.

- Give plenty of praise and encouragement.

Ways of Helping

The person may find certain tasks increasingly difficult as the dementia progresses, while others may remain much longer. Adjust any help you offer accordingly so that they can continue to make the best use of the skills they still possess. Ways of helping that may be appropriate at different times include:

- The person may be able to complete a task when it is broken down into sections, even if they can't complete it. An example of this is getting dressed. Putting the clothes out in the order they are put on may make it possible for the person to continue to dress themselves. Achieving only one or two steps of a task may give them a sense of achievement.

- Give tactful verbal reminders or simple instructions. Try to imagine that you are the person receiving the help and speak in a way that you would find helpful.

- Doing things together, such as folding clothes or drying dishes, can be helpful.

- It is very important that the person with dementia does not feel that they are being supervised or criticized in any way. The tone of voice can imply criticism as well as the actual words.

- Pointing, demonstrating, or guiding an action may sometimes be more helpful than verbal explanations when the dementia is more advanced. For example, the person may be able to brush their own hair if you start by gently guiding their hand.

Ask Advice

A person with dementia may find it hard to cope with certain tasks either because of the dementia or because of other disabilities. An occupational therapist (OT) can advise on aids and adaptations and other ways to help the person retain their independence for as long as possible. You can contact an OT through social services or through your doctor.

Any changes involving equipment or different approaches to practical tasks are more likely to be successful if they are introduced at an early stage when the person with dementia finds it possible to absorb new information.

Feeling Safe

- Feeling safe is such a basic human need that one might say our survival depends upon it. A person with dementia is likely to experience the world as an unsafe place for much of the time. We can only imagine how frightening it must be to experience the world in this way. This is why a person with dementia may try to keep as close as possible to people they recognize.

- The less anxious and stressed the person with dementia feels, the more likely they are to be able to use their skills to the best advantage. A relaxed, uncritical atmosphere is therefore very important.

- Familiar surroundings and a regular routine are reassuring for people with dementia.

- Too many conflicting sounds or too many people can add to confusion. If possible, turn off the radio or the television or, if the person needs to concentrate on something in particular, take them to a quiet place.

- A person with dementia is quite likely to be upset or embarrassed by their declining abilities or clumsiness. They will need plenty of reassurance.

- Although you need to be tactful and encouraging, sometimes the best thing when things go wrong is to have a good laugh together.

Occupation

We all need to feel useful and needed. This does not change when someone develops dementia. Carrying out appropriate activities around the home or in the garden, if you have one, is a way of enabling a person with dementia feel useful and to practice everyday skills.

285

Suggestions for chores in the home include dusting, polishing, folding clothes, laying and clearing tables, drying dishes, and sorting cutlery. Work in the garden might include digging, watering, raking, or sweeping leaves.

You will know what the person's past interests were. Look and see whether you can help them to maintain skills related to past interests. If the person used to enjoy carpentry, they may get satisfaction from sanding a piece of wood, for example. If they enjoyed cooking they may be able to advise you on a recipe or help with a particular dish.

- It is more important that the person feels useful than that they complete the task perfectly.

- If you do have to redo something, be very tactful and make sure that they are not aware of this.

- Remember to thank the person for their help.

Memory Aids

Memory aids and frequent reminders given at the appropriate stage may enable the person to practice their skills for longer. Commonsense measures such as labels on cupboards and drawers, a large calendar, a notice board for messages, notes stuck by the front door, for example, can all help in the early stages of dementia when the person is able to understand the message and to act upon it.

Social Skills

- Meeting people and getting out and about will enable people with dementia to maintain their social skills for longer. It can also help to counteract the apathy and withdrawal so common in dementia. However, remember that the person will need plenty of individual attention at social gatherings and on outings.

- Explain the situation to friends and neighbors so they will understand changes in behavior.

- Encourage the person to attend a day center if a suitable place is offered. You will both benefit from a break, even for a few hours, and a good day center will help maintain social and other skills.

- Accompany the person with dementia to places where other people go. This might be a visit to the shops, to a garden center, to a gallery, or to a park, depending on their interests.

- If the person enjoys going out for a drink or a meal, continue this for as long as possible. A word with the manager of a friendly pub, café, or restaurant can often smooth the way if there are likely to be minor embarrassments.

- Encourage the person to take a pride in their appearance so that they feel more confident. Helping the person to get dressed up before they go out or before visitors come can make it more of an occasion.

Chapter 46

Home Safety for People with Alzheimer's Disease

Introduction

Caring for a person with Alzheimer's Disease (AD) is a challenge that calls upon the patience, creativity, knowledge, and skills of each caregiver. We hope that this information will help you cope with some of these challenges and develop creative solutions to increase the security and freedom of the person with AD in your home, as well as your own peace of mind.

This chapter is for those who provide in-home care for people with AD or related disorders. Our goal is to improve home safety by identifying potential problems in the home and offering possible solutions to help prevent accidents.

We begin with a checklist to help you make each room in your home a safer environment for the person with AD. Next, we hope to increase awareness of the ways specific impairments associated with the disease can create particular safety hazards in the home. Specific home safety tips are listed to help you cope with some of the more hazardous behaviors that may occur as the disease advances. We also include tips for managing driving and planning for natural disaster safety. The chapter ends with a list of resources for family caregivers.

"Home Safety for People with Alzheimer's Disease," National Institute on Aging, National Institutes of Health, NIH Pub. 02-5179, September 2002. The National Institute on Aging gratefully acknowledges the caring staff of the Alzheimer's Disease Research Center at the University of California, San Diego, and the Alzheimer's Association of San Diego, who shared their valuable advice, experience, and expertise to create this information.

What Is Alzheimer's Disease?

Alzheimer's disease is a progressive, irreversible disease that affects brain cells and produces memory loss and intellectual impairment in as many as four million American adults. This disease affects people of all racial, economic, and educational backgrounds.

AD is the most common cause of dementia in adults. Dementia is defined as loss of memory and intellect that interferes with routine personal, social, or occupational activities. Dementia is not a disease; rather, it is a group of symptoms that may accompany certain diseases or conditions. Other symptoms include changes in personality, mood, or behavior.

Although AD primarily affects people age 65 or older, it also may affect people in their 50s and, although rarely, even younger. Other causes of irreversible dementia include multi-infarct dementia (a series of minor strokes resulting in widespread death of brain tissue), Pick's disease, Binswanger's disease, Parkinson's disease, Huntington's disease, Creutzfeldt-Jakob disease, amyotrophic lateral sclerosis (Lou Gehrig's disease), multiple sclerosis, and alcohol abuse. The recommendations in this text deal primarily with common problems in AD, but they also may apply to any of the related dementing disorders.

What Are the Symptoms of AD?

There is no "typical" person with Alzheimer's. There is tremendous variability among people with AD in their behaviors and symptoms. At present, there is no way to predict how quickly the disease will progress in any one person, nor to predict the exact changes that will occur. We do know, however, that many of these changes will present problems for caregivers. Therefore, knowledge and prevention are critical to safety.

People with AD have memory problems and cognitive impairment (difficulties with thinking and reasoning), and eventually they will not be able to care for themselves. They may experience confusion, loss of judgment, and difficulty finding words, finishing thoughts, or following directions. They also may experience personality and behavior changes. For example, they may become agitated, irritable, or very passive. Some may wander from home and become lost. They may not be able to tell the difference between day and night, and they may wake up, get dressed, and start to leave the house in the middle of the night thinking that the day has just started. They may suffer from losses that affect vision, smell, or taste.

These disabilities are very difficult, not only for the person with AD, but for the caregiver, family, and other loved ones as well. Caregivers need resources and reassurance to know that while the challenges are great, there are specific actions to take to reduce some of the safety concerns that accompany Alzheimer's disease.

General Safety Concerns

People with AD become increasingly unable to take care of themselves. However, individuals will move through the disease in their own unique manner. As a caregiver, you face the ongoing challenge of adapting to each change in the person's behavior and functioning. The following general principles may be helpful.

Think prevention. It is very difficult to predict what a person with AD might do. Just because something has not yet occurred, does not mean it should not be cause for concern. Even with the best-laid plans, accidents can happen. Therefore, checking the safety of your home will help you take control of some of the potential problems that may create hazardous situations.

Adapt the environment. It is more effective to change the environment than to change most behaviors. While some AD behaviors can be managed with special medications prescribed by a doctor, many cannot. You can make changes in an environment to decrease the hazards and stressors that accompany these behavioral and functional changes.

Minimize danger. By minimizing danger, you can maximize independence. A safe environment can be a less restrictive environment where the person with AD can experience increased security and more mobility.

Is It Safe to Leave the Person with AD Alone?

This issue needs careful evaluation and is certainly a safety concern. The following points may help you decide.

Does the person with AD:

- become confused or unpredictable under stress?

- recognize a dangerous situation; for example, fire?

- know how to use the telephone in an emergency?

- know how to get help?

- stay content within the home?

- wander and become disoriented?

- show signs of agitation, depression, or withdrawal when left alone for any period of time?

- attempt to pursue former interests or hobbies that might now warrant supervision such as cooking, appliance repair, or woodworking?

You may want to seek input and advice from a health care professional to assist you in these considerations. As Alzheimer's disease progresses, these questions will need ongoing evaluation.

Home Safety Room-by-Room

Prevention begins with a safety check of every room in your home. Use the following room-by-room checklist to alert you to potential hazards and to record any changes you need to make. You can buy products or gadgets necessary for home safety at stores carrying hardware, electronics, medical supplies, and children's items.

Keep in mind that it may not be necessary to make all of the suggested changes. This chapter covers a wide range of safety concerns that may arise, and some modifications may never be needed. It is important, however, to re-evaluate home safety periodically as behavior and abilities change.

Your home is a personal and precious environment. As you go through this checklist, some of the changes you make may impact your surroundings positively, and some may affect you in ways that may be inconvenient or undesirable. It is possible, however, to strike a balance. Caregivers can make adaptations that modify and simplify without severely disrupting the home. You may want to consider setting aside a special area for yourself, a space off-limits to anyone else and arranged exactly as you like. Everyone needs private, quiet time, and as a caregiver, this becomes especially crucial.

A safe home can be a less stressful home for the person with AD, the caregiver, and family members. You don't have to make these changes alone. You may want to enlist the help of a friend, professional, or community service such as the Alzheimer's Association.

Throughout the Home

- Display emergency numbers and your home address near all telephones.

- Use a telephone answering machine when you cannot answer calls. The person with AD often is unable to take messages or may be a target for telephone exploitation by solicitors. When the answering machine is on, turn down the phone bell to avoid disruptive ringing.

- Install smoke alarms near all bedrooms; check their functioning and batteries frequently.

- Avoid the use of flammable and volatile compounds near gas water heaters. Do not store these materials in an area where a gas pilot light is used.

- Install secure locks on all outside doors and windows.

- Hide a spare house key outside in case the person with AD locks you out of the house.

- Avoid the use of extension cords if possible by placing lamps and appliances close to electrical outlets. Tack extension cords to the baseboards of a room to avoid tripping.

- Cover unused outlets with childproof plugs.

- Place red tape around floor vents, radiators, and other heating devices to deter the person with AD from standing on or touching a hot grid.

- Check all rooms for adequate lighting.

- Place light switches at the top and the bottom of stairs.

- Stairways should have at least one handrail that extends beyond the first and last steps. If possible, stairways should be carpeted or have safety grip strips.

- Keep all medications (prescription and over-the-counter) locked. Each bottle of prescription medicine should be clearly labeled with the patient's name, name of the drug, drug strength, dosage frequency, and expiration date. Child-resistant caps are available if needed.

- Keep all alcohol in a locked cabinet or out of reach of the person with AD. Drinking alcohol can increase confusion.

- If smoking is permitted at all, monitor while the person with AD is smoking. Remove matches, cigarettes, and ashtrays. With these reminders out of sight, the person may forget the desire to smoke.

- Avoid clutter, which can create confusion and danger. Throw out/recycle newspapers and magazines regularly. Keep all walk areas free of furniture.

- Keep plastic bags out of reach. A person with AD may choke or suffocate.

- Remove all guns or other weapons from the home, or safety proof them by installing safety locks or by removing ammunition and firing pins.

- Lock all power tools and machinery in the garage, workroom, or basement.

- Remove all poisonous plants from the home. Check with local nurseries or poison control centers for a list of poisonous plants.

- Keep fish tanks out of reach. The combination of glass, water, electrical pumps, and potentially poisonous aquatic life could be harmful to a curious person with AD.

Outside Approaches to the House

- Keep steps sturdy and textured to prevent falls in wet or icy weather.

- Mark the edges of steps with bright or reflective tape.

- Consider a ramp with handrails into the home rather than steps.

- Eliminate uneven surfaces or walkways, hoses, or other objects that may cause a person to trip.

- Restrict access to a swimming pool by fencing it off with a locked gate, covering it, and keeping it closely supervised when in use.

- In the patio area, remove the fuel source and fire starters from any grills when not in use, and supervise use when the person with AD is present.

- Place a small bench or table by the entry door to hold parcels while unlocking the door.

- Make sure outside lighting is adequate. Light sensors that turn on lights automatically as you approach the house are available and may be useful. They also may be used in other parts of the home.

- Prune bushes and foliage well away from walkways and doorways.

- Consider a NO SOLICITING sign for the front gate or door.

Entryway

- Remove scatter rugs and throw rugs.

- Use textured strips or nonskid wax on hardwood floors to prevent slipping.

Kitchen

- Install childproof door latches on storage cabinets and drawers designated for breakable or dangerous items. Lock away all household cleaning products, matches, knives, scissors, blades, small appliances, and valued china.

- If prescription or nonprescription drugs are kept in the kitchen, store them in a locked cabinet.

- Remove scatter rugs and foam pads from the floor.

- Remove knobs from the stove, or install an automatic shut-off switch.

- Do not use or store flammable liquids in the kitchen. Lock them in the garage or in an outside storage unit.

- Keep a night-light in the kitchen.

- Remove or secure the family "junk drawer." A person with AD may eat small items such as matches, hardware, erasers, plastics, etc.

- Remove artificial fruits and vegetables or food-shaped kitchen magnets, which might appear to be edible.

- Insert a drain trap in the kitchen sink to catch anything that may otherwise become lost or clog the plumbing.

- Consider dismantling the garbage disposal. People with AD may place objects or their own hands in the disposal.

Bedroom

- Use a night-light.

- Use an intercom device (often used for infants) to alert you to any noises indicating falls or a need for help. This also is an effective device for bathrooms.

- Remove scatter rugs.

- Remove portable space heaters. If you use portable fans, be sure that objects cannot be placed in the blades.

- Be cautious when using electric mattress pads, electric blankets, electric sheets, and heating pads, all of which may cause burns. Keep controls out of reach.

- Move the bed against the wall for increased security, or place the mattress on the floor.

Bathroom

- Do not leave a severely impaired person with AD alone in the bathroom.

- Remove the lock from the bathroom door to prevent the person with AD from getting locked inside.

- Place nonskid adhesive strips, decals, or mats in the tub and shower. If the bathroom is uncarpeted, consider placing these strips next to the tub, toilet, and sink.

- Use washable wall-to-wall bathroom carpeting to prevent slipping on wet tile floors.

- Use an extended toilet seat with handrails, or install grab bars beside the toilet.

- Install grab bars in the tub/shower. A grab bar in contrasting color to the wall is easier to see.

- Use a foam rubber faucet cover (often used for small children) in the tub to prevent serious injury should the person with AD fall.

- Use plastic shower stools and a hand-held showerhead to make bathing easier.

- In the shower, tub, and sink, use a single faucet that mixes hot and cold water to avoid burns.

- Adjust the water heater to 120 degrees (F) to avoid scalding tap water.

- Insert drain traps in sinks to catch small items that may be lost or flushed down the drain.

- Store medications (prescription and nonprescription) in a locked cabinet. Check medication dates and throw away outdated medications.

- Remove cleaning products from under the sink, or lock them away.

- Use a night-light.

- Remove small electrical appliances from the bathroom. Cover electrical outlets. If men use electric razors, have them use a mirror outside the bathroom to avoid water contact.

Living Room

- Clear all walk areas of electrical cords.

- Remove scatter rugs or throw rugs. Repair or replace torn carpet.

- Place decals at eye level on sliding glass doors, picture windows, or furniture with large glass panels to identify the glass pane.

- Do not leave the person with AD alone with an open fire in the fireplace, or consider alternative heating sources. Remove matches and cigarette lighters.

- Keep the controls for cable or satellite TV, VCR, and stereo system out of sight.

Laundry Room

- Keep the door to the laundry room locked if possible.

- Lock all laundry products in a cabinet.

- Remove large knobs from the washer and dryer if the person with AD tampers with machinery.

- Close and latch the doors and lids to the washer and dryer to prevent objects from being placed in the machines.

Home Safety Behavior-by-Behavior

Although a number of behavior and sensory problems may accompany Alzheimer's disease, not every person will experience the disease in exactly the same way. As the disease progresses, particular behavioral changes can create safety problems. The person with AD may or may not have these symptoms. However, should these behaviors occur, the following safety recommendations may help reduce risks.

Wandering

- Remove clutter and clear the pathways from room to room to allow the person with AD to move about more freely.

- Make sure floors provide good traction for walking or pacing. Use nonskid floor wax or leave floors unpolished. Secure all rug edges, eliminate throw rugs, or install nonskid strips. The person with AD should wear nonskid shoes or sneakers.

- Place locks on exit doors high or low on the door out of direct sight. Consider double locks that require a key. Keep a key for yourself and hide one near the door for emergency exit purposes.

- Use loosely fitting doorknob covers so that the cover turns instead of the actual knob.

  Due to the potential hazard they could cause if an emergency exit is needed, locked doors and doorknob covers should be used only when a caregiver is present.

- Install safety devices found in hardware stores to limit the distance that windows can be opened.

- If possible, secure the yard with fencing and a locked gate. Use door alarms such as loose bells above the door or devices that ring when the doorknob is touched or the door is opened.

- Divert the attention of the person with AD away from using the door by placing small scenic posters on the door; placing removable gates, curtains, or brightly colored streamers across the door; or wallpapering the door to match any adjoining walls.

- Place STOP, DO NOT ENTER, or CLOSED signs in strategic areas on doors.

- Reduce clues that symbolize departure such as shoes, keys, suit-cases, coats, or hats.

- Obtain a medical identification bracelet for the person with AD with the words "memory loss" inscribed along with an emergency telephone number. Place the bracelet on the person's dominant hand to limit the possibility of removal, or solder the bracelet closed.

- Place labels in garments to aid in identification. Check with the local Alzheimer's Association about the Safe Return program.

- Keep an article of the person's worn, unwashed clothing in a plastic bag to aid in finding someone with the use of dogs.

- Notify neighbors of the person's potential to wander or become lost. Alert them to contact you or the police immediately if the individual is seen alone and on the move.

- Give local police, neighbors, and relatives a recent picture, along with the name and pertinent information about the person with AD, as a precaution should he or she become lost. Keep extra pictures on hand.

- Consider making an up-to-date home video of the person with AD.

- Do not leave a person with AD who has a history of wandering unattended.

Rummaging/Hiding Things

- Lock up all dangerous or toxic products, or place them out of the person's reach.

- Remove all old or spoiled food from the refrigerator and cup-boards. A person with AD may rummage for snacks but may lack the judgment or taste to rule out spoiled foods.

- Simplify the environment by removing clutter or valuable items that could be misplaced, lost, or hidden by the person with AD. These include important papers, checkbooks, charge cards, and jewelry.

- If your yard has a fence with a locked gate, place the mailbox outside the gate. People with AD often hide, lose, or throw away mail. If this is a serious problem, consider obtaining a post office box.

299

• Create a special place for the person with AD to rummage freely or sort (for example, a chest of drawers, a bag of selected objects, or a basket of clothing to fold or unfold). Often, safety problems occur when the person with AD becomes bored or does not know what to do.

• Provide the person with AD a safe box, treasure chest, or cupboard to store special objects.

• Close access to unused rooms, thereby limiting the opportunity for rummaging and hiding things.

• Search the house periodically to discover hiding places. Once found, these hiding places can be discreetly and frequently checked.

• Keep all trash cans covered or out of sight. The person with AD may not remember the purpose of the container or may rummage through it.

• Check trash containers before emptying them in case something has been hidden there or accidentally thrown away.

Hallucinations, Illusions, and Delusions

Due to the complex changes occurring in their brain, people with AD may see or hear things that have no basis in reality. Hallucinations come from within the brain and involve hearing, seeing, or feeling things that are not really there. For example, a person with AD may see children playing in the living room when no children exist. Illusions differ from hallucinations because the person with AD is misinterpreting something that actually does exist. Shadows on the wall may look like people, for example. Delusions are persistent thoughts that the person with AD believes are true but in reality, are not. Often, stealing is suspected, for example, but cannot be verified.

It is important to seek medical evaluation if a person with AD has ongoing disturbing hallucinations, illusions, or delusions. Often, these symptoms can be treated with medication or behavior management techniques. With all of the above symptoms, the following environmental adaptations also may be helpful.

• Paint walls a light color to reflect more light. Use solid colors, which are less confusing to an impaired person than a patterned wall. Large, bold prints (for example, florals in wallpaper or drapes) may cause confusing illusions.

- Make sure there is adequate lighting, and keep extra bulbs handy in a secured place. Dimly lit areas may produce confusing shadows or difficulty with interpreting everyday objects.

- Reduce glare by using soft light or frosted bulbs, partially closing blinds or curtains, and maintaining adequate globes or shades on light fixtures.

- Remove or cover mirrors if they cause the person with AD to become confused or frightened.

- Ask if the person can point to a specific area that is producing confusion. Perhaps one particular aspect of the environment is being misinterpreted.

- Vary the home environment as little as possible to minimize the potential for visual confusion. Keep furniture in the same place.

- Have the person with AD avoid watching violent or disturbing television programs. The person with AD may believe the story is real.

- Do not confront the person with AD who becomes aggressive. Withdraw and make sure you have access to an exit as needed.

Impairment of the Senses

Alzheimer's disease can cause changes in a person's ability to interpret what they see, hear, taste, feel, or smell, even though the sense organs may still be intact. The person with AD should be evaluated periodically by a physician for any such changes that may be correctable with glasses, dentures, hearing aids, or other treatments.

Vision

People with AD may experience a number of changes in visual abilities. For example, they may lose their ability to comprehend visual images. Although there is nothing physically wrong with their eyes, people with AD may no longer be able to interpret accurately what they see due to changes in their brain. Also, their sense of perception and depth may be altered. These changes can cause safety concerns.

- Create color contrast between floors and walls to help the person see depth. Floor coverings are less visually confusing if they are a solid color.

- Use dishes and placemats in contrasting colors for easier identification.

- Mark the edges of steps with brightly colored strips of tape to outline changes in elevation.

- Place brightly colored signs or simple pictures on important rooms (the bathroom, for example) for easier identification.

- Be aware that a small pet that blends in with the floor or lies in walkways may be a hazard. The person with AD may trip over a small pet.

Smell

A loss or decrease in smell often accompanies Alzheimer's disease.

- Install good quality smoke detectors and check them frequently. The person with AD may not smell smoke or may not associate it with danger.

- Keep refrigerators clear of spoiled foods.

Touch

People with AD may experience loss of sensation or may no longer be able to interpret feelings of heat, cold, or discomfort.

- Adjust water heaters to 120 degrees (F) to avoid scalding tap water. Most hot water heaters are set at 150 degrees (F), which can cause burns.

- Color code separate water faucet handles, with red for hot and blue for cold.

- Place a sign on the oven, coffee maker, toaster, crock-pot, iron, or other potentially hot appliances that says DO NOT TOUCH or STOP! VERY HOT. The person with AD should not use appliances without supervision. Unplug appliances when not in use.

- Use a thermometer to tell you whether the water in the bathtub is too hot or too cold.

- Remove furniture or other objects with sharp corners or pad them to reduce potential for injury.

Taste

People with AD may lose taste sensitivity. As their judgment declines, they also may place dangerous or inappropriate things in their mouth.

- If possible, keep a spare set of dentures. If the person keeps removing dentures, check for correct fit.

- Keep all condiments such as salt, sugar, or spices away from easy access if you see the person with AD using excess amounts. Too much salt, sugar, or spice can be irritating to the stomach or cause other health problems.

- Remove or lock up medicine cabinet items such as toothpaste, perfume, lotions, shampoos, rubbing alcohol, or soap, which may look and smell like edible items to the person with AD.

- Consider a childproof latch on the refrigerator, if necessary.

- Keep the poison control number by the telephone. Keep a bottle of Ipecac (vomit inducing) available but use only with instructions from poison control or 911.

- Keep pet litter boxes inaccessible to the person with AD. Do not store pet food in the refrigerator.

- Learn the Heimlich maneuver or other techniques to use in case of choking. Check with your local Red Cross for more information and instruction.

Hearing

People with AD may have normal hearing, but they may lose their ability to interpret what they hear accurately. This may result in confusion or over-stimulation.

- Avoid excessive noise in the home such as having the stereo and the TV on at the same time.

- Be sensitive to the amount of noise going on outside, and close windows or doors, if necessary.

- Avoid large gatherings of people in the home if the person with AD shows signs of agitation or distress in crowds.

- Check hearing aid batteries and functioning frequently.

Driving

Driving is a complex activity that demands quick reactions, alert senses, and split-second decision-making. For a person with AD, driving becomes increasingly more difficult. Memory loss, impaired judgment, disorientation, impaired visual and spatial perception, slow reaction time, diminished attention span, inability to recognize cues such as stop signs and traffic lights can make driving particularly hazardous.

People with AD who continue to drive can be a danger to themselves, their passengers, and the community at large. As the disease progresses, they lose driving skills and must stop driving. Unfortunately, people with AD often cannot recognize when they should no longer drive. This is a tremendous safety concern. It is extremely important to have the impaired person's driving abilities carefully evaluated.

Warning Signs of Unsafe Driving

Often, it is the caregiver, a family member, neighbor, or friend who becomes aware of the safety hazards. If a person with AD experiences one of more of the following problems, it may be time to limit or stop driving.

Does the person with AD:

- get lost while driving in a familiar location?
- fail to observe traffic signals?
- drive at an inappropriate speed?
- become angry, frustrated, or confused while driving?
- make slow or poor decisions?

Please do not wait for an accident to happen. Take action immediately.

Explaining to the person with AD that he or she can no longer drive can be extremely difficult. Loss of driving privileges may represent a tremendous loss of independence, freedom, and identity. It is a significant concern for the person with AD and the caregiver. The issue of not driving may produce anger, denial, and grief in the person with AD, as well as guilt and anxiety in the caregiver. Family and concerned professionals need to be both sensitive and firm. Above all, they should be persistent and consistent.

The doctor of a person with AD can assist the family with the task of restricting driving. Talk with the doctor about your concerns. Most people will listen to their doctor. Ask the doctor to advise the person with AD to reduce his or her driving, go for a driving evaluation or test, or stop driving altogether. An increasing number of States have laws requiring physicians to report AD and related disorders to the Department of Motor Vehicles. The Department of Motor Vehicles then is responsible for retesting the at-risk driver. Testing should occur regularly, at least yearly.

When dementia impairs driving and the person with AD continues to insist on driving, a number of different approaches may be necessary.

Work as a team with family, friends, and professionals and use a single, simple explanation for the loss of driving ability such as: "You have a memory problem, and it is no longer safe to drive." "You cannot drive because you are on medication." or "The doctor has prescribed that you no longer drive."

- Have the doctor write on a prescription pad DO NOT DRIVE. Ask the doctor to write to the Department of Motor Vehicles or Department of Public Safety saying this person should no longer drive. Show the letter to the person with AD as evidence.

- Offer to drive.

- Walk when possible, and make these outings special events.

- Use public transportation or any special transportation provided by community organizations. Ask about senior discounts or transportation coupons. The person with AD should not take public transportation unsupervised.

- Park the car at a friend's home.

- Hide the car keys.

- Exchange car keys with a set of unusable keys. Some people with AD are in the habit of carrying keys.

- Place a large note under the car hood requesting that any mechanic call you before doing work requested by the person with AD.

- Have a mechanic install a "kill switch" or alarm system that disengages the fuel line to prevent the car from starting.

- Consider selling the car and putting aside the money saved from insurance, repairs, and gasoline for taxi funds.

- Do not leave a person with AD alone in a parked car.

Natural Disaster Safety

Natural disasters come in many forms and degrees of severity. They seldom give warning, and they call upon good judgment and ability to follow through with crisis plans. People with AD are at a serious disadvantage. Their impairments in memory and reasoning severely limit their ability to act appropriately in crises.

It is always important to have a plan of action in case of fire, earthquake, flood, tornado, or other disasters. Specific home safety precautions may apply and environmental changes may be needed. The American Red Cross is an excellent resource for general safety information and preparedness guides for comprehensive planning. If there is a person with AD in the home, the following precautions apply:

- Get to know your neighbors, and identify specific individuals who would be willing to help in a crisis. Formulate a plan of action with them should the person with AD be unattended during a crisis.

- Give neighbors a list of emergency numbers of caregivers, family members, and primary medical resources.

- Educate neighbors beforehand about the person's specific disabilities, including inability to follow complex instructions, memory loss, impaired judgment, and probable disorientation and confusion. Give examples of some of the simple one-step instructions that the person may be able to follow.

- Have regular emergency drills so that each member of the household has a specific task. Realize that the person with AD cannot be expected to hold any responsibility in the crisis plan and that someone will need to take primary responsibility for supervising the individual.

- Always have at least an extra week's supply of any medical or personal hygiene items critical to the person's welfare, such as:
    - food and water
    - medications

- incontinence undergarments

- hearing aid batteries

- glasses

- Be sure that the person with AD wears an identification bracelet stating "memory loss" should he or she become lost or disoriented during the crisis. Contact your local Alzheimer's Association chapter and enroll the person in the Safe Return program.

- Under no circumstances should a person with AD be left alone following a natural disaster. Do not count on the individual to stay in one place while you go to get help. Provide plenty of reassurance.

Who Would Take Care of the Person with AD If Something Happened to You?

It is important to have a plan in case of your own illness, disability, or death.

- Consult a lawyer regarding a living trust, durable power of attorney for health care and finances, and other estate planning tools.

- Consult with family and close friends to decide who will take responsibility for the person with AD. You also may want to seek information about your local public guardian's office, mental health conservator's office, adult protective services, or other case management services. These organizations may have programs to assist the person with AD in your absence.

- Maintain a notebook for the responsible person who will be assuming caregiving. Such a notebook should contain the following information:

  - emergency numbers

  - current problem behaviors and possible solutions

  - ways to calm the person with AD

  - assistance needed with toileting, feeding, or grooming

  - favorite activities or food

• Preview board and care or long-term care facilities in your community and select a few as possibilities. If the person with AD is no longer able to live at home, the responsible person will be better able to carry out your wishes for long-term care.

Conclusion

Home safety takes many forms. This chapter focuses on the physical environment and specific safety concerns. But the home environment also involves the needs, feelings, and lifestyles of the occupants, of you the caregiver, your family, and the person with AD. Disability affects all family members, and it is crucial to maintain your emotional and physical welfare in addition to a safe environment.

We encourage you to make sure you have quiet time, time out, time to take part in something you enjoy. Protect your own emotional and physical health. Your local Alzheimer's Association chapter can help you with the support and information you may need as you address this very significant checkpoint in your home safety list. You are extremely valuable and as you take on a commitment to care for a person with AD, please take on the equally important commitment to care for yourself.

Additional Resources

Several organizations offer caregivers information about AD. To learn more about support groups, services, research, and additional publications, you may wish to contact the following groups.

Alzheimer's Association
225 North Michigan Avenue
Suite 1700
Chicago, IL 60601-7633
Toll-free: 800-272-3900
Phone: 312-335-8700
Fax: 312-335-1110
TTY: 312-335-8882
Website: http://www.alz.org
E-mail: info@alz.org

The Alzheimer's Association is a nonprofit organization that supports families and caregivers of people with Alzheimer's disease. Local chapters provide referrals to local resources and services and sponsor support groups and educational programs. Online and print versions of publications also are available. In addition, the Association offers the SAFE RETURN program to help in the identification and safe, timely return of people with Alzheimer's disease and related dementias who wander and become lost. The Association maintains a national photo/information database and staffs a 24-hour toll-free emergency crisis line.

Alzheimer's Disease Education and Referral (ADEAR) Center

P.O. Box 8250
Silver Spring, MD 20907-8250
Toll-free: 800-438-4380 (English, Spanish)
Phone: 301-495-3311
Fax: 301-495-3334
Website: http://www.alzheimers.org
E-mail: adear@alzheimers.org

This service of the National Institute on Aging is funded by the Federal government. It offers information and publications on diagnosis, treatment, patient care, caregiver needs, long-term care, education and training, and research related to AD. Publications and videos can be ordered through the ADEAR Center or via the website.

American Red Cross

2025 E. Street NW
Washington, DC 20006
Phone: 1-800-435-7669
Website: www.redcross.org
E-mail: info@usa.redcross.org

The Red Cross offers health information, health services, disaster relief, and emergency services to the public. Local chapters provide programs for older people, including safety courses and home nurse care instruction.

Children of Aging Parents

1609 Woodbourne Road
Suite 302A
Levittown, PA 19057
Toll-Free: 800-227-7294
Phone: 215-945-6900

Children of Aging Parents, *continued*
Fax: 215-945-8720
Website: http://www.caps4caregivers.org

This nonprofit group provides information and materials for adult children caring for their older parents. Caregivers of people with Alzheimer's disease also may find this information helpful.

Eldercare Locator
Toll-Free: 800-677-1116
Website: www.eldercare.gov

The Eldercare Locator is a nationwide, directory assistance service helping older people and their caregivers locate local support and resources for older Americans. It is funded by the Administration on Aging (AoA). The AoA Alzheimer's disease Resource Room contains information for families, caregivers, and professionals about AD, caregiving, working with and providing services to people with AD, and support services.

Family Caregiver Alliance
690 Market St., Suite 600
San Francisco, CA 94104
Toll-Free: 800-445-8106
Phone: 415-434-3388
Fax: 415-434-3508
Website: www.caregiver.org
E-mail: info@caregiver.org

The community-based nonprofit organization offers support services for those caring for adults with AD, stroke, traumatic brain injuries, and other cognitive disorders. Programs and services include an information clearinghouse.

Well Spouse Foundation
63 West Main Street, Suite H
Freehold, NJ 07728
Toll-Free: 800-838-0879
Website: www.wellspouse.org

This nonprofit membership organization gives support to wives, husbands, and partners of the chronically ill and/or disabled. Well Spouse publishes the bimonthly newsletter *Mainstay*.

On the Internet

Ageless Design
Website: www.agelessdesign.com

Consultation services, architectural design review, books, articles, brochures, pamphlets, and audiotapes are provided by this organization.

Elder Care Online
Website: www.ec-online.net

Information, education and support for caregivers, safety advice, and links to additional caregiver resources are featured on this website maintained by Prism Innovations, Inc.

Chapter 47

Caregiving: Routine Concerns

Caring for a person with Alzheimer's disease (AD) at home is a difficult task and can become overwhelming at times. Each day brings new challenges as the caregiver copes with changing levels of ability and new patterns of behavior. Research has shown that caregivers themselves often are at increased risk for depression and illness, especially if they do not receive adequate support from family, friends, and the community.

One of the biggest struggles caregivers face is dealing with the difficult behaviors of the person they are caring for. Dressing, bathing, eating—basic activities of daily living—often become difficult to manage for both the person with AD and the caregiver. Having a plan for getting through the day can help caregivers cope. Many caregivers have found it helpful to use strategies for dealing with difficult behaviors and stressful situations. Following are some suggestions to consider when faced with difficult aspects of caring for a person with AD.

"Caregiver Guide: Tips for Caregivers of People with Alzheimer's Disease," National Institute on Aging, National Institutes of Health, NIH Pub. No. 01-4013, April 2002. The National Institute on Aging gratefully acknowledges the following Alzheimer's Disease Centers for their valuable contributions of information in preparation of this Caregiver Guide: Duke University Joseph and Kathleen Bryan Alzheimer's Disease Research Center, and the Johns Hopkins University Alzheimer's Disease Center.

Dealing with the Diagnosis

Finding out that a loved one has Alzheimer's disease can be stressful, frightening, and overwhelming. As you begin to take stock of the situation, here are some tips that may help:

• Ask the doctor any questions you have about AD. Find out what treatments might work best to alleviate symptoms or address behavior problems.

• Contact organizations such as the Alzheimer's Association and the Alzheimer's Disease Education and Referral (ADEAR) Center for more information about the disease, treatment options, and caregiving resources. Some community groups may offer classes to teach caregiving, problem-solving, and management skills.

• Find a support group where you can share your feelings and concerns. Members of support groups often have helpful ideas or know of useful resources based on their own experiences. Online support groups make it possible for caregivers to receive support without having to leave home.

• Study your day to see if you can develop a routine that makes things go more smoothly. If there are times of day when the person with AD is less confused or more cooperative, plan your routine to make the most of those moments. Keep in mind that the way the person functions may change from day to day, so try to be flexible and adapt your routine as needed.

• Consider using adult day care or respite services to ease the day-to-day demands of caregiving. These services allow you to have a break while knowing that the person with AD is being well cared for.

• Begin to plan for the future. This may include getting financial and legal documents in order, investigating long-term care options, and determining what services are covered by health insurance and Medicare.

Communication

Trying to communicate with a person who has AD can be a challenge. Both understanding and being understood may be difficult.

- Choose simple words and short sentences and use a gentle, calm tone of voice.

- Avoid talking to the person with AD like a baby or talking about the person as if he or she weren't there.

- Minimize distractions and noise—such as the television or radio—to help the person focus on what you are saying.

- Call the person by name, making sure you have his or her attention before speaking.

- Allow enough time for a response. Be careful not to interrupt.

- If the person with AD is struggling to find a word or communicate a thought, gently try to provide the word he or she is looking for.

- Try to frame questions and instructions in a positive way.

Bathing

While some people with AD don't mind bathing, for others it is a frightening, confusing experience. Advance planning can help make bath time better for both of you.

- Plan the bath or shower for the time of day when the person is most calm and agreeable. Be consistent. Try to develop a routine.

- Respect the fact that bathing is scary and uncomfortable for some people with AD. Be gentle and respectful. Be patient and calm.

- Tell the person what you are going to do, step by step, and allow him or her to do as much as possible.

- Prepare in advance. Make sure you have everything you need ready and in the bathroom before beginning. Draw the bath ahead of time.

- Be sensitive to the temperature. Warm up the room beforehand if necessary and keep extra towels and a robe nearby. Test the water temperature before beginning the bath or shower.

- Minimize safety risks by using a handheld showerhead, shower bench, grab bars, and nonskid bath mats. Never leave the person alone in the bath or shower.

315

- Try a sponge bath. Bathing may not be necessary every day. A sponge bath can be effective between showers or baths.

Dressing

For someone who has AD, getting dressed presents a series of challenges: choosing what to wear, getting some clothes off and other clothes on, and struggling with buttons and zippers. Minimizing the challenges may make a difference.

- Try to have the person get dressed at the same time each day so he or she will come to expect it as part of the daily routine.

- Encourage the person to dress himself or herself to whatever degree possible. Plan to allow extra time so there is no pressure or rush.

- Allow the person to choose from a limited selection of outfits. If he or she has a favorite outfit, consider buying several identical sets.

- Arrange the clothes in the order they are to be put on to help the person move through the process.

- Provide clear, step-by-step instructions if the person needs prompting.

- Choose clothing that is comfortable, easy to get on and off, and easy to care for. Elastic waists and Velcro enclosures minimize struggles with buttons and zippers.

Eating

Eating can be a challenge. Some people with AD want to eat all the time, while others have to be encouraged to maintain a good diet.

- Ensure a quiet, calm atmosphere for eating. Limiting noise and other distractions may help the person focus on the meal.

- Provide a limited number of choices of food and serve small portions. You may want to offer several small meals throughout the day in place of three larger ones.

- Use straws or cups with lids to make drinking easier.

- Substitute finger foods if the person struggles with utensils. Using a bowl instead of a plate also may help.

- Have healthy snacks on hand. To encourage eating, keep the snacks where they can be seen.

- Visit the dentist regularly to keep mouth and teeth healthy.

Activities

What to do all day? Finding activities that the person with AD can do and is interested in can be a challenge. Building on current skills generally works better than trying to teach something new.

- Don't expect too much. Simple activities often are best, especially when they use current abilities.

- Help the person get started on an activity. Break the activity down into small steps and praise the person for each step he or she completes.

- Watch for signs of agitation or frustration with an activity. Gently help or distract the person to something else.

- Incorporate activities the person seems to enjoy into your daily routine and try to do them at a similar time each day.

- Take advantage of adult day services, which provide various activities for the person with AD, as well as an opportunity for caregivers to gain temporary relief from tasks associated with caregiving. Transportation and meals often are provided.

Exercise

Incorporating exercise into the daily routine has benefits for both the person with AD and the caregiver. Not only can it improve health, but it also can provide a meaningful activity for both of you to share.

- Think about what kind of physical activities you both enjoy, perhaps walking, swimming, tennis, dancing, or gardening. Determine the time of day and place where this type of activity would work best.

- Be realistic in your expectations. Build slowly, perhaps just starting with a short walk around the yard, for example, before progressing to a walk around the block.

- Be aware of any discomfort or signs of overexertion. Talk to the person's doctor if this happens.

- Allow as much independence as possible, even if it means a less-than-perfect garden or a scoreless tennis match.

- See what kinds of exercise programs are available in your area. Senior centers may have group programs for people who enjoy exercising with others. Local malls often have walking clubs and provide a place to exercise when the weather is bad.

- Encourage physical activities. Spend time outside when the weather permits. Exercise often helps everyone sleep better.

Incontinence

As the disease progresses, many people with AD begin to experience incontinence, or the inability to control their bladder and/or bowels. Incontinence can be upsetting to the person and difficult for the caregiver. Sometimes incontinence is due to physical illness, so be sure to discuss it with the person's doctor.

- Have a routine for taking the person to the bathroom and stick to it as closely as possible. For example, take the person to the bathroom every three hours or so during the day. Don't wait for the person to ask.

- Watch for signs that the person may have to go to the bathroom, such as restlessness or pulling at clothes. Respond quickly.

- Be understanding when accidents occur. Stay calm and reassure the person if he or she is upset. Try to keep track of when accidents happen to help plan ways to avoid them.

- To help prevent nighttime accidents, limit certain types of fluids—such as those with caffeine—in the evening.

- If you are going to be out with the person, plan ahead. Know where restrooms are located, and have the person wear simple, easy-to-remove clothing. Take an extra set of clothing along in case of an accident.

Sleep Problems

For the exhausted caregiver, sleep can't come too soon. For many people with AD, however, nighttime may be a difficult time. Getting the person to go to bed and stay there may require some advance planning.

- Set a quiet, peaceful tone in the evening to encourage sleep. Keep the lights dim, eliminate loud noises, even play soothing music if the person seems to enjoy it.

- Try to keep bedtime at a similar time each evening. Developing a bedtime routine may help.

- Encourage exercise during the day and limit daytime napping.

- Restrict access to caffeine late in the day.

- Use night lights in the bedroom, hall, and bathroom if the darkness is frightening or disorienting.

Hallucinations and Delusions

As the disease progresses, a person with AD may experience hallucinations and/or delusions. Hallucinations are when the person sees, hears, smells, tastes, or feels something that is not there. Delusions are false beliefs that the person cannot be dissuaded of.

- Sometimes hallucinations and delusions are a sign of a physical illness. Keep track of what the person is experiencing and discuss it with the doctor.

- Avoid arguing with the person about what he or she sees or hears. Try to respond to the feelings he or she is expressing, and provide reassurance and comfort.

- Try to distract the person to another topic or activity. Sometimes moving to another room or going outside for a walk may help.

- Turn off the television set when violent or disturbing programs are on. The person with AD may not be able to distinguish television programming from reality.

- Make sure the person is safe and does not have access to anything he or she could use to harm anyone.

Wandering

Keeping the person safe is one of the most important aspects of caregiving. Some people with AD have a tendency to wander away from their home or their caregiver. Knowing what to do to limit wandering can protect a person from becoming lost.

319

- Make sure that the person carries some kind of identification or wears a medical bracelet. If he or she gets lost and is unable to communicate adequately, this will alert others to his or her identity and medical condition.

- Keep a recent photograph or videotape of the person with AD to assist police if the person becomes lost.

- Keep doors locked. Consider a keyed deadbolt or an additional lock up high or down low on the door. If the person can open a lock because it is familiar, a new latch or lock may help.

- Be sure to secure or put away anything that could cause danger, both inside and outside the house.

Home Safety

Caregivers of people with AD often have to look at their homes through new eyes to identify and correct safety risks. Creating a safe environment can prevent many stressful and dangerous situations.

- Install secure locks on all outside windows and doors, especially if the person is prone to wandering. Remove the locks on bathroom doors to prevent the person from accidentally locking himself or herself in.

- Use childproof latches on kitchen cabinets and any place where cleaning supplies or other chemicals are kept.

- Label medications and keep them locked up. Also make sure knives, lighters and matches, and guns are secured and out of reach.

- Keep the house free from clutter. Remove scatter rugs and anything else that might contribute to a fall. Make sure lighting is good both inside and out.

- Consider installing an automatic shut-off switch on the stove to prevent burns or fire.

Driving

Making the decision that a person with AD is no longer safe to drive is difficult, and it needs to be communicated carefully and sensitively.

Even though the person may be upset by the loss of independence, safety must be the priority.

- Look for clues that safe driving is no longer possible, including getting lost in familiar places, driving too fast or too slow, disregarding traffic signs, or getting angry or confused.

- Be sensitive to the person's feelings about losing the ability to drive, but be firm in your request that he or she no longer do so. Be consistent—don't allow the person to drive on "good days" but forbid it on "bad days."

- Ask the doctor to help. The person may view the doctor as an "authority" and be willing to stop driving. The doctor also can contact the Department of Motor Vehicles and request that the person be reevaluated.

- If necessary, take the car keys. If just having keys is important to the person, substitute a different set of keys.

- If all else fails, disable the car or move it to a location where the person cannot see it or gain access to it.

Visiting the Doctor

It is important that the person with AD receive regular medical care. Advance planning can help the trip to the doctor's office go more smoothly.

- Try to schedule the appointment for the person's best time of day. Also, ask the office staff what time of day the office is least crowded.

- Let the office staff know in advance that this person is confused. If there is something they might be able to do to make the visit go more smoothly, ask.

- Don't tell the person about the appointment until the day of the visit or even shortly before it is time to go. Be positive and matter-of-fact.

- Bring along something for the person to eat and drink and any activity that he or she may enjoy.

- Have a friend or another family member go with you on the trip, so that one of you can be with the person while the other speaks with the doctor.

Coping with Holidays

Holidays are bittersweet for many AD caregivers. The happy memories of the past contrast with the difficulties of the present, and extra demands on time and energy can seem overwhelming. Finding a balance between rest and activity can help.

- Keep or adapt family traditions that are important to you. Include the person with AD as much as possible.

- Recognize that things will be different, and have realistic expectations about what you can do.

- Encourage friends and family to visit. Limit the number of visitors at one time, and try to schedule visits during the time of day when the person is at his or her best.

- Avoid crowds, changes in routine, and strange surroundings that may cause confusion or agitation.

- Do your best to enjoy yourself. Try to find time for the holiday things you like to do, even if it means asking a friend or family member to spend time with the person while you are out.

Visiting a Person with AD

Visitors are important to people with AD. They may not always remember who the visitors are, but just the human connection has value. Here are some ideas to share with someone who is planning to visit a person with AD.

- Plan the visit at the time of the day when the person is at his or her best. Consider bringing along some kind of activity, such as something familiar to read or photo albums to look at, but be prepared to skip it if necessary.

- Be calm and quiet. Avoid using a loud tone of voice or talking to the person as if he or she were a child. Respect the person's personal space and don't get too close.

- Try to establish eye contact and call the person by name to get his or her attention. Remind the person who you are if he or she doesn't seem to recognize you.

- If the person is confused, don't argue. Respond to the feelings you hear being communicated, and distract the person to a different topic if necessary.

- If the person doesn't recognize you, is unkind, or responds angrily, remember not to take it personally. He or she is reacting out of confusion.

Choosing a Nursing Home

For many caregivers, there comes a point when they are no longer able to take care of their loved one at home. Choosing a residential care facility—a nursing home or an assisted living facility—is a big decision, and it can be hard to know where to start.

- It's helpful to gather information about services and options before the need actually arises. This gives you time to explore fully all the possibilities before making a decision.

- Determine what facilities are in your area. Doctors, friends and relatives, hospital social workers, and religious organizations may be able to help you identify specific facilities.

- Make a list of questions you would like to ask the staff. Think about what is important to you, such as activity programs, transportation, or special units for people with AD.

- Contact the places that interest you and make an appointment to visit. Talk to the administration, nursing staff, and residents.

- Observe the way the facility runs and how residents are treated. You may want to drop by again unannounced to see if your impressions are the same.

- Find out what kinds of programs and services are offered for people with AD and their families. Ask about staff training in dementia care, and check to see what the policy is about family participation in planning patient care.

- Check on room availability, cost and method of payment, and participation in Medicare or Medicaid. You may want to place your name on a waiting list even if you are not ready to make an immediate decision about long-term care.

- Once you have made a decision, be sure you understand the terms of the contract and financial agreement. You may want to have a lawyer review the documents with you before signing.

- Moving is a big change for both the person with AD and the caregiver. A social worker may be able to help you plan for and adjust to the move. It is important to have support during this difficult transition.

For More Information

Several organizations offer information for caregivers about AD. To learn more about support groups, services, research, and additional publications, you may wish to contact the following:

Alzheimer's Association
225 North Michigan Avenue, Suite 1700
Chicago, IL 60601-7633
Toll-Free: 800-272-3900
Phone: 312-335-8700
Fax: 312-335-1110
TTY: 312-335-8882
Website: http://www.alz.org
E-mail: info@alz.org

This nonprofit association supports families and caregivers of patients with AD. Almost 300 chapters nationwide provide referrals to local resources and services, and sponsor support groups and educational programs. Online and print versions of publications are also available at the website.

Alzheimer's Disease Education and Referral (ADEAR) Center
P.O. Box 8250
Silver Spring, MD 20907-8250
Toll-Free: 800-438-4380 (English, Spanish)
Phone: 301-495-3311
Fax: 301-495-3334
Website: http://www.alzheimers.org
E-mail: adear@alzheimers.org

This service of the National Institute on Aging is funded by the Federal Government. It offers information and publications on diagnosis, treatment, patient care, caregiver needs, long-term care, education and training, and research related to AD. Staff answer telephone and written requests and make referrals to local and national resources. Publications and videos can be ordered through the ADEAR Center or via the website.

Children of Aging Parents
1609 Woodbourne Road
Suite 302A
Levittown, PA 19057
Toll-Free: 800-227-7294
Phone: 215-945-6900
Fax: 215-945-8720
Website: http://www.caps4caregivers.org

This nonprofit group provides information and materials for adult children caring for their older parents. Caregivers of people with Alzheimer's disease also may find this information helpful.

Eldercare Locator
Toll-Free: 800-677-1116
Website: www.eldercare.gov

The Eldercare Locator is a nationwide, directory assistance service helping older people and their caregivers locate local support and resources for older Americans. It is funded by the Administration on Aging (AoA), which also provides a caregiver resource called *Because We Care—A Guide for People Who Care.* The AoA *Alzheimer's Disease Resource Room* contains information for families, caregivers, and professionals about AD, caregiving, working with and providing services to persons with AD, and where you can turn for support and assistance.

Family Caregiver Alliance
690 Market Street
Suite 600
San Francisco, CA 94104
Toll-Free: 800-445-8106
Phone: 415-434-3388
Fax: 415-434-3508
Website: www.caregiver.org
E-mail: info@caregiver.org

Family Caregiver Alliance is a community-based nonprofit organization offering support services for those caring for adults with AD, stroke, traumatic brain injuries and other cognitive disorders. Programs and services include an Information Clearinghouse for FCA's publications.

National Institute on Aging (NIA)
P.O. Box 8057
Gaithersburg, MD 20898-8057
Toll-Free: 800-222-2225 (NIA Information Center)
TTY: 800-222-4225
Phone: 301-496-1752
Website: http://www.nia.nih.gov

The National Institute on Aging (NIA) offers a variety of information about health and aging, including the *Age Page* series and the NIA Exercise Kit, which contains an 80-page exercise guide and 48-minute closed-captioned video. Caregivers can find many *Age Pages* on the web site.

Simon Foundation for Continence
Box 835-F
Wilmette, IL 60091
Toll-Free: 800-237-4666
Website: http://www.simonfoundation.org

The Simon Foundation for Continence helps individuals with incontinence, their families, and the health professionals who provide their care. The Foundation provides books, pamphlets, tapes, self-help groups, and other resources.

Well Spouse Foundation
63 West Main Street, Suite H
Freehold, NJ 07728
Toll-Free: 800-838-0879
Website: http://www.wellspouse.org

Well Spouse is a nonprofit membership organization that gives support to wives, husbands, and partners of the chronically ill and/or disabled. Well Spouse publishes the bimonthly newsletter, *Mainstay*.

Chapter 48

Tips for Coping with Caregiving Challenges

Alzheimer's disease can cause a person to exhibit unusual and unpredictable behaviors that challenge caregivers, including severe mood swings, verbal or physical aggression, combativeness, repetition of words, and wandering. These behavioral changes can lead to frustration and tension, for both people with Alzheimer's and their caregivers. It is important to remember that the person is not acting this way on purpose, and to analyze probable causes and develop care adjustments.

Common Causes of Behavior Changes

- Physical discomfort caused by an illness or medications.
- Overstimulation from a loud or overactive environment.
- Inability to recognize familiar places, faces, or things.
- Difficulty completing simple tasks or activities.
- Inability to communicate effectively.

Tips for Responding to Challenging Behaviors

- Stay calm and be understanding.
- Be patient and flexible.

"Caregiving Challenges," is reprinted with permission of the Alzheimer's Association. For additional information, call the Alzheimer's Association national toll-free number, 800-272-3900, or visit their website at www.alz.org. © 2002 Alzheimer's Association. All rights reserved.

- Don't argue or try to convince the person.
- Acknowledge requests and respond to them.
- Try not to take behaviors personally.
- Accept the behavior as a reality of the disease and try to work through it.

Exploring Causes and Solutions

It is important to identify the cause of the challenging behavior and consider possible solutions.

Identify and Examine the Behavior

- What was the undesirable behavior? Is it harmful to the individual or others?
- What happened before the behavior occurred?
- Did something trigger the behavior?

Explore Potential Solutions

- Is there something the person needs or wants?
- Can you change the surroundings? Is the area noisy or crowded? Is the room well-lighted?
- Are you responding in a calm, supportive way?

Try Different Responses in the Future

- Did your response help?
- Do you need to explore other potential causes and solutions? If so, what can you do differently?

Agitation

The term agitation is used to describe a large group of behaviors associated with Alzheimer's disease. As the disease progresses, most people with Alzheimer's experience agitation in addition to memory loss and other thinking symptoms.

Agitated Behaviors

In the early stages of the disease, people with Alzheimer's may experience personality changes such as irritability, anxiety, or depression.

As the disease progresses, other symptoms may occur, including sleep disturbances, delusions (firmly held belief in things that are not real), hallucinations (seeing, hearing, or feeling things that are not there), pacing, constant movement or restlessness, checking and rechecking door locks or appliances, tearing tissues, general emotional distress, and uncharacteristic cursing or threatening language.

Possible Causes of Agitation

Agitation may be caused by a number of different medical conditions and drug interactions or by any circumstances that worsen the person's ability to think. Situations that may lead to agitated behavior include moving to a new residence or nursing home, other changes in the environment or caregiver arrangements, misperceived threats, or fear and fatigue resulting from trying to make sense out of a confusing world.

Treating Agitation

A person exhibiting agitated behavior should receive a thorough medical evaluation, especially when agitation comes on suddenly. The treatment of agitation depends on a careful diagnosis, determination of the possible causes, and the types of agitated behavior the person is experiencing. With proper treatment and intervention, significant reduction or stabilization of the symptoms can often be achieved.

There are two distinct types of treatments for agitation: behavioral interventions and prescription medications. Behavioral treatments should be tried first. In general, steps to managing agitation include (1) identifying the behavior, (2) understanding its cause, and (3) adapting the caregiving environment to remedy the situation.

Preventing Agitation

General caregiving strategies to prevent or reduce agitated behaviors include the following:

- Create a calm environment: remove stressors, triggers, or danger; move person to a safer or quieter place; change expectations; offer security object, rest, or privacy; limit caffeine use; provide opportunity for exercise; develop soothing rituals; and use gentle reminders.

- Avoid environmental triggers: noise, glare, insecure space, and too much background distraction, including television.

- Monitor personal comfort: check for pain, hunger, thirst, constipation, full bladder, fatigue, infections, and skin irritation; ensure a comfortable temperature; be sensitive to fears, misperceived threats, and frustration with expressing what is wanted.

- Simplify tasks and routines.

- Allow adequate rest between stimulating events.

- Use lighting to reduce confusion and restlessness at night.

Identifying Agitation Triggers

Correctly identifying what has triggered agitated behavior can often help in selecting the best behavioral intervention. Often the trigger is some sort of change in the person's environment:

- change in caregiver

- change in living arrangements

- travel

- hospitalization

- presence of house guests

- bathing

- being asked to change clothing.

During an Episode of Agitation

- **Do:** redirect the person's attention, back off and ask permission, use calm positive statements, reassure, slow down, use visual or verbal cues, add light, offer guided choices between two options, focus on pleasant events, offer simple exercise options, or limit stimulation.

- **Do not:** raise voice, take offense, corner, crowd, restrain, rush, criticize, ignore, confront, argue, reason, shame, demand, condescend, force, explain, teach, show alarm, or make sudden movements out of the person's view.

- **Say:** May I help you? Do you have time to help me? You're safe here. Everything is under control. I apologize. I'm sorry that you are upset. I know it's hard. I will stay until you feel better.

Safety Measures

- Equip doors and gates with safety locks.

- Remove guns from the person's environment.

Combativeness

When a person with Alzheimer's disease is frustrated, scared, or unable to communicate, he or she may become aggressive and even combative.

Possible Causes

Combativeness can be caused by many factors, including physical discomfort, environmental factors, and poor communication. If the person you are caring for is exhibiting combativeness, consider the following:

Physical Discomfort

- Is the person tired because of inadequate rest or sleep?

- Are medications causing side effects?

- Is the person unable to let you know he or she is experiencing pain?

Environmental Factors

- Is the person overstimulated by loud noises, an overactive environment, or physical clutter?

- Does the person feel lost or abandoned?

Poor Communication

- Are you asking too may questions or making too many statements at once?

- Are your instructions simple and easy to understand?

- Is the person picking up on your own stress and irritability?

- Are you being negative or critical?

331

Caregiving Tips

- Identify signs of frustration. Look for early signs of frustration during activities such as bathing, dressing, or eating, and respond in a calm and reassuring tone.

- Don't take the behavior personally. The person isn't necessarily angry with you. He or she may have misunderstood the situation or be frustrated with lost abilities caused by the disease.

- Avoid teaching. Avoid elaborate explanations and arguments. Be encouraging and don't expect the person to do more than he or she can.

- Use distractions. If the person is frustrated because he or she can't unbutton a shirt, distract the person with another activity. After some time has passed you can return to helping the person unbutton the shirt.

- Communicate directly with the person. Avoid expressing anger or impatience in your voice or physical action. Instead use positive, accepting expressions, such as "don't worry" or "thank you." Also use touch to reassure and comfort the person. For example, put your arm around the person or give him or her a kiss.

- Decrease level of danger. Assess the level of danger—for yourself and the person with Alzheimer's. You can often avoid harm by simply stepping back and standing away from the person. If the person is headed out of the house and onto the street, be more assertive.

- Avoid using restraint or force. Unless the situation is serious, avoid physically holding or restraining the person. He or she may become more frustrated and cause personal harm.

Hallucinations

A hallucination is a false perception of objects or events involving the senses. When a person with Alzheimer's disease has a hallucination, he or she sees, hears, smells, tastes, or feels something that isn't there. The person may see the face of a former friend in a curtain or may hear people talking.

If the hallucination doesn't cause problems for you, the person, or other family members, you may want to ignore it. However, if they happen continuously, consult a physician to determine if there is an underlying physical cause. Also, have the person's eyesight and hearing checked, and make sure the person wears his or her glasses and hearing aid on a regular basis.

Offer Reassurance

- Respond in a calm, supportive manner.

- A gentle tap on the shoulder may turn the person's attention toward you.

- Look for the feelings behind the hallucinations. You might want to say, "It sounds as if you're worried," or "I know this is frightening for you."

- Avoid arguing with the person about what he or she sees.

Use Distractions

- Suggest that you take a walk or sit in another room. Frightening hallucinations often subside in well-lit areas where other people are present.

- Try to turn the person's attention to music, conversation, or activities you enjoy together.

Modify the Environment

- Check for noises that might be misinterpreted, such as noise from a television or an air conditioner. Look for lighting that casts shadows, reflections, or distortions on the surfaces of floors, walls, and furniture.

- Cover mirrors with a cloth or remove them if the person thinks that he or she is looking at a stranger.

Incontinence

It is common for persons with Alzheimer's disease to experience loss of bladder and/or bowel control. This can be caused by:

- **Medical conditions.** The person may have a urinary tract infection, constipation, or a prostate problem. Other illnesses, such as diabetes and stroke, and medication side effects may also trigger incontinence.

- **Fear.** The person may fear that an embarrassing accident may occur. This fear may cause him or her to visit the bathroom more times than necessary.

- **Abrupt movement.** Urine release may be caused by a sneeze, laugh, or cough. Weak pelvic muscles in women can also cause uncontrollable loss of urine.

- **Dehydration.** Withholding fluids when a person starts to lose bladder control may compound the problem. Dehydration can create urinary tract infections that lead to incontinence.

- **Diuretics.** Certain beverages, such as coffee, cola, and tea, may contribute to incontinence.

- **Environment.** The person may be having trouble finding the bathroom or getting to it in time because it is too far away.

- **Clothing.** Zippers and buttons on clothing could be making it difficult for the person to undress.

If incontinence is a new problem, consult your doctor to rule out potential causes such as a urinary tract infection, weak pelvic muscles, or medications. If the problem continues, try to:

- **Provide visual cues.** Signs may assist an individual in finding the bathroom. Placing colored rugs on the bathroom floor and lid covers on the toilet may help the bathroom stand out. Avoid having items nearby that can be mistaken for a toilet, such as a trash can.

- **Monitor incontinence.** Identify when accidents occur and plan accordingly. For example, if they happen every two hours, get the person to the bathroom before that time. To help control incontinence at night, limit the intake of liquids after dinner and in the evening.

- **Remove obstacles.** Make sure clothing is easy for the individual to remove. Clothing with Velcro™ may be easier for the person to remove than clothing with buttons.

- **Provide reminders.** Because the person with Alzheimer's may forget to use the bathroom, you may need to remind him or her periodically. Also watch for visible cues such as restlessness or facial expressions that may indicate the person needs to use the bathroom.

- **Be supportive.** Help the person with Alzheimer's retain a sense of dignity despite incontinence problems. A reassuring attitude will help lessen feelings of embarrassment.

Sleeplessness and Sundowning

Sleeping problems experienced by persons with Alzheimer's and caregiver exhaustion are two of the most common reasons people with Alzheimer's are eventually placed in nursing homes. Some studies indicate that as many as 20 percent of persons with Alzheimer's will, at some point, experience periods of increased confusion, anxiety, agitation, and disorientation beginning at dusk and continuing throughout the night.

While experts are not certain how or why these behaviors occur, many attribute them to late-day confusion, or "sundowning," caused by the following factors:

- end-of-day exhaustion (mental and physical)

- an upset in the "internal body clock," causing a biological mix-up between day and night

- reduced lighting and increased shadows

- disorientation due to the inability to separate dreams from reality when sleeping

- less need for sleep, which is common among older adults.

Tips for Reducing Evening Agitation and Nighttime Sleeplessness

- **Plan more active days.** A person who rests most of the day is likely to be awake at night. Discourage afternoon napping and plan activities, such as taking a walk, throughout the day.

- **Monitor diet.** Restrict sweets and caffeine consumption to the morning hours. Serve dinner early, and offer only a light meal before bedtime.

- **Seek medical advice.** Physical ailments, such as bladder or incontinence problems, could be making it difficult to sleep. Your doctor may also be able to prescribe medication to help the person relax at night.

335

- **Change sleeping arrangements.** Allow the person to sleep in a different bedroom, in a favorite chair, or wherever it's most comfortable. Also, keep the room partially lit to reduce agitation that occurs when surroundings are dark or unfamiliar.

Nighttime restlessness doesn't last forever. It typically peaks in the middle stages, then diminishes as the disease progresses. In the meantime, caregivers should make sure their home is safe and secure, especially if the person with Alzheimer's wanders. Restrict access to certain rooms or levels by closing and locking doors, and install tall safety gates between rooms. Door sensors and motion detectors can be used to alert family members when a person is wandering.

Once the person is awake and upset, experts suggest that caregivers:

- approach their loved one in a calm manner
- find out if there is something he or she needs
- gently remind him or her of the time
- avoid arguing or asking for explanations
- offer reassurance that everything is all right and everyone is safe.

Unpredictable Situations

People with Alzheimer's disease can act in different and unpredictable ways. It is important to remember that the person is not acting this way on purpose. Whatever the behavior, try to identify the cause and possible solution.

Bold Behavior

The person with Alzheimer's disease may forget that he or she is married and begin to flirt or make inappropriate advances toward members of the opposite sex.

If the person is engaging in unusual, inappropriate behavior, try to distract the person with another activity or lead them into a private place. Avoid getting angry or laughing at the person.

Inappropriate Dressing

The person may forget how to dress or take clothes off at inappropriate times and in unusual settings. For example, a woman may remove a blouse or skirt simply because it is too tight or uncomfortable.

Help the person dress by laying out clothes in the order they need to be put on. Choose clothing that is simple and comfortable.

Shoplifting

The person with Alzheimer's may not understand or remember that merchandise must be paid for. He or she may casually walk out of the store without paying—unaware of any wrongdoing.

Have your loved one carry a wallet-size card that states that he or she is memory-impaired. This may prevent the person with Alzheimer's disease from feeling embarrassed.

Paranoia

The person may become easily jealous and suspicious. For example, a man may think his wife has a boyfriend if he sees her with their son. A person with Alzheimer's may also misinterpret an unfamiliar face as someone who is a thief.

If the person makes accusations or becomes extremely suspicious, don't waste time arguing. Try to distract the person with another activity or reassure him or her with a hug or touch.

Wandering

An individual with Alzheimer's is likely to wander at some point during the disease. Identifying the cause of the behavior can help eliminate or reduce its occurrence.

Causes

Wandering can be caused by several factors, including:

- Medication side effects
- Stress
- Confusion related to time
- Restlessness
- Agitation
- Anxiety
- Inability to recognize familiar people, places, and objects
- Fear arising from the misinterpretation of sights and sounds

- Desire to fulfill former obligations, such as going to work or looking after a child.

Tips for Reducing Wandering Behavior

- Encourage movement and exercise to reduce anxiety, agitation, and restlessness.

- Involve the person in productive daily activities, such as folding laundry or preparing dinner.

- Remind the person that he or she is in the right place.

- Reassure the person if he or she feels lost, abandoned, or disoriented.

Tips for Protecting Your Loved One from Wandering

- Enroll the person in the Alzheimer's Association's Safe Return Program, a nationwide identification system designed to assist in the safe return of people who become lost when wandering.

- Inform your neighbors of the person's condition and keep a list of their names and telephone numbers.

- Keep your home safe and secure by installing deadbolt locks on exterior doors and limiting access to potentially dangerous areas.

- Be aware that the person may not only wander by foot but also by car or by other modes of transportation.

Tips for Preparing for Emergencies

- Keep a list of emergency phone numbers and addresses of the local police and fire departments, hospitals, and poison control as well as Safe Return help lines.

- Check fire extinguishers and smoke alarms, and conduct fire drills regularly.

Chapter 49

Communication and Dementia

Losing the ability to communicate can be one of the most frustrating and difficult problems for people with Alzheimer's disease or other dementias which affect language. As the disease progresses, the person experiences a gradual lessening of their ability to communicate. They find it more and more difficult to express themselves clearly and take in what is being said, and carers find it an increasing struggle to understand what the person with dementia is feeling or trying to say.

Some Changes You May Notice in the Person with Dementia

- They may have difficulty finding a word and say a related word instead of the one that is lost.

- They may not be able to understand what you are saying or only be able to grasp part of it.

- They may talk fluently but not make sense.

- Writing and understanding the written word will also deteriorate.

- They may be able to talk of the distant past but not of recent events.

"Communication in Dementia," © 2002 Alzheimer's Disease and Related Disorders Association of NWS (New South Wales), Inc.; reprinted with permission. Additional information is available online at www.alznsw.asn.au.

- They may lose the normal social conventions of conversation and interrupt, ignore another speaker, not respond when spoken to or become very self-centered.

- They may have difficulty expressing emotions appropriately.

Here Are Some Suggestions to Help with Communication Problems

Be Flexible

- Remember that each person is unique and each relationship is different so it is a question of trying things out to discover what works best for you.

- Talk to other carers and health care professionals and see what works for them.

- Don't expect too much: keep modifying your expectations at each stage so that they remain realistic.

- Remember that words are not the only form of communication: you will need to rely more heavily on non-verbal cues such as the tone of voice, touch, and the way you move to convey how you feel when the person you are caring for begins to have difficulty understanding conversation.

- Listen for and learn to recognize the feelings and emotions rather than the words.

Preserve Self Esteem

- Try not to talk down to the person or to treat them as a child: conversation should be simple, but remain on an adult level.

- Continue sharing activities and pastimes with the person and show them you value them.

- People still retain their feelings and emotions even though they may not understand what is being said, so do everything you can to preserve their dignity and self-esteem.

- Never discuss the person in front of others as if they were not present, even if you think they do not understand.

Ways of Talking

- Remain calm and talk in a gentle, matter-of-fact way; keep sentences short and simple, focusing on one idea at a time, talk about specific events that may be remembered or everyday things like weather.

- Allow plenty of time for what you have said to be interpreted.

- Speak slowly and clearly without raising your voice.

- Repeating a point using different words can be helpful.

- Incorporating information in your conversation which tells the person where they are, what is happening around them and who they are with, can make them feel more secure and less confused.

- Use orienting names whenever you can such as "your son, Jack."

- Try to tune into the feelings rather than the content of the conversation; don't attempt complex discussions: keep information simple.

The Right Environment

- Avoid competing noises or activities such as TV or radio.

- Make sure glasses, hearing aids and dentures are all correctly prescribed and well-fitting.

- If you are able to remain still and with the person while you are talking to them, it will be easier for them to follow you and will show you are prepared to work at trying to understand them.

- Always try to move slowly and quietly.

- Maintaining regular routines helps minimize confusion and this can assist communication.

- Sit or squat beside a seated person—never stand above; make eye contact.

- When talking in a group make sure the person is not on the end of the row. It is better to place the person so that the conversation is around them and they will not feel "left out."

Simplifying Activities

- Break down an instruction into simple activities: for example, name the next item to be put on as they get dressed rather than suggest they put on their clothes.

- As the condition worsens, break tasks into even smaller steps.

- Explain what you are doing at each step along the way; focus on familiar tasks; introducing new tasks can be confusing.

- Make it easy for the person to join in a conversation by asking questions that need only a "yes" or "no" answer, e.g. "It's very cold for this time of the year isn't it?"

Finding Words

- If the person has difficulty finding a word, ask them to explain in a different way or guess at their meaning and ask if you are correct.

- If they can't think of the right word, try giving clues instead of immediately supplying it, e.g. "cup of ....". You can also try giving a description, e.g., "You clean your teeth with it." You can ask them to show you what they are referring to. Pointing to something will often help the person get the message across.

Verbal Abuse

- Avoid upsetting arguments or allowing your own stress and exasperation to show.

- Use distraction when possible to help overcome upsets and frustration.

- Arguments over mistaken ideas should be avoided. If the person insists they have seen a TV program a million times before, even after you have pointed out that it is a first run, say something such as "Oh, well, I don't think I have seen it before. It's interesting, isn't it?" Your arguments will only end up frustrating you and probably upsetting the person.

Encourage Laughter

- Use laughter; humor is a great safety valve to overcome a mistake or misunderstanding.

Body Language

- Pointing or demonstrating can help a person to understand what you are saying; touching and holding their hand may help keep their attention and show them you care.

- Try to maintain eye contact when speaking and listening.

Asking Questions

- Avoid too many choices: present only one option at a time.

- Ask questions which require only yes/no responses and give them plenty of time to respond.

- Try to be tactful when the person asks the same questions over and over again.

Aids to Communicating

- Showing and touching physical objects and pictures may help with memory and assist conversation.

- Music can be an excellent way of communicating; it can help a person recall words and express feelings.

- Old photos can be used to stimulate memories and recall events.

Chapter 50

Outings for People with Dementia

Many families ask for guidance or suggestions on appropriate outings for their loved one with dementia, but there are no easy answers. Because the person's interests, likes, and dislikes often change during the course of the disease, the caregiver is left with the challenge of finding new activities to engage or entertain the person.

In creating such activities, caregivers should first ask, "Whose needs am I trying to meet?" then establish goals to fill the needs of that person—the person with dementia.

For example, try not to continue the relationship as it was by preserving familiar activities your loved one can no longer take part in. Some familiar activities can be continued for a long time into the disease, as long as they are adapted to the person's changing abilities. Caregivers who know and are sensitive to the needs of their loved one can continue to make sound judgements about what works and what doesn't.

Be careful not to take the roles of "patient" and "caregiver" and only tend to daily needs such as eating and bathing. Without thinking, you

"Personalize Outings for Persons with Dementia," by Dorothy Seman, RN, MS, NHA, Clinical Coordinator, Alzheimer's Family Care Center (Chicago, IL), an adult day care center for people with dementia that is a collaborative effort between the Rush Alzheimer's Disease Center and the Veterans Affairs Chicago Health System. © 2003 Dorothy Seman. Reprinted with permission. Additional information about Alzheimer's disease and other dementias is available at the website of the Rush Alzheimer's Disease Center at http://www.rush.edu/patients/radc/.

345

might fall into the habit of meeting your needs at the expense of your loved one, or vice versa.

When considering outside activities or outings for you and your loved one, think about simple goals you hope to accomplish, such as:

- Getting some exercise and fresh air

- Being together in a relaxed setting

- Doing something enjoyable or interesting

- Feeling love and support from relatives and friends

After setting these goals, keep the following in mind:

- Plan activities that were enjoyable in the past, and begin making any changes based on interest and tolerance.

- Avoid activities with crowds, such as popular sporting events.

- Go to places at times when there are fewer people and prompt, personal service, such as an early lunch or dinner at a familiar restaurant.

- Limit time spent on one activity. Activities that last longer than a few hours are often too taxing.

- Consider activities that are flexible enough to permit a change of plans, such as leaving a party early.

- Plan activities that don't require much concentration, but have some ability to hold the person's attention. Try visiting a pet store, zoo, or flower show.

- Allow the person to participate according to ability. Don't demand more than he or she is capable of. For example, "Come on, you remember your sister-in-law, Barbara."

- Enjoy simple activities: A walk to the park or an ice cream store, a visit to a church or temple, a quiet drive through a forest preserve, a walk along the lake front, a stop at the local playground.

- Be creative in trying things that might be unusual, but workable, such as a trip to a garage sale, a swim at the local YMCA, or a leisurely stop at a local bakery.

Most activities are meaningful for persons with dementia because of the supportive relationship they share with their caregiver. As the disease progresses, many individuals rely on familiar people and the newly adapted, now familiar routines in their life. Repeat community outings that the person with dementia enjoys.

Remember that a break in routine, though refreshing for the caregiver, may produce stress and discomfort for the person with dementia. For many people with dementia, familiarity, not variety, is the spice of life.

—by Dorothy Seman, M.S., R.N.

Chapter 51

Understanding Wandering

What Is Wandering?

Wandering refers to the need to keep on the move. It is often seen in people with Alzheimer's disease.

- The wandering behavior may appear to be aimless or confused, or it may be focused on getting to a particular destination or pursuing a particular goal.

- Wandering may occur at any time of the day or night, and may take the person out of the home.

- Wandering outdoors can expose the person to such dangers as traffic or unsafe weather conditions.

What causes wandering?

- Wandering is a common behavior for a person with Alzheimer's disease.

- It is a direct result of physical changes in the brain.

- Short-term memory loss and inability to reason or to make judgments contribute to wandering behavior.

Text in this chapter is from "Understanding Wandering," "Reasons for Wandering," "What to Do If Wandering Happens," and "Reuniting after an Episode of Wandering," © 2002 Alzheimer Society of Canada. Reprinted with permission from the Alzheimer Society of Canada. For more information visit the website at www.alzheimer.ca.

349

How can wandering be managed?

- In itself, wandering is not a harmful behavior.

- When done in a safe environment, it can be a healthy outlet for a person with Alzheimer's disease.

- Channeling wandering into a safe activity involves looking at all the potential triggers of the behavior.

- By determining what may be contributing to the behavior, it may then be possible to figure out ways to manage it.

Reasons for Wandering

A person with Alzheimer's disease may wander for a variety of reasons. She may be:

- too hot or too cold.

- hungry or in pain.

- trying to recreate a situation from her past, such as going to work or catching a bus.

As a caregiver, pinpointing the reason behind wandering can be a challenging task, especially when verbal communication has become difficult. Looking at non-verbal clues may help you establish the reason for the wandering:

- Is there a pattern to the behavior?

- Does the wandering appear aimless or confused?

- Is there a particular purpose to the wandering?

Being able to find the pattern of wandering can help you identify why the person wanders. Once this is determined, you can begin to put strategies in place to manage the behavior.

Following are some of the types of wandering associated with Alzheimer's disease and some possible reasons for the behavior.

Aimless Wandering

- Non-focused walking with little or no direction or destination.

- It may take place because the person is bored or needs to exercise.

- It may be the person's response to feeling stress or physical discomfort.

Purposeful Wandering

- Goal-oriented wandering.

- The person may appear to be searching for something or trying to return to familiar surroundings from her past.

- She may be looking for security and reassurance in her life.

- She may have a physical need, such as hunger or the need to use the washroom.

Night-Time Wandering

- Night hours are often a time for wandering.

- Broken sleep patterns may cause restlessness and disorientation in the middle of the night.

- Confusion about time may also cause the person to be unaware of the difference between day and night.

- She may wake, get out of bed and go to the kitchen to look for something to eat or try to get dressed.

Industrious Wandering

- The person may incorporate repetitive behavior into her wandering.

- In her need to keep busy, she may continue habits, or recreate schedules or routines established long ago, such as trying to go to work or catch a bus.

What to Do If Wandering Happens

It's not easy to remain calm and think clearly when a loved one has wandered. Keep in mind that you are not alone and that others are there to help you.

351

The following are general strategies that may be helpful in the event that a person with Alzheimer's disease wanders away from home.

Check Common Areas

- Try and get a sense of how long the person has been gone.

- Look inside the house, including the basement, before expanding your search to the outdoors.

- Check to see if any items such as luggage, car keys or credit cards are missing. These may provide clues to her whereabouts.

- If you live in a rural area, do not search on your own. You may endanger yourself and complicate the search for the police.

Contact the Police

- Contact the police when a loved one has wandered.

- Once the police arrive, share any records you have which may help in the search.

- Let the police know about any medical conditions, or medications the person is taking.

- Provide them with a recent photograph.

- If you know of any areas that she may have wandered to, share these with the police.

Mobilize Support

- If you will be involved in the search for the person, ensure someone stays at home in case the individual returns.

- At the same time, alert friends and neighbors that the person has wandered away.

Reuniting After an Episode of Wandering

A person with Alzheimer's disease who has been found wandering will often be anxious and confused. Using the following communication strategies may help to calm the person and encourage her return home.

Approach Calmly

- Approach the person in a casual manner, making sure that she sees you coming.

- If the person does not wish to return home immediately, walk a short distance with her while speaking in a calm, normal tone of voice.

Provide Reassurance

- Reassure the person about where she is and why.

- Let her know that you have been worried about her and will be happy to see her return home.

- Talk to her about familiar things that may trigger a response to return home. An invitation to have a cup of tea or feed the dog may be enough to prompt the person to go home with you.

- The person may be determined to reach a particular location. If possible, consider taking her there right away or at a later date.

Keep Your Perspective

- The whole experience of wandering can be extremely stressful. Remember that the behavior is a part of Alzheimer's disease. Neither you nor the person is to blame.

- Once the person is safely home again, it is natural to want to ensure that wandering does not happen again. The steps you take to prevent a recurrence should focus on prevention. Keep in mind that restraints should never be used as they can have serious effects on the emotional and physical well-being of the person.

Chapter 52

Coping with Changes in Intimate Relationships

Intimacy in Alzheimer's Disease

Spring is in the air and thoughts of love and romance fill the hearts of many and brighten their days. Uncomfortable feelings of regret and loneliness may surface, however, for those who diligently "give care" to their loved ones with Alzheimer's disease but are disturbed by their lowered expectations for intimacy and closeness. Many caregivers would rather withdraw and hide than confront these conflicting needs for distance and intimacy especially when a partner may have difficulty recognizing who you are and remembering the nature of the relationship.

We all carry with us a history of close relationships when our intimacy needs were met, challenged, and/or unfulfilled, sometimes all

The beginning text in this chapter reprinted with permission from "Intimacy in Alzheimer's Disease," by Naomi Nelson, Ph.D., former Director of Education for the Alzheimer's Disease Center (ADC) in the Department of Neurology, Baylor College of Medicine. For additional Information about how the ADC helps patients and families through research, patient care, and education, contact ADC, 6550 Fannin Street, Smith Tower, #1801, Houston, TX 77030, 1-713-798-6660, or visit the website at http://www.bcm.tmc.edu/neurol/struct/adrc/adrc1.html. © 1999 Department of Neurology, Baylor College of Medicine. Text under the heading "Intimacy and Sexuality Issues in Dementia: A Guided List of Resources," is from a document by the same name, © 2002 Alzheimer's Disease and Related Disorders Association of NWS (New South Wales), Inc.; reprinted with permission. Additional information is available online at www.alznsw.asn.au.

at the same time. Caring for a loved one with Alzheimer's disease usually makes the memories of those past intimate encounters more special, but at the same time, present and future needs for intimacy may become confusing. Someone has suggested that the best definition of intimacy can be understood by changing the order of the syllables to read ci-in-ta-my, meaning "see into me." Intimacy then becomes a sharing of one's deepest self with another who can respond, but who also appreciates our uniqueness and vulnerability. Unfortunately, such an explanation of intimacy is too often disrupted by the changes inherent in Alzheimer's disease.

There are numerous threats to intimacy even under the best of circumstances. Feelings of anger, guilt, resentment, and despair can distance individuals from one another. Relationships may change because of divorce, family and economic problems, communication difficulties, mistrust, and feelings of low self-esteem. In the midst of these relationship upheavals may come the devastating effects of Alzheimer's disease. The recognition of intimacy needs and continuation of a close relationship becomes even more of a challenge.

It has been simply stated that Alzheimer's disease changes everything. And it does. Alzheimer's disease has been characterized as a relationship of separation with no hope for further connection. For example, partners with Alzheimer's disease may be unable to recognize that the person providing their care is also their spouse. These individuals may also have an increased or diminished interest in physical closeness. The well partner may also be changing and his/her spouse may no longer be attractive in an intimate way resulting in conflicting feelings of obligation and resentment.

What may help those who are struggling with changes in their intimate relationships?

As with all aspects of Alzheimer's disease, there are no specific rules, but some suggestions from caregivers and professionals may help:

- Try to confront your own needs for intimacy. Only after being clear about those needs can you face the challenges created by a relationship with someone who has Alzheimer's disease.

- Consider that the changes in intimacy are part of many other losses and adaptations that accompany Alzheimer's disease. If some earlier losses are not acknowledged or resolved, the intimacy issues may seem more pronounced and/or more confusing.

- Talk with a good friend or professional about your tense feelings about wanting to "let go and hang on" at the same time. Few of us willingly want to face our emotional reactions when a previous relationship is no longer recognizable. Allow yourself a wide range of feelings for grieving about the changes and losses.

- Acknowledge your understandable needs for communication, affection, physical touching, and closeness. Treasure those moments with your loved one when such needs can be genuinely experienced. Receiving and giving personal affection may be one of the few ways your loved one can communicate with you.

- Remember your loved one as a person who happens to have Alzheimer's disease. Find someone to talk with who will understand the complexities of your needs for intimacy and the special needs of your loved one. You need support in your role of "giving care."

Intimacy and Sexuality Issues in Dementia: A Guided List of Resources

This resources list is one in a series prepared in the information resources center, Alzheimer's Australia NSW. Resources lists are updated on an annual basis. The list is intended to provide an understanding of material available in the information resources center on intimacy and sexuality issues. It follows a slightly different format to other resources lists in the same series, because there is no HelpNote to accompany it. For each section a brief discussion of issues is followed by a suggested list of resources. This is a select bibliography and does not cover all the resources available in the information resources center.

What Is Intimacy and How Is It Affected by Dementia?

Intimacy is a natural need of human life from birth and throughout life. It is the giving and receiving of love and affection, caring touch, empathic understanding, comfort in times of need, and a feeling of safety in relationships. The need for closeness is a very important part of people's lives. However, for all of us the way in which we express our need for intimacy, will vary with our individual characters and life experiences.

People with dementia continue to need caring, safe relationships, and touch. However, they too will vary in their individual ways giving and receiving affection, and in the way in which their dementing

357

condition affects that capacity. For example, some people with dementia may dislike being touched, and changes may need to be made in the way in which closeness and affection are expressed. As a result of the disease process some people with dementia may also become demanding and insensitive to the needs of others and less able to provide caring support for their family and partners. This can be a great source of loss and distress for carers.

Sexuality—the feeling of sexual desire and its expression though sexual activity—is also a natural expression of a human need. However, for most people it goes beyond the narrow concept of sexual intercourse, and is bound up with many of the broader expressions of intimacy, including physical closeness, kissing, and hugging.

People with dementia may experience a variety of changes in their expression of sexuality. Some continue to desire sexual contact, others may lose interest in sexual activity and others may for a short time display inappropriate sexual behavior. These changes also carry an emotional cost for carers.

Despite the fact that our humanity is inextricably bound up with our need for intimacy and our sexuality, the literature of aging, long term care, and dementia has tended to avoid these topics or to cover them with unhelpful brevity. However, there are some helpful resources available.

Couple and Family Carer Issues of Intimacy and Sexuality

The need for closeness does not cease when one partner develops a dementing illness, but changes may be felt in the way the need is expressed. For some couples, sexual activity is unaffected in the early stages of the disease process, and they may even feel more loving and close. Other couples may be able to keep their relationship affectionate despite a decrease in the quality of sexual activity. Later in the disease more major adjustments may be required.

Resources which may help clarify these issues include:

- Alzheimer's challenges couples' closest ties. *Alzheimer's Association National Newsletter*, 15(2), Summer 1995, pp. 1, 7. [Format: Journal article]—This looks at some of the ways in which Alzheimer's disease can affect couple relationships. It includes quotes from carers and makes suggestions about dealing with inappropriate behaviors.

- *Alzheimer's disease: a guide for families* / Lenore S. Powell, Katie Courtice.—Reading, Mass.: Addison-Wesley, © 1983, pp.

64–67, 126–128.—Discusses the changes in the quality of the couple relationship and the effects which may be felt by family carers, as well as inappropriate behaviors which can occur.

- *Alzheimer's disease: coping with a living death* / Robert T. Woods.—Souvenir Press, 1989, pp. 83–85. [Format: Book]—This includes a broad look at changes to the marital relationship and suggests that carers who are experiencing difficulties seek professional counseling.

- *A thousand tomorrows: intimacy, sexuality and Alzheimer's.*— Terra Nova, 1995. [Format: Video]—In this video couples discuss the changes Alzheimer's disease has brought to their relationships, in terms of intimacy and sexuality. An excellent video for carers and support groups.

There are also some resources which address the concerns of family members other than partners. These include:

- *The 36-hour day: a family guide to caring for persons with Alzheimer's disease, related dementing illnesses, and memory loss in later life* / Nancy L. Mace, Peter V. Rabins.—Rev. ed.— Baltimore: Johns Hopkins University Press, © 1991, pp. 130– 133, 279–281. [Format: Book]—This book for family carers discusses inappropriate sexual behavior in the home and in nursing homes. It points out that these behaviors are actually rare in people with a dementing illness.

- *Sexuality and dementia: carers' perspective* / Dementia Services Development Centre.—Stirling: Dementia Services Development Center, [1996?]. [Format: Video]—In this video a group of carers, (three spouse carers and one woman who cares for her mother) discuss the effects of dementia on relationships, affectionate behavior and sexuality.

Intimacy and Sexuality in Residential Care

- Assessments of institutionalized dementia patients' competencies to participate in intimate relationships / Peter A. Lichtenberg and Deborah M. Strzepek. *The Gerontologist*, 30(1), 1990, pp. 117– 120. [Format: Journal article in special interest folder]—This paper describes the assessment technique used to assist staff in determining whether to allow particular residents to develop affectionate and/or sexual relationships.

- *Dementia with dignity* / Barbara Sherman.—Rev. ed.—Sydney: McGraw-Hill, 1994, pp. 103–107. [Format: Book]—Gives a good discussion of some issues concerning sexuality and dementia, with practical case examples. The section on handling problem behavior (pp. 66–75) is also relevant.

- Intimacy: nursing home resident issues and staff training / Carly R. Hellen. *American Journal of Alzheimer's Disease*, March/April 1995, 10(2), pp. 12–17. [Format: Journal article]—Despite the title of the article, this paper looks mainly at issues surrounding sexuality in nursing homes. It makes suggestions for gathering preadmission information, dealing with excessive masturbation, working with families and staff training.

- Management of sexual relationships among elderly residents of long-term care facilities / by Meredith Wallace. *Geriatric Nursing*, 13(6), 1992, pp. 308–311. [Format: Journal article in special interest folder]—This paper describes a protocol for assessment and management of relationships between residents in long term care. It is not dementia specific.

- *Sexuality and dementia: a guide* / by Carole Archibald. Illustrated by Anne Rodger.—Stirling, UK: University of Stirling, 1994. [Format: Book]—This book would be very useful in staff training. It provides a practical framework for addressing issues of sexuality in long term care. Case studies for discussion are included. This can be used with the kit "Sexuality and dementia: video and training handbook."

- *Sexuality and dementia: video [and] training handbook* / Carole Archibald, Alan Chapman.—Stirling: Dementia Services Development Centre, 1994. [Format: Video; Book]—A good training video for staff. Discussion points are highlighted by vignettes. A framework for dealing with 'problem' situations is suggested. It is suggested that this be used in conjunction with the book "Sexuality and dementia: a guide".

- Sexuality and sexual needs of the person with dementia / Carole Archibald. IN *The new culture of dementia care* / Edited by Tom Kitwood and Sue Benson.—Loughton, Essex: Hawker Publications, 1995. pp. 35–39. [Format: Book chapter]—A positive and well written paper which describes an approach to sexuality issues. The problem-solving approach addresses the needs of the person with dementia, family carers, other residents and staff.

- Sexuality in the special care unit / Edna L. Ballard. IN *Special care programs for people with dementia* / Edited by Stephanie B. Hoffman, Mary Kaplan.—Baltimore: Health Professions Press, 1996, pp. 79–99.—This discussion of the issues surrounding sexuality and intimacy is well written and thoughtful. Quotes from carers illustrate the points the author is making and practical guidelines are given.

- 'Sex'? Not my grandmother! / Barbara Sherman. IN *Practical solutions in dementia care* / Alzheimer's Association Australia.—[Brisbane]: Alzheimer's Association Australia, 1995. pp. 62 + [Tape 2]. [Format: Conference proceedings summary; Audiocassette contents]—A good discussion of the way in which sexual attitudes may affect caring in a long term care setting. Issues raised include masturbation, the need for couples to have the opportunity to continue to their intimacy, and the way in which people with dementia may perceive care by staff to have a sexual connotation. Case studies are presented on the audiocassette.

- What kind of love is this? / by Athena H. McLean. *The Sciences*, 34(5), 1994, pp. 36–39. [Format: Journal article in special interest folder]—A broad look at the issues involved in relationships between residents in long term care, which suggests that staff evaluation be based on emotional/affective memory as well as cognitive capacity.

Management of Inappropriate Sexual Behavior

Some people with dementia may retain sexual desires despite advancing dementia. Where the person with dementia is able to satisfy these needs appropriately, this does not present a problem. However, there are some circumstances where their behavior will be, or will be perceived to be, a problem. Literature in this area suggests that some behavior which is interpreted as sexually inappropriate may have another explanation. For example, a person rearranging their clothing may need to go to the toilet. Whatever the explanation for their behavior, it may help to remember that the underlying cause is always found in the changes to the brain caused by the dementia. They are not deliberately seeking to hurt or annoy others. In many cases too, gently discouraging the behavior or redirecting the person with dementia to another activity may be sufficient. Some of the resources listed earlier in this resources list may have information on this topic. Additional resources are:

- Management of sexually disinhibited behavior by a dementia patient / P. Alexopoulos. *Australian Journal on Ageing*, August 1994, 13(3), pp. 119. [Format: Journal article]—This case study describes the successful use of cues to modify inappropriate sexual behavior in resident with vascular dementia.

- *Person to person* / by Tom Kitwood and Kathleen Bredin.— Loughton, Essex: Gale Centre, 1992, pp. 49–50. [Format: Book]—This brief discussion suggests a gentle and accepting approach to the problems raised by sexually inappropriate behavior.

Intimacy and Sexuality Issues for Health Professionals

- *Alzheimer's disease and marriage: an intimate account* / Lore K. Wright.—Newbury Park, Ca.: Sage Publications, © 1993.—This book discusses the results of 3 years research contrasting the experiences of healthy older couples with the lives of couples with one partner affected by Alzheimer's disease. Quotes directly taken from the in-depth interviews are given, and the topics covered include companionship, affection and sexuality.

- *Questions of intimacy: video and guidelines* / Alzheimer's Association Victoria. Video produced by Open Channel. Guidelines written by Wendy Taylor, Maria Pavlou and Delys Sargent.— Hawthorn, Vic.: Alzheimer's Association Victoria, 1995. [Format: Kit; Video; Book]—This kit aims to promote discussion among counselors and carers of people with dementia on issues of intimacy and sexuality and to develop competencies in health professionals to work in that area. It covers intimacy more than sexuality. It is primarily helpful for professional counselors, residential care staff and educators. It may also be helpful in a support group setting.

- Sexual behavioral changes in Alzheimer disease / Christian Derouesne...[et al]. *Alzheimer Disease & Associated Disorders*, Summer 1996, 10(2), pp. 86–92. [Format: Journal article]—The aim of this study was to assess the frequency and type of sexual behavioral changes in a group of people with Alzheimer's disease living in the community.

- Sexuality/intimacy and how we talk about 'it' / Wendy Taylor. IN *Practical solutions in dementia care* / Alzheimer's Association Australia.—[Brisbane]: Alzheimer's Association Australia, 1995.

pp. 70 + [Tape 2]. [Format: Conference proceedings summary; Audiocassette contents]—Discusses the need for counselors and other health professionals to be trained in personal awareness and sensitive handling of intimacy and sexuality issues, to assist carers in an exploration of their needs and concerns.

- Sexuality and sexual counseling for couples where a partner has dementia / Hugh Woolford. IN *Practical solutions in dementia care* / Alzheimer's Association Australia.—[Brisbane]: Alzheimer's Association Australia, 1995. pp. 77 + [Tape 2]. [Format: Conference proceedings summary; Audiocassette contents]—This conference paper highlights issues the fact that many older couples still enjoy an active sexual relationship. Difficulties created by cognitive impairment in one partner are then discussed. The author also touches on his experience of dealing with sexuality issues in support groups.

- *The young mind: issues in relation to young people and dementia* / Prepared by Stephen Freeth.—North Ryde, NSW: Alzheimer's Association Australia, 1994, p. 27. [Format: Book]— Briefly discusses the effects on marital relationships and sexuality which were found in discussions with carers of people with early onset dementia.

Resources which Cover the Issue of Sexuality in Older Age Include

- *The challenge of ageing* / Edited by M.W. Shaw.—Edinburgh: Churchill Livingstone, 19, pp. 14–15.—This is a brief but positive look at the right of older people to have their sexual needs recognized.

- *The heart has no wrinkles* / Producer: Adrienne Parr. Director: Wendy Thompson.—Crows Nest, NSW: Health Media, Department of Health, NSW, 1988. [Format: Video]—Intended for use as a trigger for discussion of aging and sexuality. It is set in a long term care facility but is not dementia specific. However, the principles which it demonstrates of respecting the need of older people to have their dignity, right to privacy and right to relationships respected are still applicable.

- Sexuality and the ageing: a review of the current literature / Billye Kay, James N. Neelley. *Sexuality and Disability*, 5(1), Spring 1982, pp. 38–46. [Format: Journal article]—This article does not discuss dementia, but presents a useful discussion of the facts and myths concerning sexual changes and sexual needs in older adults.

• Lecture 6: Sexuality and the elderly—debunking the myths / Lecturer: Lyn Lillington. IN *Counseling the elderly* [audiocassette] / Continuing Education, University of New South Wales. Lecturer: Murray Lloyd...[et al].—Kensington, NSW: University of New South Wales, [Format: Audiocassette contents]—Relates research on sexuality and aging, and looks at factors which may affect sexual functioning in older adults.

Chapter 53

Caregiver Stress

What is caregiving?

Caregiving means caring for others, whether friends or relatives, who have health problems or disabilities and need help. Caregivers provide many kinds of help to care receivers, from grocery shopping to helping with daily tasks such as bathing, dressing, and eating. Most people who need help from caregivers are elderly.

- About one fourth of American families are caring for an older family member, an adult child with disabilities, or a friend.

- According to recent surveys, more than seven million persons are informal caregivers to older adults. Caregivers include spouses, adult children, and other relatives and friends. Other surveys found that almost 26 million family caregivers provide care to adults (aged 18+) with a disability or chronic illness, and five million informal caregivers provide care for older adults aged 50+ with dementia.

- Studies show that more than half of caregivers are women. Care receivers are about half women and half men.

"Caregiver Stress," The National Women's Health Information Center, Office on Women's Health, Department of Health and Human Services. This FAQ has been reviewed by Susan G. Kornstein, M.D. of the Virginia Commonwealth University, reviewed August 2002.

- The average amount of time that caregivers spend on caregiving is about 20 hours per week. Even more time is required when the care receiver has multiple disabilities.

- Caring for a person with disabilities can be physically demanding, especially for older caregivers, who make up half of all caregivers.

- One third of all caregivers describe their own health as fair to poor.

- Caregivers often worry that they will not outlive the person for whom they are caring.

- Caregivers often suffer from depression. Caregivers are also more likely to become physically ill.

What is caregiver stress?

Caregiver stress is a daily fact of life for many caregivers. Caregiving often takes a great deal of time, effort, and work. Many caregivers struggle to balance caregiving with other responsibilities including full-time jobs and caring for children. Constant stress can lead to "burnout" and health problems for the caregiver. Caregivers may feel guilty, frustrated, and angry from time to time.

Caregivers often need help caring for an elderly or disabled care receiver. Sometimes other family members or friends and neighbors are able to help, but many caregivers do most or all of the caregiving for a loved one alone. Research has shown that caregivers often are at increased risk for depression and illness. This is especially true if they do not receive enough support from family, friends, and the community.

Caring for a person with Alzheimer's disease (AD) or other kinds of dementia at home can be overwhelming. The caregiver must cope with declining abilities and difficult behaviors. Basic activities of daily living often become hard to manage for both the care receiver and the caregiver. As the disease worsens, the care receiver usually needs 24-hour care.

What can caregivers do to prevent stress and burnout?

Caregivers can call upon others for support and assistance. Other family members, friends, and neighbors may be able to help in different ways. It may not be easy to ask for help, and you may need to make very specific requests. But getting help from others will benefit you and the person you are caring for.

Respite care can be a good way to get a break (respite) from constant caregiving. If other caregivers aren't available to fill in for the main caregiver, respite care services may be available in the community.

As a caregiver, you can take steps to take care of your own health:

- Eat a healthy diet rich in fruits, vegetables and whole grains and low in saturated fat. Ask your health care provider about taking a multivitamin as well.

- Try to get enough sleep and rest.

- Find time for some exercise most days of the week. Regular exercise can help reduce stress and improve your health in many ways.

- See your health care provider for a checkup. Talk to your provider about symptoms of depression or illness that you may be having. Get counseling if needed.

- Stay in touch with friends. Social activities can help keep you feeling connected and help with stress. Faith-based groups can offer support and help to caregivers.

- Find a support group for other caregivers in your situation (such as caring for a person with dementia). Many support groups are available online through the internet.

What is the National Family Caregiver Support Program (NFCSP)?

The National Family Caregiver Support Program (NFCSP) is a federally-funded program through the Older Americans Act. It helps states provide services to help family caregivers. These services include:

- Information to caregivers about available services

- Help to caregivers in gaining access to services

- Individual counseling, organization of support groups, and caregiver training

- Respite care

- Supplemental services, on a limited basis, to complement the care provided by caregivers.

367

How can I find out about caregiving resources in my community?

There are resources with staff who can help you figure out whether and what kinds of assistance you and your care receiver may need.

The local Area Agency on Aging (AAA) is one of the first resources you should contact when help is needed caring for an older person. Almost every state has one or more AAAs, which serve local communities, older residents, and their families. In a few states, the State Unit or Office on Aging serves as the AAA. Local AAAs are generally listed in the city or county government sections of the telephone directory under "Aging" or "Social Services."

You can also call the National Eldercare Locator, a toll-free service funded by the Administration on Aging (AoA), at 800-677-1116. The Eldercare Locator can help you find your local or state AAA. Eldercare Locator operators are available Monday through Friday, 9:00 a.m. to 8:00 p.m., Eastern Time. When contacting the Locator, callers should have the address, zip code, and county of residence for the person needing assistance. The Eldercare Locator is also available online at http://www.eldercare.gov.

If your family member has a limited income, he or she may be eligible for AAA services including homemaker home health aide services, transportation, home-delivered meals, chore and home repair as well as legal assistance. These government-funded services are often targeted to those most in need. While there are no income criteria for many services, sometimes you may have more service options if you can pay for private help. AAAs can direct you to other sources of help for older persons with limited incomes such as subsidized housing, food stamps, Supplemental Security Income, and Medicaid.

Supportive services for the person needing care can include both in-home and community-based services, such as:

- Transportation
- Meals
- Personal and in-home care services
- Home health care
- Cleaning and yard work services
- Home modification
- Senior centers
- Respite services including adult day care.

If you are an employee covered under the federal Family and Medical Leave Act, if you meet the eligibility requirements, you are entitled to take up to 12 weeks of unpaid leave during any one-year to care for certain relatives.

What kind of paid help is available for home health care? Is there government support for this?

People with low incomes may be eligible for AAA services including homemaker home health aide services and other services. Check with your local or state AAA or the Eldercare Locator service (see resources below). Government-funded services are often targeted to those most in need. While there are no income criteria for many services, sometimes you may have more service options if you can pay for private help.

If you decide to hire a home care worker, you will need to decide how much help your older relative needs. Will several hours a day be enough, does he or she need help all day until the family returns home, or does your relative live alone and need round the clock care? You also need to decide what type of home care worker your relative needs. Home care personnel include:

- Housekeeper or chore worker is supervised by the person hiring them and performs basic household tasks and light cleaning.

- A homemaker or personal care worker is supervised by an agency or you and provides personal care, meal planning and household management and medication reminders.

- A companion or live-in is supervised by an agency or you and provides personal care, light housework, exercise, companionship, and medication reminders.

- A home health aide, certified nurse assistant, or nurses aide is supervised by an agency's registered nurse. Services include personal care; help with transfers, walking, and exercise; household services that are essential to health care; and assistance with medicines.

Nonprofit and for profit home care agencies recruit, train, and pay the worker. You pay the agency.

Home health care agencies focus on the medical aspects of care and provide trained health care personnel, such as nurses and physical therapists. Medicare may pay for their services.

369

Who is eligible for Medicare home health care services?

To get Medicare home health care, a person must meet all of these four conditions:

- A doctor must decide that the person needs medical care in the home and make a plan for care at home.

- The person must need at least one of the following: intermittent (and not full time) skilled nursing care, or physical therapy, or speech language pathology services; or continue to need occupational therapy.

- The person must be homebound. This means that he or she is normally unable to leave home. Being homebound means that leaving home is a major effort. When the person leaves home, it must be infrequent, for a short time, or to get medical care, or to attend religious services.

- The home health agency caring for the person must be approved by the Medicare program.

For more information about Medicare, call 800-MEDICARE or visit the Medicare website (http://www.medicare.gov).

Will Medicaid help pay for home health care?

Medicaid is a joint federal and state program that helps with medical costs for some people with low incomes and limited resources. To qualify for Medicaid, you must have a low income and few savings or other assets. Medicaid coverage differs from state to state. In all states, Medicaid pays for basic home health care and medical equipment. Medicaid may pay for homemaker, personal care, and other services that are not paid for by Medicare.

For more information about what Medicaid covers for home health care in your state, call your state medical assistance office. If you need the telephone number for your state, call 800-MEDICARE.

For More Information

For more information, call the National Women's Health Information Center at 800-994-9662 or contact the following organizations.

Administration on Aging
One Massachusetts Avenue
Washington, DC 20201
Phone: 202-619-0724
Fax: 202-401-7620
Website: www.aoa.gov
E-mail: AoAInfo@aoa.gov

Alzheimer's Association
225 North Michigan Avenue, Suite 1700
Chicago, IL 60601-7633
Toll-free: 800-272-3900
Phone: 312-335-8700
Fax: 312-335-1110
TTY: 312-335-8882
Website: http://www.alz.org
E-mail: info@alz.org

Family Caregiver Alliance
690 Market St., Suite 600
San Francisco, CA 94104
Toll-Free: 800-445-8106
Phone: 415-434-3388
Fax: 415-434-3508
Website: www.caregiver.org
E-mail: info@caregiver.org

National Family Caregivers Association
10400 Connecticut Avenue, #500
Kensington, MD 20895-3944
Toll-Free: 800-896-3650
Fax: 301-942-2302
Website: http://www.nfcacares.org
E-mail: info@nfcacares.org

Chapter 54

When You Need Assistance with Caregiving

The 21st century will be marked by a dramatic increase in the size of the older population as the baby boom generation ages. An increase in older adults will mark a corresponding increase in dementing illnesses such as Alzheimer's disease, Parkinson's disease, and stroke. These disorders affect not only the individual, but can also be devastating to the family. Already, millions of working adults are juggling the competing demands of caring for a chronically ill or disabled parent, raising a family, and managing a career.

If you are a caregiver, you are not alone. An estimated one out of four U.S. households is involved in caring for a loved one aged 50 or older. As many as 12.8 million Americans of all ages need assistance from others to carry out everyday activities. While there is no reliable estimate of the number of family caregivers, at least 7 million Americans are caring for a parent at any given time.

Between one-third to one-half of all caregivers are also employed outside the home. Working caregivers sacrifice leisure time, and often suffer stress-related illnesses. Negative effects on working caregivers include time lost from work, lower productivity, quitting a job

"Fact Sheet: Work and Eldercare," prepared by Family Caregiver Alliance in cooperation with California's Caregiver Resource Centers, a statewide system of resource centers serving families and caregivers of brain-impaired adults. Funded by the California Department of Mental Health. Printed September 1999. All rights reserved. © 1999 Family Caregiver Alliance; reprinted with permission. For more information from Family Caregiver Alliance, visit www.caregiver.org.

to give care, lost career opportunities, and lower future earnings. Eventually, some 12 percent quit their jobs to provide care full-time. Work disruptions due to employee caregiving responsibilities result in productivity losses of $1,142 per year per employee.

Getting Started

A range of community resources exist to help caregivers and their impaired loved ones. The arrangements can be informal (for example, your family, friends, and neighbors) or formal (service agencies and programs). In assessing your family's needs consider the following:

- Make a list of what you need help with and the times you need it. For example, I need someone to keep my mother company and prepare her meals during work hours, or I need someone to give Dad a ride to the senior center on Tuesdays and Thursdays at 9:00 a.m.

- Consider what level of care is needed (companion, chore work, nursing) and whether the care can be delivered at home or at an adult day care center.

- Consult your or your parents' insurance policy to see if any coverage is available. Determine how much money you and your family can afford to spend on outside resources. (Generally, long-term care is not covered by health insurance policies.)

- Explore care options in your community or near your parent's home.

Finding Community Resources

Information and Referral (I&R): These are services to help you locate programs and services in your community. Senior or community I&R services maintain lists of resources, by geographic area, to help you get started in finding the services you need. In addition, if you have access to the internet, there are a growing number of resource listings, news groups, and chat groups where you can seek out information on your own. Even if your parent lives far away, you can find services to help.

Informal Arrangements

There may be chores that can be done by friends, family, neighbors, or church members. Simple tasks include preparing meals, providing rides, helping with grocery shopping or laundry, providing reassuring phone calls, or companionship for your relative. Local senior centers or colleges often have programs for community volunteers.

A family meeting can be very helpful in discussing difficult medical and legal issues. Identifying needs, airing concerns, and delegating tasks should be done in an open, supportive environment where all necessary family members can be involved.

To work through certain family dynamics or conflicts, an outside person can be useful. A geriatric care manager can be hired to help the family and caregiver make a care plan and, if need be, to help with care arrangements and monitoring. This may be especially helpful if your ill parent lives far from you.

In-Home Care

Home care can be either formal (home care agency or personal attendant) or informal (friend, family, or volunteer). If no medical or personal care is needed, any caring, responsible person may be suitable. An ad can be placed in your local community or college newspaper to search for a responsible part-time companion and chore worker. If care involves toileting or bathing, you will need a person who is trained and competent. Similarly, if lifting the person and/or a wheel chair is necessary, be sure the worker is physically able do the work. Always check references carefully.

If medications are to be dispensed, or nursing care is required, you will likely need a licensed vocational nurse (LVN). A registered nurse (RN) is needed only when more complex medical care is necessary (such as treating wounds, or managing a ventilator). Medicare may be able to cover medically necessary part-time care for a home-bound older person.

Adult Day Care

Adult day care centers provide a therapeutic environment for older adults outside the home. They provide social services and activities in a safe, supportive environment. Depending on the program, health and therapeutic care may or may not be available. It is important to check eligibility criteria. Some centers may not accept participants who are disruptive, have other health problems, or are incontinent. Participants generally attend several hours per day, up to five days a week. Transportation to and from the adult day care center may also be provided.

375

Other Community Resources

In California, Caregiver Resource Centers (CRCs) provide a range of supportive services to family caregivers of brain-impaired adults (for example, Alzheimer's, Parkinson's, stroke, traumatic brain injury, Parkinson's disease). CRCs help caregivers with information, educational programs, and emotional support, as well as planning for and arranging services for a brain-impaired loved one.

Other community services include case management services, home-delivered meals, transportation services, temporary overnight care, hospice (for terminally ill individuals), and support groups (for either the caregiver or the ill individual). Your local I&R service can help you locate these.

Residential Placement

When a parent can no longer be cared for at home, it may be necessary to consider a residential facility. Arriving at this decision can be quite painful. Both you and your parents are likely to have strong feelings about nursing homes. You may want to discuss the decision with other family members, a counselor, or spiritual advisor.

Ultimately, it is important to evaluate your parent's current living situation and carefully assess how care needs can be met. Concerns about safety, your parent's ability to be left alone, medical needs, and adequate help for basic daily activities (for example, eating, dressing, toileting, bathing, moving around) should be considered. In addition, the daily strain on the caregiver should not be ignored. If you, your sibling or parent is the primary caregiver, it is vital to recognize when caregiving demands exceed what is humanly possible. If you determine home is no longer a viable option, it is time to look at residential placements.

Residential care options are not limited to what most people refer to as nursing homes. A range of options exist for residential care. For maximum independence, senior residences or assisted living facilities offer apartment-style living with additional services such as meals, house cleaning, transportation, recreational activities, and, sometimes, an on-call nurse.

Residential care facilities (RCFs; also called board and care homes), are group homes for individuals who cannot live alone, but do not need skilled nursing. These facilities offer help with personal care and hygiene, meals, social interaction with others, and bedside care. They have 24-hour staff in case of emergencies. RCFs do not accept Medicaid

(Medi-Cal in California) reimbursement since medical care is not administered.

Skilled nursing facilities (SNF) provide nursing care to residents and must be equipped to administer medications, injections and provide other nursing functions. SNFs do not typically provide rehabilitative care (for example, physical or speech therapy). Medicare will pay for up to 100 days of medically-necessary skilled nursing care in a SNF. Medicare pays 100% of the first 20 days. As of 1998, days 21–100 require a $95.50 per day co-payment. Medicare will not pay for "custodial care."

Some nursing homes and hospitals have special care units for individuals with Alzheimer's disease. These facilities should provide specialized care, trained staff, and secured premises. Since there is currently no federal care standard for special units, it is important to obtain information on staff credentials, resident-to-staff ratio, and the specific services offered to ensure that the unit provides a clear benefit.

Legal/Financial Issues

If a parent becomes cognitively impaired, you are likely to face a host of new legal issues. Typical concerns include:

- Who will manage the confused person's money;

- Who will make important health care decisions; and

- How to plan for long-term care.

An attorney can help you plan for the financial aspects of your parent's long-term care needs. At a minimum, a suitable attorney should have experience in estate and financial planning, probate, and wills. In addition, it is helpful for your attorney to be familiar with public benefits (for example, Medicaid—or Medi-Cal in California), Social Security, special needs trusts, tax planning, and housing and health care contracts. Some ways to locate an attorney include: your local County Bar Association (attorney referral service), senior legal aide, or a personal recommendation from a friend or fellow support group member.

Surrogate decision-making for a person with memory loss can be difficult and emotionally-charged. The process can be simplified significantly, however, if your parent has completed a durable power of attorney (DPA) and a durable power of attorney for health care

(DPAHC). These two very different documents enable your parent to designate another person to manage his/her finances and health care decisions. To complete a DPA or DPAHC, the person must be mentally competent at the time the documents are signed. The legal authority to make surrogate decisions will begin only when and if the person becomes incompetent. It is a good idea to have DPA and DPAHC forms reviewed by an experienced attorney to ensure that the person's wishes are clearly expressed and the information is complete.

In the case where your parent is already suffering from dementia and does not have the capacity to make decisions, you may need to obtain a conservatorship. A conservatorship provides the legal authority to manage a person's finances, estate, personal affairs, assets, and medical care. In order to obtain a conservatorship, a friend, family member, or public official must petition the court with facts about why the individual can no longer manage financial or personal affairs. At a hearing, the judge determines what special powers may be granted to the conservator. Conservatorships tend to be complex; the legal agreements are court supervised and the conservatee's (impaired person's) assets and income become part of the public record. In addition, prospective conservators may face substantial costs for court, legal, investigator, and conservator's fees.

Handling Stress

Caring for an ill or disabled parent can be particularly challenging while juggling the competing demands of work, family, and caregiving. It is important to get the emotional and practical support you need to cope with the stress of being a caregiver. Taking care of yourself will help ensure that you are physically and emotionally able to care for your impaired parent.

- Obtain up-to-date information. For example, Caregiver Resource Centers have a variety of caregiver-related fact sheets and other materials to help you make informed decisions.

- Ask for help. Don't try to do everything yourself. A sibling, relative, or friend may be able to help you. Some organizations offer specialized care planning guidance to help you get through the "maze" of long-term care options.

- When highly stressed, consider joining a support group or speaking with a professional therapist.

- Be patient. There may be good days and bad days. Learn how to communicate effectively with your parent without laying blame. It will take some time to arrange services that address all needs.

- Give yourself a break. Remember to schedule some time to relax. "Respite care" is designed to allow a break for the caregiver, and can last an hour, a day, or even a week. Check your local resources.

What Employers Can Do

Eldercare is now recognized by a growing number of employers. Support for employees who have caregiving responsibilities can take a variety of forms:

- Employers can offer "cafeteria style" employee benefits which allow employees to select supplemental dependent care coverage to reimburse costs for in-home care or adult day care. Benefits also should cover therapeutic counseling for the employee to help cope with the stresses of caregiving.

- Human Resource or employee assistance program staff can provide information on helpful Internet sites, local I&R services, or resource centers.

- Larger businesses can organize in-house caregiver support groups or coordinate with local community groups or hospitals so that employees can attend an outside support group.

- One of the most critical benefits for an employee with caregiving responsibilities is time. Flexible work hours, family illness days, and leave time are key. Data from the Bureau of National Affairs (1993) found that flexible scheduling improved job performance, decreased lateness and employee turnover, and increased job satisfaction.

- Companies with 50 or more employees must comply with the Family and Medical Leave Act (FMLA), which allows for up to 12 weeks of unpaid leave to care for a seriously ill parent, spouse, or child, while protecting job security. Smaller firms can use the FMLA guidelines to provide support for individual employees.

379

- Other ideas include holding a company "caregiver fair" or a series of lunchtime seminars on issues such as hiring a home care attendant, or coping skills for caregivers. Employers can establish a telephone hot-line, or publish a list of key contacts in their employee newsletter.

- Offer private long-term care insurance coverage for employees, their spouses, and dependents.

Resource

Family Caregiver Alliance
690 Market St., Suite 600
San Francisco, CA 94104
Toll-Free: 800-445-8106
Phone: 415-434-3388
Fax: 415-434-3508
Website: www.caregiver.org
E-mail: info@caregiver.org

Family Caregiver Alliance supports and assist caregivers of brain-impaired adults through education, research, services, and advocacy.

FCA's information Clearinghouse covers current medical, social, public policy, and caregiving issues related to brain impairments. Information on a broad range of subjects is available through FCA Fact Sheets and other publications or at our website.

Credits

Enright, R., and Friss, L. (1987) *Employed Caregivers of Brain-Impaired Adults: An Assessment of the Dual Role*, Final report submitted to the Gerontological Society of America, prepared for Family Caregiver Alliance, San Francisco, CA.

Kratch, P. and Brooks, J.A. (1995) Identifying the Responsibilities and Needs of Working Adults Who are Primary Caregivers, *Journal of Gerontological Nursing*, October: 41-50.

Metropolitan Life Insurance Company (1997) *The Met Life Study of Employer Costs for Working Caregivers*, Westport, CT: MetLife Mature Market Group, June 1997.

National Alliance for Caregiving and AARP (1997) *Family Caregiving in the U.S.: Findings from a National Survey*, Washington, D.C.

Scharlach, A. (1999) *Caregiving in the 21ˢᵗ Century*, Testimony before a Joint Legislative Hearing of the California Senate Subcommittee on Aging and Long-Term Care and the Assembly Committee on Aging and Long-Term Care, February 2, 1999, Sacramento, CA.

US General Accounting Office (1994) *Long-Term Care: Diverse Growing Population Includes Millions of Americans of All Ages* (GAO/HEHS-95-26, November 7, 1994)

Wagner, D.L. & Neal, M.B. (1994) *Caregiving and Work: Consequences, Correlates, and Workplace Responses*, Educational and Gerontology 20:645-63.

Witrogen McLeod, B. (1995) Eldercare, Prime Social Issue of the 21ˢᵗ Century. *San Francisco Examiner*, August 21, 1995.

Chapter 55

How Do I Hire a Home Care Employee?

Introduction

Today, one in four American families cares for an older relative, friend, or neighbor. An estimated 25 to 40 percent of women care for both their older relatives and their children. Half of all caregivers also work outside the home. It is no wonder then that caregivers often need help. Depending on your work, living, and family arrangements, there are a number of things you can do to make caregiving easier.

Ways to Make Caregiving Easier

- **Work Options and On-the-Job Training Programs:** If you are a working caregiver, it is important to discuss your needs with your employer. Telecommuting, flextime, job sharing, or rearranging your schedule can help to minimize stress. Increasingly, companies are offering resource materials, counseling, and training programs to help caregivers.

- **Involving Older Children:** Older children living at home may be able to assist you and/or your older family member. Such responsibility, provided it is not overly burdensome, can help young people become more empathic, responsible, and self-confident and give you needed support.

Excerpted from, "Because We Care: A Guide for People Who Care," U.S. Administration on Aging (AOA), 2002. The full text of this document is available online on the AOA website at www.aoa.gov.

• **Asking Other Family Members to Help:** You can and should ask other family members to share in caregiving. A family conference can help sort out everyone's tasks and schedules. Friends and neighbors also may be willing to provide transportation, respite care, and help with shopping, household chores or repairs.

Sources of Information

If you need additional information and assistance in caring for your older relative or friend, you can contact:

• The National Eldercare Locator, funded by the Administration on Aging. Eldercare Locator advisors can direct you to agencies and organizations that can assist you. When calling the Eldercare Locator at 1-800-677-1116, please provide the older person's address and ZIP code.

• The Area Agency on Aging (AAA) serving your older relative or friend's community can provide information about in-home and community services. Information also is available about benefit and assistance programs for older persons with limited incomes. These include:

  • Subsidized housing

  • Food stamps

  • Supplemental Security Income

  • Medicaid

  • The Qualified Medicare Beneficiary program, which covers the cost of the Part A and B insurance premiums, deductibles, and coinsurance for low-income older persons.

In addition, the AAA can direct you to senior center and adult day programs. These programs are particularly helpful to working caregivers who want a safe environment with planned activities for their older relative.

• Senior centers serve active older persons and those who have minor problems with mobility and activities of daily living.

• Adult day programs serve older persons with serious mobility limitations, dementia, or medical conditions that require daily attention.

- Many AAA's have a registry of home care workers from which you can recruit directly as well as information on home care agencies and volunteer groups that provide help.

- Hospital or Nursing Home Discharge Planners also can refer you to home care agencies and home care workers.

Determining the Type of Care You Need

If you decide to hire a home care employee, you need to determine how much and what type of help your older relative needs. Following are descriptions of some of the types of home care personnel:

- Housekeepers or chore workers may be supervised by the person hiring them and perform basic household tasks and light cleaning. Chore workers often do heavier types of cleaning such as washing widows and other heavy cleaning.

- A homemaker may be supervised by an agency or you and provides meal preparation, household management, personal care, and medication reminders.

- A home health aide, certified nurse assistant, or nurse's aide, often referred to as home health care workers, are supervised by a home care agency's registered nurse and provides personal care, help with bathing, transfers, walking, and exercise; household services that are essential to health care; and assistance with medications. They report changes in the patient's condition to the RN or therapist, and complete appropriate records.

Sometimes, home care employees take on several of the roles described above.

General Eligibility Requirements for Home Care Benefits

Medicare may pay for home health care services through a certified home health care agency, if a physician orders these services. Home health care agencies focus on the medical aspects of care and provide trained health care personnel, including nurses and physical therapists. For a patient to be eligible for services paid for under Medicare, she must need skilled nursing assistance, or physical, speech, and/or occupational therapy. Home health care workers are a supplement to this care and usually help the older person for three hours a day, several days a week.

If your older family member or friend needs additional hours of care or requires custodial care, she may be eligible for services under Medicaid. The state where she resides determines if her income and assets qualify her for Medicaid covered services. Otherwise, you or your older relative must cover the cost of having a home care worker.

Home care agencies, which can be nonprofit or for-profit, recruit, train, and pay the worker. You pay the agency. Social service agencies, in addition to home care services, may provide an assessment of the client's needs by a nurse or social worker, and help with the coordination of the care plan. If services are being covered under Medicare, your doctor, care manager, or discharge planner will probably make arrangements for a home health care agency.

Selecting an Agency

If you select an agency, ask the following questions. Those questions starred with an asterisk should also be asked, if you are hiring the home care employee.

1. What type of employee screening is done?

2. Who supervises the employee?

3. What types of general and specialized training have the employees received?

4. Who do you call if the employee does not come?

5. What are the fees and what do they cover?

6. Is there a sliding fee scale?

7. What are the minimum and maximum hours of service?

8. Are there limitations in terms of tasks performed or times of the day when services are furnished?

Unless your older friend or relative needs care for a limited number of hours each day, the rates charged by home care agencies for homemaker, home health aide services, and van services for transportation are often beyond the means of middle income families. If this is the case, you may want to explore the option of hiring a home care employee directly.

Hiring a Home Care Employee

Avenues for hiring home care aides include:

- Asking other caregivers for referrals

- Going to senior or other employment services

- Contacting agencies that assist displaced homemakers and others entering the job market

- Advertising in the newspapers

Screen home care employees carefully to ensure that they have the necessary qualifications, training, and or temperament.

Interviewing Applicants

Your interview with a prospective home care employee should include a full discussion of the client's needs and limitations, with a written copy of the job description; the home care worker's experience in caregiving and his or her expectations.

Special Points to Consider

- If the older person needs to be transferred from a wheelchair, make sure that the aide knows how to do this safely. If the aide does not know how to bathe a person in bed or transfer, but is otherwise qualified, it may be possible to provide the necessary training, but make sure she can do it before hiring her.

- Do not try to hire someone on a 7-day-a-week basis. No employee can remain a good employee for long if she does not have time for her personal needs and interests. Additionally, aides who live in or sleep over cannot be expected to be on call 24-hours a day. If your older relative needs frequent help or supervision during the night, you should hire a second home care aide, or have a family member fill in.

- If your older relative needs a considerable amount of help, live-in help may be available, which can be less expensive than hourly or per day employees. However, keep in mind that you will be providing food and lodging and that it may be more difficult to dismiss live-in aides, especially if they do not have alternative housing available. It also is important to ensure that the aide has her own living quarters, and that she has some free time during the day, sufficient time to sleep, and days off.

References

Have applicants fill out an employment form that includes their:

- full name
- address
- phone number
- date of birth
- social security number
- educational background
- work history
- references

Ask to see their licenses and certificates, if applicable, and personal identification including their social security card, driver's license, or photo ID.

Thoroughly check their references. Ask for the names, addresses, phone numbers, and dates of employment for previous employers, and be certain to contact them. If there are substantial time gaps in their employer references, it could indicate that they have worked for people who were not satisfied with their performance. It is best to talk directly to former employers rather than accepting letters of recommendation. With the applicant's permission, it is also possible to conduct a criminal background check.

Job Expectations

When hiring a home care aide, it is important to list the job tasks and to ask applicants to check those they are willing to perform. You should also discuss:

- vacations
- holidays
- absences
- lateness

- benefits and wages
- the amount of notification time each of you should give if the employment is terminated

If you work and are heavily dependent on the home care assistant, emphasize the importance of being informed as soon as possible if she is going to be late or absent so that you can make alternative arrangements. It is helpful to keep a list of home care agencies, other home care workers, neighbors, or family members who can provide respite care, if needed.

Be Clear About

- the employee's salary
- when he or she will be paid
- reimbursement for money the aide may spend out of pocket

Needed Information

When hiring a home care assistant, it is helpful to spend a day with him or her, so that you can go through the daily routine together. At the very least you need to inform the home care worker, both verbally and in writing, about the older person's:

- likes and dislikes
- special diets and restrictions
- problems with mobility
- illnesses and signs of an emergency
- possible behavior problems and how best to deal with them
- therapeutic exercises
- medications, when they are taken, and how to reorder them
- dentures, eye glasses, and any prosthesis

Also provide information, verbally and in writing, about:

- how you can be contacted
- contacts in case of an emergency
- security precautions and keys
- clothing

- medical supplies, where they are kept, and how they are used

- food, cooking utensils, and serving items

- washing and cleaning supplies and how they are used

- light bulbs, flash lights and the location of the fuse box

- the location and use of household appliances

Transportation

If free or low-cost transportation is not available, try to hire some-one who drives since this saves you substantial amounts of money in taxi or commercial van ride fares. If the home care employee is going to drive your family car, you must inform your insurance company, and provide a copy of the aide's driver's license to your insurance agent. Your insurance company will check to see if the license has been revoked, suspended, or if the aide has an unsatisfactory driving history. If the home care assistant has a car, discuss use of her car on the job and insurance coverage.

Insurance and Payroll

Check with your insurance company about coverage for a home care employee, and contact the appropriate state and federal agencies concerning social security taxes, state and federal withholding taxes, unemployment insurance, and workman's compensation.

If you do not want to deal with these somewhat complicated withholdings from the employee's salary, payroll preparation services can issue the employee's check with the necessary withholdings for a fee.

Some home care aides work as contractors. Even in these cases, you must report their earnings to the Internal Revenue Service. Before employing an aide on a contract basis, consult your financial advisor or tax preparer to make certain that you are following the IRS rules that govern contract workers, since there can be a fine line between who is considered to be an employee versus a contractor.

Ensuring Security

Regardless of who cares for your elderly relative, protect your private papers and valuables by putting them in a locked file cabinet, safe deposit box, or safe.

- Make arrangements to have someone you trust pick up the mail, or have it sent to a post box where you can pick it up.

- Check the phone bill for unauthorized calls, and, if necessary, have a block placed on 900 numbers, collect calls, and long-distance calls. You can always use a prepaid calling card for long distance calls.

- Protect checkbooks and credit cards. Never make them available to anyone you do not thoroughly trust.

- Review bank, credit card statements, and other bills at least once a month, and periodically request credit reports from a credit report company. Your bank can provide you with the names and addresses of these companies.

- If you do leave valuable possessions in the house, it is best to put locks on cabinets and closets and to have an inventory with photographs.

Protecting Against, Identifying, and Handling Abuse

Although abusive situations are not common, you must be alert to the possibility. They are one of the primary reasons why it is so important to carefully check the references of a prospective home care aide. You can help to prevent abuse situations by:

- Ensuring that the home care assistant thoroughly understands what the position entails, your care receiver's medical problems and limitations, as well as behavior that could lead to stressful situations.

- Ensuring that the home care aide is not overburdened.

- Keeping the lines of communication fully open so that you can deal with potential problems.

Following are possible signs of abuse or neglect:

- Personality changes in your older relative or friend

- Whimpering, crying, or refusing to talk

- Unexplained or repeated bruises, fractures, burns, or pressure sores

391

- Weight loss

- An unkempt appearance

- Poor personal hygiene

- Dirty or disorganized living quarters

- Confusion, excessive sleeping, or other signs of inappropriate sedation

If you suspect that an abusive situation exists, don't wait for it to be tragically confirmed. Find a way to check either by talking to the older person in a safe situation or, if necessary, by installing monitoring devices. If you witness, or are told by a reliable source, about neglect; physical abuse; emotional abuse, including yelling, threatening, or overly controlling, possessive behavior, which often involves isolating the older person from others; seek help, if necessary, and replace the home care aide as quickly as possible. If the situation appears serious, remove your care receiver from the premises and place him or her with another family member or in a facility that offers respite care. Always ensure that your relative is safe before confronting or dismissing the worker, especially if you are concerned about possible retaliation.

Once you have ensured your relative's safety, report the aide to Adult Protective Services so they can take appropriate actions to prevent the aide from gaining employment with other vulnerable elders. If the abuse is of a serious nature including, serious neglect, physical injury, sexual abuse, or the misuse of the funds of the older person, you should also contact the police.

Supervising a Home Care Worker

Once you have hired a home care worker, make sure that the lines of communication are fully open and that both you and the worker have a clear understanding of the job responsibilities to the older person and to each other. Explain what you want done and how you would like it done, keeping in mind that the home care employee is there to care for the older person and not the rest of the family.

If the home care worker lives in, try to ensure that he or she has living quarters that provide you, the older person, and the assistant the maximum amount of privacy possible.

Once the home care aide is on the job, periodic and/or ad hoc meetings can be held to discuss any problems the home care assistant or the older person may have with the arrangement and to find ways to resolve them. It is important to be positive and open in your approach to resolving difficulties. In most cases, they can be corrected.

However, if, after repeated attempts, you find that major problems are not resolved satisfactorily it may be best to terminate the relationship, and seek another home care employee. During this time, it may be necessary for your older relative to reside temporarily in a long-term care facility or for you to hire an aide through an agency. It is best to have reserve funds on hand should such an emergency arise.

While home care may not be less expensive than nursing home care or assisted living, it offers older people the opportunity to remain at home. What is more, it affords a degree of flexibility and choice for the at-risk elderly that few other living arrangements can provide.

Chapter 56

Housing Options to Consider

When Your Care Receiver Lives with You

American society is often a muddle of contradictions, and this is certainly true when it comes to families. On the one hand, we cherish the concept of the extended family and laud the ideal of multiple generation households. On the other we cherish our privacy and fiercely defend our independence. It is thus important for you, your relative or friend, and other family members to weigh the pro's and con's of living together. This is especially true if you are working or have other family responsibilities. You will need to consider these before you enter into an arrangement that may or may not be the best option for you and your care receiver.

Pro's and Con's

It is probably best for everyone involved to discuss what you imagine the pro's and con's of living together to be. Every family's situation is unique. Listed below are some of the benefits and drawbacks that may result. It is important for your relative or friend to take part in the decision, and to be a valued and contributing member of the family with meaningful roles, whenever possible.

On the plus side:

Excerpted from "Because We Care: A Guide for People Who Care," U.S. Administration on Aging (AOA), 2002. The full text of this document is available online on the AOA website at www.aoa.gov.

1. If your care receiver needs considerable care, you will save the expense of a long-term care facility or, at least, some in-home services.

2. You know that your care receiver is getting the best possible care because you are either providing it yourself or directly overseeing the care.

3. You will be able to make major decisions that can give you a sense of empowerment.

4. You will have more time to spend with your family member or friend.

5. Your children will have an opportunity to spend more time with their grandparent(s) or other older relative, have an important lesson in compassion and responsibility, learn about their roots, and develop a sense of family continuity.

6. If your care receiver is fairly healthy, he or she may help with household tasks, and/or with the children.

On the other side:

1. You may have less time for yourself and/or other family members and if you work you may find conflicts between your job and caregiving responsibilities. Some employment versus caregiving responsibilities may be relieved, especially in light of the technology revolution that is taking place, where telecommuting may now be an option.

2. Depending on your lifelong relationship, you may find that you and/or your relative resent changes in your relationship that may take place.

3. You will lose at least some of your privacy.

4. Other family members may resent the new arrangement.

5. There may be less space for everyone in the family.

6. You may find that hands-on caregiving is too physically and/or emotionally demanding.

If you decide that you do want to live together, you might want to try it on a trial basis, if possible. You might consider renting or subletting your care receiver's home on a short-term basis so that he or she has the option of returning home if the new arrangement does not work out to everyone's satisfaction.

You will want to consider what, if any, physical changes need to be made to your residence and how much they will cost.

Will Intergenerational Living Work in Your Home?

As a guide, you may want to ask the following questions:

1. Is your home large enough so that everyone can have privacy when they want it?

2. Is there a separate bedroom and bath for your family member, or can you create an accessory apartment?

3. Are these rooms on the first floor? If not, can your relative climb stairs safely?

4. Can you add to or remodel your home to provide a first-floor bedroom and bath?

5. Do you need to add safety features such as ramps and better lighting?

6. Does the bathroom have a shower, is it large enough to accommodate a wheelchair, if needed, and can safety features, such as grab bars, be installed to prevent falls?

7. Are door openings wide enough for a wheel chair?

You also may want to set some ground rules for privacy.

Sharing Time Together

Obviously, if you want your care receiver to live with you, you will want to share times together.

1. Set aside times to talk.

2. Involve your care receiver, if possible, in family outings and social events.

3. Invite other family and friends to your home, and let them know that you are available to come to their house as well. All of them will not respond, but some will.

397

4. Even errands, such as shopping, can be something of a social event, and give your relative a chance to participate in decision making.

At the same time, you want to ensure that other family members do not feel that they have been "displaced" and that they are as important to you as ever.

What Housing Options Are Available?

There are many times when it is not possible for a caregiver and care receiver to live together.

• The level of care that your spouse, relative, or friend needs may require highly skilled health care personnel on a regular basis. In this case, an extended care facility, such as assisted living or a nursing home, may be a better care alternative.

• Your relative or friend may live in another town and does not want to move.

• There may not be room in your home, or family members, including your relative, may not want to live together.

Whatever the reasons, living in different housing does not mean that you cannot be a good caregiver. You and your relative will, however, need to make arrangements for additional help and/or services as needed—either in his or her present home or in a new housing arrangement.

Points to Consider When Choosing Housing and Living Arrangements

When providing services to older persons who have limitations in their mobility and multiple needs, the type of housing and living arrangements you choose become critical keys in assuring that they get the care they need. Housing and care in this instance go hand in hand. There are many types of housing arrangements available for older persons, and they often overlap in the types of care and services they provide.

Before making a housing choice, you and your older relative should assess present needs and envision, as best as possible, how these needs may change in the future.

398

- What options will be open to you if the need for more supportive housing and living arrangements arises?

- Will your family member need to move to another care arrangement?

- Are these facilities available in the community, and how much will they cost?

- How are you going to pay for housing and services now and in the future?

- If you enter into housing that requires a substantial deposit at the time of admission, will some of the money be returned if your relative decides to leave?

- What guarantees do you have that the facility is financially secure?

You and your older relative will want to ask these questions before making a decision about moving into a new housing arrangement. If this arrangement involves a large entrance fee or deposit or the signing of a contract, you also will want to consult a lawyer before making the commitment.

Guidelines for Choosing Housing Options

Regardless of what the facility is called, check it out thoroughly before making a decision. The types of facilities listed below range from informal home-share arrangements to commercial enterprises, government-sponsored facilities, and housing options administered by nonprofit organizations. Some are licensed or accredited, others are not.

- Accreditation is an evaluation of a facility's operation against a set of standards. The Continuing Care Accreditation Commission— a membership organization of continuing care communities—is one such organization.

- Licensing is an evaluation of a facility's operation in accordance with government regulations. About half of the states currently regulate assisted living facilities.

- Many skilled and intermediate care nursing facilities are accredited to accept patients under the Medicare and/or Medicaid programs, which means that they must meet certain standards and provide certain services.

Regardless of these considerations, you are responsible, in large part, for ensuring that the facility is the right one for your spouse, relative, or friend.

Even if you are not thinking about housing options in the foreseeable future, it is wise to have several in mind in case an emergency arises and you need temporarily care for your relative. Home care agencies often do not have staff available to fill in on short notice, and you may need the services of a long-term care facility.

You can:

• Start your preliminary search by phone.

• Visit those facilities that have the services your care receiver wants and needs.

• Take your older relative to see the facility. Better yet, visit several and let your relative make the final choice, if at all possible.

If your relative is able to make sound decisions, and does not like any of the housing options or does not want to move into a facility after visiting several, keep looking or further explore the possibility of home care in her home or yours. Use a check list (this check list can be used as a general guide for all types of housing) to ensure that the housing arrangement is the right one for your relative.

Types of Housing and Living Arrangements

Listed below are types of housing and living arrangements, what they generally offer, and for whom they are intended. Added to these considerations are those of costs. While some housing options are modestly priced, others, especially those that are for-profit, tend to be expensive.

• Retirement communities are planned towns with a range of housing, services, and care options.

• Continuing care communities offer varying levels of care in the same building or on the same campus. When selecting a continuing care retirement community or retirement community, remember they may encompass everything from housing for independent living to assisted living and skilled nursing home care. Therefore, it may be difficult to identify what is offered simply because a facility has a certain name. These communities are usually designed for older persons with substantial financial resources.

- ECHO (Elder Cottage Housing Opportunity) housing is a self-contained housing unit temporarily placed on a relative's lot that is suitable for older persons who are largely self-sufficient.

- Accessory apartments are self-contained apartments in the care receiver's home, your home or the home of another caregiver. Designed for older persons who may be largely self-sufficient or need help with housekeeping, cooking, and personal care—commonly referred to as activities of daily living (ADL's).

- Shared housing can be in the home of the older person or in some else's home. Common areas, such as kitchens and dining rooms, are shared. This type of housing offers the older home-owner added income or the older renter an inexpensive place to live. It may offer companionship, and the possibility of having someone else around, at least part of the time, to help out with chores or in case of emergencies, but this depends on the persons sharing the house. This type of arrangement can work well for those elderly who are independent, but who would welcome a little extra income and/or help. It is important, however, to check the person's references carefully before making a decision.

- Congregate senior housing usually offers small apartments. Some offer group meals and social activities. They are designed for persons who are largely independent and do not need personal care or help with activities of daily living.

- Adult foster care is usually provided in private homes—often by the owner of the residence. The home usually provides meals, housekeeping and sometimes personal care and assistance with ADL's.

- Senior group homes are located in residential neighborhoods and offer meals, housekeeping, and usually some personal care and assistance with Activities of Daily Living (ADL's). Usually a caregiver is on site, with medical personnel making periodic visits.

- Both adult foster care and group homes may be referred to as board and care homes or residential care facilities.

- Assisted living may provide everything, including skilled nursing care. Others provide only personal care, assistance with ADLs, and/or social activities. These may also be called retirement homes or residential care facilities to name a few.

- Nursing homes provide an array of services including 24-hour skilled medical care for total care patients; custodial care; therapy for patients convalescing from hospitalizations; and personal care and help with activities of daily living for persons with dementia, chronic health, and/or mobility problems.

Chapter 57

End-Stage Alzheimer's Disease: The Long Goodbye

The final stage of Alzheimer's disease is often called "the long goodbye," and it can be one of the most difficult stages for the patient's family and caregivers. Multiple medical and ethical issues arise during this time. The focus of the patient's primary care physician often shifts from treating the disease to preventing and alleviating unnecessary pain and suffering for the patient and family.

End-stage Alzheimer's disease is marked by progressive loss of motor abilities that can cause increasing difficulty with speech and communication. Patients might be unable to recognize close family members, and may need greater assistance with walking and transferring from bed. Often, patients are unable to chew or swallow and can become incontinent of bowel and bladder. This can be a time of great emotional turmoil and grief as the decision-making burden is transferred from patients to their families and loved ones.

Careful planning and open communication between physicians and caregivers will provide patients with comfort and dignity during the final stages of the battle.

Medical Complications

Alzheimer's disease may progress from onset of symptoms to end-stage in 8 to 10 years, with a great amount of variability from person

"End-Stage Alzheimer's: The Long Goodbye," by Diana Kerwin, MD, Assistant Professor, Medical College of Wisconsin Department of Medicine, Division of Geriatrics and Gerontology, April 2003. Reprinted with permission of Medical College of Wisconsin HealthLink, www.healthlink.mcw.edu. © 2003 Medical College of Wisconsin.

to person. Due to the loss of motor abilities and resulting immobility, patients will have greater needs for assistance. If currently living at home, they might need to be placed in an assisted-living residence or nursing home with professional caregivers who specialize in caring for residents with dementia. Families might decide instead to initiate home health care to assist with the care of their loved ones. Problems with swallowing and immobility, in particular, can place patients at risk for medical complications that are often the cause of death in Alzheimer's patients.

The most common medical complications of Alzheimer's patients include pneumonia, blood clots, weight loss, malnutrition, and skin and bladder infections. Medical intervention to treat these complications can cause more pain and discomfort. Those with severe dementia might be unable to understand and cooperate with the treatment, so it is essential for families and physicians to weigh the risks and benefits of all medical interventions. The most important aspects of care during this stage are to honor patients' wishes and to maintain their comfort and dignity.

Advance Directives

Planning for the final stages of Alzheimer's disease should begin at the time of diagnosis. The diagnosis of dementia often causes fear and anxiety about what will happen in the future, and early planning and a proactive approach helps to alleviate these fears. A better understanding of what to expect as Alzheimer's disease progresses can help patients and their families make informed decisions regarding care, and ensure that patients' wishes are understood and honored if and when the time comes that they can no longer participate in the decision-making.

A living will, advance directives, and arrangements for a "Power of Attorney for Health Care" and "Power of Attorney for Finance" are extremely important issues to address as early as possible. If you are not familiar with these issues, your local Alzheimer's Association chapter can refer you to attorneys who specialize in this type of planning and help to guide you through the process.

Hospice Care

In the past, hospice care was identified as care for terminally ill cancer patients. However, the principles of hospice, to provide comfort and reassurance to dying patients and support for families during a time of grief and bereavement, can be applied to all during the final stages of disease. Hospice care can be invaluable whether patients are at home, in an assisted-living residence, or in a nursing home.

In 1982, Medicare created a hospice nursing home benefit when it was recognized that hospice care in nursing homes was not a duplication of end-stage care, but a valuable supplement. There are guidelines regarding when to initiate hospice care and it is important for families and physicians to discuss them. Hospice care guidance during the final stages of Alzheimer's disease can provide support for both patients and families, and help to preserve the comfort and dignity of your loved ones as they reach the end of their "long goodbye."

— by Diana Kerwin, MD. Assistant Professor
Medical College of Wisconsin Department of Medicine
Division of Geriatrics and Gerontology

Additional Reading

1. *The 36-Hour Day*, N. Mace and P. Rabins, Baltimore, MD: Johns Hopkins University Press, 1991.

2. *Alzheimer's: A Caregiver's Guide and Sourcebook.* H. Gruetzner, New York: John Wiley & Sons, Inc.

Part Six

Alzheimer's Disease Research

Chapter 58

Alzheimer's Disease: The Search for Causes

One of the most important parts of unraveling the Alzheimer's disease (AD) mystery is finding out what causes the disease. What makes the disease process begin in the first place? What makes it worse over time? Why does the number of people with the disease increase with age? Why does one person develop it and another remain healthy?

Some diseases, like measles or pneumonia, have clear-cut causes. They can be prevented with vaccines or cured with antibiotics. Others, such as diabetes or arthritis, develop when genetic, lifestyle, and environmental factors work together to cause a disease process to start. The importance of each one of these factors may be different for each individual.

AD fits into this second group of diseases. We don't yet fully understand what causes AD, but we know it develops because of a complex series of events that take place in the brain over a long period of time. Many studies are exploring the factors involved in the cause and development of AD.

Genetic Factors at Work in AD

In the last few years, painstaking detective work by scientists has paid off in discoveries of genetic links to the two main types of AD.

From "AD Research—Finding New Answers and Asking Better Questions," excerpted from "Alzheimer's Disease: Unraveling the Mystery," Alzheimer's Disease Education and Referral (ADEAR) Center, a service of the National Institute on Aging, NIH Pub. No. 02-3782, October 2002. The full text of this document is available online at www.alzheimers.org/unraveling/index.htm.

One type is the more rare, early-onset Alzheimer's disease. It usually affects people aged 30 to 60. Some cases of early-onset disease are inherited and are called familial AD (FAD). The other is late-onset Alzheimer's disease. It is the most common form and occurs in those 65 and older.

DNA, Chromosomes, and Genes: The Body's Amazing Control Center

The nucleus of almost every human cell contains a vast chemical information database. This database carries all the instructions the cell needs to do its job. This database is DNA. DNA exists as two long, intertwined, thread-like strands packaged in units called chromosomes. Each cell has 46 chromosomes in 23 pairs. Chromosomes are made up of four chemicals, or bases, arranged in various sequence patterns. People inherit material in each chromosome from each parent.

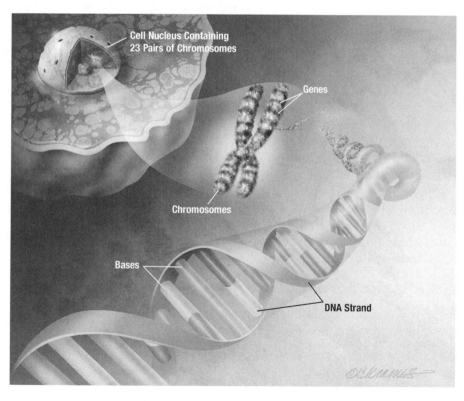

Figure 58.1. DNA, Chromosomes, and Genes.

Each chromosome has many thousands of segments, called genes. The sequence of bases in a gene tells the cell how to make specific proteins. Proteins determine the physical characteristics of living organisms. They also direct almost every aspect of the organism's construction, operation, and repair. Even slight alterations in a gene can produce an abnormal protein, which, in turn, can lead to cell malfunction, and eventually, to disease. Any rare change in a gene's DNA that causes a disease is called a mutation. Other more common (or frequent) changes in a gene's DNA don't automatically cause disease, but they can increase the chances that a person will develop a particular disease. When this happens, the changed gene is called a genetic risk factor.

Genes and Early-Onset Alzheimer's Disease

Over the past several decades, researchers working on AD realized that some cases, particularly of early-onset AD, ran in families. This led them to examine DNA samples from such families to see whether they had some genetic trait in common. Chromosomes 21, 14, and 1 became the focus of attention. The scientists found that some families have a mutation in selected genes on these chromosomes. On chromosome 21, the mutation causes an abnormal amyloid precursor protein (APP) to be produced. On chromosome 14, the mutation causes an abnormal protein called presenilin 1 to be produced. On chromosome 1, the mutation causes yet another abnormal protein to be produced. This protein, called presenilin 2, is very similar to presenilin 1. Even if only one of these genes inherited from a parent contains a mutation, the person will almost inevitably develop early-onset AD. This means that in these families, children have about a 50-50 chance of developing the disease if one of their parents has it.

Even though early-onset AD is very rare and mutations in these three genes do not play a role in the more common late-onset AD, these findings were crucial because they showed that genetics was indeed a factor in AD, and they helped to identify some key players in the AD disease process. Importantly, they showed that mutations in APP can cause AD, highlighting the key role of beta-amyloid in the disease. Many scientists believe that mutations in each of these genes cause an increased amount of the damaging beta-amyloid to be made in the brain.

The findings also laid the foundation for many other studies that have pushed back the boundaries of our knowledge and created new possibilities for future treatment. For example, in the last several years, a series of highly sophisticated experiments have shown that presenilin may actually be one of the enzymes (substances that cause or speed up a chemical reaction) that clips APP to form beta-amyloid (the protein fragment that is the main component of AD plaques). This discovery has helped clarify how presenilins might be involved in the early stages of AD. It has also given scientists crucial new targets for drug therapy and has spurred many new studies in the test tube, in animals, and even in people.

A Different Genetic Story in Late-Onset Alzheimer's Disease

While some scientists were focused on the role of chromosomes 21, 14, and 1 in early-onset AD, others were looking elsewhere to see if they could find genetic clues for the late-onset form. By 1992, these investigators had narrowed their search to a region of chromosome 19. At the same time, other colleagues were looking for proteins that bind to beta-amyloid. They were hoping to clarify some of the steps in the very early stages of the disease process. They found that one form of a protein called apolipoprotein E (apoE) did bind quickly and tightly to beta-amyloid. They also found that the gene that produces apoE was located in the same region of chromosome 19 pinpointed by the geneticists. This finding led them to suggest that one form of this gene was a risk factor for late-onset Alzheimer's disease.

Other studies since then have shown that the gene that produces apoE comes in several forms, or alleles—e2, e3, and e4. The apoE e2 allele is relatively rare and may provide some protection against the disease. If AD does occur in a person with this allele, it develops later in life. ApoE e3 is the most common allele. Researchers think it plays a neutral role in AD. ApoE e4 occurs in about 40 percent of all AD patients who develop the disease in later life. It is not limited to people whose families have a history of AD, though. AD patients with no known family history of the disease are also more likely to have an apoE e4 allele than persons who do not have AD. Dozens of studies have confirmed that the apoE e4 allele increases the risk of developing AD. These studies have also helped to explain some of the variation in the age at which AD develops. However, inheriting an apoE e4 allele doesn't mean that a person will definitely develop AD. Some people with one or two apoE e4 alleles never get the disease and others who do develop AD do not have any apoE e4 alleles.

Although we still don't exactly know how apoE e4 increases AD risk, one theory is that when its protein product binds quickly and tightly to beta-amyloid, the normally soluble amyloid becomes insoluble. This may mean that it is more likely to be deposited in plaques.

While scientists are working to understand more fully the apoE gene and its role in AD, they have also identified regions on other chromosomes that might contain genetic risk factors. For example, in 2000, three teams of scientists, using three different strategies, published studies showing that chromosome 10 has a region that may contain several genes that might increase a person's risk of AD. Identifying these genes is one important step in the research process that will lead to new understanding about the ways in which changes in protein structures cause the disease process to begin and the sequence of events that occurs as the disease develops. Once they understand these processes, scientists can search for new ways to diagnose, treat, or even prevent AD.

Other Factors at Work in AD

Even if genetics explains some of what might cause AD, it doesn't explain everything. So, researchers have looked at other possibilities that may reveal how the Alzheimer's disease process starts and develops.

Beta-Amyloid

We still don't know whether beta-amyloid plaques cause AD or whether they are a by-product of the disease process. We do know, however, that forming beta-amyloid from APP is a key process in AD. That's why finding out more about beta-amyloid is an important avenue of ongoing AD research. Investigators are studying:

- The nature of beta-amyloid
- Ways in which it is toxic to neurons
- Ways in which plaques form and are deposited
- Ways in which beta-amyloid and plaques might be reduced in the brain

Tau

In the last few years, scientists have been giving an increasing amount of attention to tau, the other hallmark of Alzheimer's disease.

This protein is commonly found in nerve cells throughout the brain. In AD, tau undergoes changes that cause it to gather together abnormally in tangled filaments in neurons. In studying tau and what can go wrong, investigators have found that tau abnormalities are also central to other rare neurodegenerative diseases. These diseases, called tauopathies, include frontotemporal dementia, Pick's disease, supranuclear palsy, and corticobasal degeneration. They share a number of characteristics, but also each have distinct features that set them apart from each other and from AD. Characteristic signs and symptoms include changes in personality, social behavior, and language ability; difficulties in thinking and making decisions; poor coordination and balance; psychiatric symptoms; and dementia. Recent advances include the discovery of mutations in the tau gene that cause one tauopathy called frontotemporal dementia with parkinsonism linked to chromosome 17 (FTDP-17). The development of several mouse models that produce tau tangles, will allow researchers to address the many questions that remain about these diseases. The development of a "double transgenic" mouse that has both tau tangles and beta-amyloid plaques will also lead to further insights about AD.

Cardiovascular Risk Factors

Several recent studies in populations have found a possible link between factors related to cardiovascular disease and AD. One of these studies found that elevated levels of an amino acid called homocysteine, a risk factor for heart disease, are associated with an increased risk of developing AD. The relationship between AD and homocysteine is particularly interesting because blood levels of homocysteine can be reduced by increasing intake of folic acid and vitamins B_6 and B_{12}. In fact, in other studies, scientists have shown that folic acid may protect against nerve cell loss in brain regions affected by AD. Investigators have also found that the use of statins, the most common type of cholesterol-lowering drugs, is associated with a lower risk of developing AD.

Oxidative Damage from Free Radicals

Another promising area of investigation relates to a long-standing theory of aging. This theory suggests that over time, damage from a kind of molecule called a free radical can build up in neurons, causing a loss in function. Free radicals can help cells in certain ways, such as fighting infection. However, too many can injure cells because they

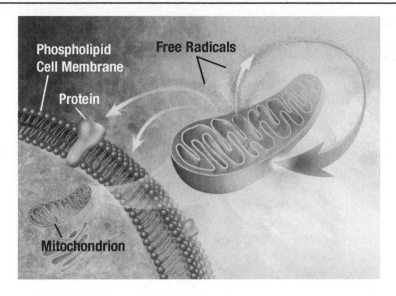

Figure 58.2. *Free radicals may play a role in loss of memory function.*

are very active and can readily change other nearby molecules, such as those in the neuron's cell membrane or in DNA. The resulting molecules can set off a chain reaction, releasing even more free radicals that can further damage neurons. This kind of damage is called oxidative damage. It may contribute to AD by upsetting the delicate machinery that controls the flow of substances in and out of the cell. The brain's unique characteristics, including its high rate of metabolism and its long-lived cells, may make it especially vulnerable to oxidative damage over the lifespan. Some epidemiological and laboratory studies suggest that anti-oxidants from dietary supplements or food may provide some protection against developing AD. Other studies suggest that low calorie diets may protect against the development of AD by slowing down metabolic rates.

Inflammation

Another set of hints about the causes of AD points to inflammation in the brain. This process is part of the immune system and helps the body react to injury or disease. Fever, swelling, pain, or redness in other parts of the body are often signs of inflammation. Because cells and compounds that are known to be involved in inflammation

415

are found in AD plaques, some researchers think it may play a role in AD.

They disagree, though, on whether inflammation is a good or a bad thing. Some think it is harmful—that it sets off a vicious cycle of events that ultimately causes neurons to die. Evidence from many studies supports this idea.

Other scientists believe that some aspects of the inflammatory process may be helpful—that they are part of a healing process in the brain. For example, certain inflammatory processes may play a role in combating the accumulation of plaques. Many studies are now underway to examine the different parts of the inflammatory process more fully and their effects on AD.

Brain Infarction

We've all heard the sensible advice about ways to live a long and healthy life: eat right, exercise, don't smoke, wear a seat belt. All of these habits can help prevent heart attacks, stroke, and injuries. This advice may even have some relevance for AD as well. Results from one long-term study of aging and AD show that participants who had evidence of stroke in certain brain regions had more symptoms of dementia than could be explained by the number of plaques and tangles in their brain tissue. These findings suggest that damage to blood vessels in the brain may not be enough to cause AD, but that it could make AD clinical symptoms worse.

Chapter 59

Mentally Stimulating Activities May Reduce Alzheimer's Risk

In recent years, many of us have come to believe that doing cross-word puzzles or playing cards might ward off a decline in memory or help us maintain "brainpower" as we age. Now, a new study suggests there might be some truth to the use-it-or-lose-it hypothesis.

The study, by scientists at the Rush Alzheimer's Disease Center and Rush-Presbyterian-St. Luke's Medical Center in Chicago, IL, appearing in the February 13, 2002, *Journal of the American Medical Association*, found that more frequent participation in cognitively stimulating activities is associated with a reduced risk of Alzheimer's disease (AD). The research looked at everyday activities like reading books, newspapers or magazines, engaging in crosswords or card games, and going to museums among participants in the Religious Orders Study, an ongoing examination of aging among older Catholic nuns, priests, and brothers from several groups across the U.S. On a scale measuring cognitive activity—with higher scores indicating more frequent activity—a one-point increase in cognitive activity corresponded with a 33 percent reduction in the risk of AD.

The examination of cognitively stimulating activities and risk of AD was conducted by Robert S. Wilson, Ph.D., and colleagues at the Rush Alzheimer's Disease Center, including David A. Bennett, M.D., principal investigator for the Religious Orders Study, and Denis A. Evans, M.D., director of the National Institute on Aging (NIA)-supported

"Use It Or Lose It? Study Suggests Mentally Stimulating Activities May Reduce Alzheimer's Risk," NIH News Release, National Institute on Aging, February 12, 2002.

Rush Alzheimer's Disease Center. The NIA is part of the National Institutes of Health, Department of Health and Human Services.

The findings are likely to strike a chord among middle-aged and older people interested in preserving cognitive health. "We are asked constantly about this use-it-or-lose-it approach to maintaining memory," says Elisabeth Koss, Ph.D., Assistant Director of the NIA's Alzheimer's Disease Centers Program. "This study provides important new evidence that there may be something to the notion of increased cognitive activity and reduced risk of Alzheimer's disease. Further research should help better sort out whether cognitive activities can be prescribed to reduce risk of AD and why that may be so."

The study followed over 700 dementia-free participants age 65 and older for an average of 4.5 years from their initial assessments. At baseline and then yearly, some 21 cognitive tests were administered to assess various aspects of memory, language, attention, and spatial ability. At the initial evaluations, participants also were asked about time typically spent in seven common activities that significantly involve information processing—viewing television; listening to the radio; reading newspapers or magazines; reading books; playing games such as cards, checkers, crosswords, or other puzzles; and going to museums. The frequency of participating in each activity was rated on a five-point scale, with the highest point assigned to participating in an activity every day or about every day and the lowest point to engaging in an activity once a year or less.

During the follow-up period, 111 people in the study developed AD. In comparing the levels of cognitive activity with diagnosis of AD, the researchers found that the frequency of activity was related to the risk of developing AD. For each one point increase in the participants' scores on the scale of cognitive activities, the risk of developing AD decreased by 33 percent. On average, compared with someone with the lowest activity level, the risk of disease was reduced by 47 percent among those whose frequency of activity was highest.

The researchers also looked at general cognitive decline among the participants. Over the period of the study, the group of older people showed modest age-related declines on several types of memory and information processing tests. There were lower rates of decline, however, in working memory, perceptual speed, and episodic memory among people who did more cognitively stimulating activities.

What accounts for the association between cognitively stimulating activities and reduced risk of cognitive decline and AD is unclear. It may be, some scientists theorize, that cognitive activities are protective in some way. Some speculate that repetition might improve

418

the efficiency of certain cognitive skills and make them less vulnerable to the brain damage in AD. Or, some kind of compensatory mechanisms might be at work, strengthening information processing skills to help compensate for age-related declines in other cognitive areas. The study does not, however, eliminate the possibility that people who develop AD in future years may be less prone, years before, to engage in cognitively stimulating activities. Notes Wilson, "The associations among cognitive activity, Alzheimer's disease, and cognitive function are extremely complex. Additional study, including testing some of these activities as cognitive interventions, will help to tell us whether such enjoyable and easy-to-do activities could be employed in some way to reduce the risk of memory decline and loss." Because the participants in the study have agreed to brain donation, the investigators hope to be able to determine the mechanism underlying the association between cognitive activities and cognitive decline.

More than 900 older Catholic clergy from 40 groups across the U.S. are participating in the Religious Orders Study. All participants have agreed to annual memory testing and brain donation at the time of death. "We are grateful for the remarkable dedication and altruism of this unique group of people," says Bennett. "I expect we will learn a great deal more from them, as we look for insights into how the brain functions with age."

About the National Institute on Aging

The NIA leads the federal effort to support and conduct research on aging and on AD. The Rush Alzheimer's Disease Center is one of 29 NIA-supported Alzheimer's Disease Centers across the U.S. which conduct basic, clinical, and social and behavioral research on dementia and AD. NIA also sponsors the Alzheimer's Disease Education and Referral (ADEAR) Center, which provides information on AD research to the public, health professionals, and the media. ADEAR can be contacted toll free at 1-800-438-4380 weekdays during business hours or by visiting its website, http://www.alzheimers.org/. Press releases, fact sheets, and other general information materials on aging and aging research can be viewed at the NIA's home website, http://www.nia.nih.gov.

Chapter 60

Can Lifestyle Choices and Habits Delay Alzheimer's Disease Symptoms?

Lifestyle and Habits That May Delay or Prevent Alzheimer's Disease

Researchers have identified a number of factors that may predispose us to developing Alzheimer's disease. Some of these, like our family histories and genes, are impossible for us to change. Still, there are some factors we can affect. These range from things we can control relatively easily such as aluminum exposure to those, such as education level or marital status, which are more difficult to change.

Alcohol and Tobacco Consumption

While some studies have suggested that either alcohol or tobacco consumption may increase the risk of developing Alzheimer's disease, others have not. A study conducted by the Harvard School of Public Health looked at more than 500 older residents of East Boston and found that mild to moderate alcohol intake did not increase the incidence of Alzheimer's disease, and neither did smoking.

A French study sought to determine if smoking or alcohol intake might possibly be protective against the development of Alzheimer's disease, as some earlier research had suggested. Although preliminary interpretations of the data they collected implied that wine drinking was protective, broadening the population studied to include those in long-term care facilities showed that wine drinking offered no protection. Smoking was similarly found to be of no help in preventing Alzheimer's disease. Indeed, both habits were found to increase the risks of some mental decline with aging.

Education

Early data suggested that those with less education were more likely to develop Alzheimer's disease. The Framingham Study, a decades-long, ongoing study of the health of a population in a town outside Boston, found that education, or a lack of it, was not by itself a risk factor for Alzheimer's disease, but that the increased rate of smoking and other risks for stroke found in those with less education may account for the increased incidence of Alzheimer's disease among the less educated.

Another study of the East Boston population, this one conducted by researchers from the Rush Institute on Aging in Chicago, found that the risk of developing Alzheimer's disease declined 17% for each year of education a person had. A French study of nearly 3,000 older persons found that lower education levels correlated with higher risks for Alzheimer's disease, as well.

Marital Status

A Greek study comparing 65 people with Alzheimer's disease to 69 without it found that being married reduced the risk of developing Alzheimer's disease. A French study of nearly 4,000 older adults found that the risk of Alzheimer's disease was higher in those who had never married.

Estrogen Use

While some studies have suggested that postmenopausal estrogen use reduces the risk of developing Alzheimer's disease, a 2000 study published in the *Journal of the American Medical Association* that compared the effects of estrogen on the cognitive functioning of women with mild Alzheimer's disease found that estrogen provided no benefit. The authors of the study suggested that perhaps estrogen replacement therapy is protective of the healthy brain, but of less value to the brain that has already begun to deteriorate due to Alzheimer's disease. In other words, they believe that estrogen may prevent, but not reverse the disease. This area remains a source of controversy, and more studies are underway to determine estrogen's actual benefit. [Editor's note: Updated information about hormone replacement therapy and Alzheimer's disease is included in Chapter 63.]

Risk Factors for Cerebral Ischemia

Cerebral ischemia is a term that means a decrease in blood flow to the brain. Research indicates that damage to the blood vessels that deliver blood, oxygen, and nutrients to the brain can increase the risk of Alzheimer's disease. Some of the causes of that damage are:

- Atherosclerosis (or hardening of the arteries)
- Atrial fibrillation (an abnormal heart rhythm that increases the risk of strokes caused by blood clots lodging in the circulation of the brain)
- Coronary artery disease (blockages in the blood vessels that supply the heart)
- Hypertension (high blood pressure)
- Diabetes

All of these conditions can contribute to a higher risk of stroke, and stroke and Alzheimer's disease occur in the same people quite often, though their co-incidence has not been rigorously studied. Some scientists suggest that treating or preventing those conditions that cause stroke is prudent not only to reduce the risk of stroke, but to possibly reduce the risk of developing Alzheimer's disease as well.

Head Injury

A study done at Duke University reviewing the medical records of World War II veterans revealed that their risk of developing Alzheimer's disease was increased if they had suffered serious head injury in young adulthood. The risk of Alzheimer's disease or dementia was twice as high for those with a history of moderate head injury (loss of consciousness or amnesia for 30 minutes to 24 hours) and four times as high for those with a history of severe head injury (loss of consciousness for more than 24 hours).

Aluminum Exposure

Over two decades ago, scientists found a high level of aluminum in the brains of those with Alzheimer's disease. Whether this metal contributes to the disease or simply collects in the lesions caused by the disease is still not clear. We take aluminum in through our drinking water, our diets (particularly in baked goods that use aluminum additives), and over-the-counter medications, such as antacids and buffered aspirin. Aluminum might also enter our bodies through foods cooked in aluminum cookware. The manufacturers of newer pots and pans made with anodized aluminum state that such pots do not permit leaching of aluminum into foods.

Chapter 61

Does Aluminum Play a Role in Causing Alzheimer's Disease?

Aluminum

- Aluminum is one of several factors scientists are investigating in the search for a cause of Alzheimer's disease.

- The role of aluminum in the body and the brain is not well understood.

- Scientists disagree as to whether or not there is a connection between aluminum and Alzheimer's disease.

What is aluminum?

We usually think of aluminum as a light silvery metal used to make pots and pans, airplanes, or tools, but it also has a non-metallic form. It is this form of aluminum that makes up eight per cent of the earth's surface.

Where is it found?

In the Environment

Aluminum in its non-metallic form is found everywhere:

"Causes of Alzheimer Disease: Aluminum," © 2002 Alzheimer Society of Canada. Reprinted with permission from the Alzheimer Society of Canada (www.alzheimer.ca).

- naturally in the foods we eat

- in drinking water both as a natural component and in some municipalities as an additive

- in the water treatment process

- in many food products, added during manufacturing

- in many cosmetics

- in drugs, to make them more effective or less irritating

- in the air we breathe as a result of dry soil, smoke, and sprays

In the Body

Aluminum is always present in the body, but its role is not fully understood. Very little of the aluminum taken in by a healthy individual is actually absorbed; most is flushed out of the body by the kidneys.

What has lead some scientists to believe there is a connection between aluminum and Alzheimer's disease?

Aluminum has been linked with dementia and Alzheimer's disease in particular by several studies. Like with many scientific theories, there remain many unanswered questions.

- Some scientists have found more aluminum than normal in the brains of people with Alzheimer's disease. Much debate goes on about the specific techniques used for measurement:

  - Are they sensitive enough?

  - Because aluminum is so plentiful, are the tissue samples being contaminated by aluminum in the environment?

- Several studies report that people who live in areas with low levels of aluminum in the drinking water have less chance of developing Alzheimer's disease than those who live where levels of aluminum in the drinking water are higher. These studies have raised numerous questions:

  - How much water does each individual drink?

  - How much aluminum do they ingest from other sources, i.e., food, cosmetics, drugs?

426

- How do scientists determine if people have Alzheimer's disease?

- How is the aluminum measured in the drinking water?

- A form of dementia that developed in people on artificial kidney machines was found to be caused by high concentrations of aluminum in the fluid used by the machines. The dementia was eliminated by reducing the aluminum concentration in the fluids. This type of dementia was not Alzheimer's disease.

At present so little is known about the underlying cell changes in Alzheimer's disease that definitive statements about any toxic substance, such as aluminum, cannot be made with any certainty.

So, what about the pots and pans?

Aluminum pots and pans contribute only very small amounts of aluminum to foods that are cooked in them. The amount does increase when food is acidic (for example, tomatoes, rhubarb).

There is no proof that the use of such utensils plays a significant role in the development of Alzheimer's disease.

Chapter 62

Brain Injury and Alzheimer's Disease: What Is the Link?

Although more than forty years have passed since British neurosurgeon McDonald Critchley described severe memory problems in a sample of boxers—presumably the result of repeated head trauma—the relationship between brain injury and Alzheimer's disease has proven difficult to unravel. For years, there was scant evidence that head injuries endured by non-boxers posed an increased risk for Alzheimer's disease; although epidemiologic studies linking the two conditions began appearing in the 1980s, negative studies continue to be published with enough frequency to ensure that the issue remains controversial. And while recent reports have revealed in some injured brains neuropathologic changes that bear a remarkable resemblance to Alzheimer's disease, the interpretation and implications of these findings remain uncertain.

Nonetheless, some researchers believe that decoding the Alzheimer's disease/brain injury connection will have implications far beyond the possibility of warding off dementia in head trauma patients. "It gives you insight into what may be the base mechanism for Alzheimer's disease," said Gareth W. Roberts, BSc, PhD, MBA, who coauthored several studies on the relationship between the two conditions before becoming Chief Executive Officer of the Cambridge, UK bioinformatics firm Proteom. "And once you have a feeling for what the core pathologic process is, you can ask, 'What kinds of things might stop that?'"

From "Brain Injury and Alzheimer's Disease—What's Is the Link," by Peter Doskoch, in *Neurology Reviews*, Vol. 8, No. 12, December 2000. Reprinted with permission of Clinicians Group—A Jobson Company.

Other investigators envision similarly lofty applications. "I look upon head injury [research] as a paradigm for understanding environmental risk factors for neurodegenerative diseases in general," said John Q. Trojanowski, MD, PhD, Professor of Pathology and Laboratory Medicine at the University of Pennsylvania. For most patients, he noted, environmental factors are likely to far outweigh genetic influences in the etiology of neurodegenerative disease. "I think if we can 'crack' head trauma, it will open up ways of thinking about other environmental causes of these diseases."

What Happens after Brain Injury?

Recent studies have provided "very strong evidence that there is a connection between head trauma and at least some of the pathology of Alzheimer's disease," Dr. Trojanowski said. For example, in a report at the recent World Alzheimer Congress 2000, Steven T. DeKosky, MD, and colleagues at the University of Pittsburgh Medical Center reported findings from neocortical samples taken from brain injury patients one and three days after injury. The samples, which were obtained by surgical resection and compared with postmortem samples from neurologically normal controls, revealed increases in amyloid precursor protein (APP), apolipoproteins E and D, and ß-amyloid (Aß). Many of the Aß deposits "had morphologic characteristics of classic amyloid plaques in Alzheimer's disease," Dr. DeKosky and colleagues reported.

Several studies have found that Aß deposition occurs in a third of fatal head injury cases, even in children who survived only a few hours. The Aß is generally distributed throughout the brain; its presence does not correlate with cerebral contusions, increased intracranial pressure, or intracranial hematomas. Neurofibrillary tangles may also occur. The nature of pathology depends in part on injury severity—tangles do not seem to occur after mild trauma—but "I don't think there's much insight into how severe the injury has to be" to trigger Alzheimer's disease-like pathology, Dr. Trojanowski said.

These changes make sense, Dr. Roberts said, if one accepts the view that Alzheimer's disease is largely an inflammatory process. APP is found in synapses, he noted, and "one of the things we do know happens after brain injury is synaptic remodeling." Moreover, electron microscopy shows that synapses are involved in amyloid plaque formation. This may be a repair process of some sort, he said, but "instead of being shut down when it is appropriate, it just carries on. It becomes a bit like arthritis, where mechanisms that should help you instead become chronically activated and disabling."

It should be noted, however, that the neuropathology of brain injury is by no means a carbon copy of the changes that occur in Alzheimer's disease. For example, levels of growth inhibitory factor are increased in reactive astrocytes in experimentally induced brain injury, whereas these levels are reduced throughout the brain in Alzheimer's disease. Moreover, the neocortical distribution of neurofibrillary tangles is more superficial in former boxers with dementia pugilistica, or punch drunk syndrome, than in Alzheimer's disease patients.

How Large Is the Risk?

Despite the array of pathologic evidence linking the disorders, the relationship between Alzheimer's disease and head injury remains unsettled from an epidemiologic standpoint. Findings reported last year from the Rotterdam Study, for example, found no increased risk of Alzheimer's disease in subjects with a history of head injury. Nonetheless, positive studies outnumber negative ones, and head injury is "becoming more accepted as being associated with the risk of Alzheimer's disease," said Brenda L. Plassman, PhD, Director of the Program in Epidemiology of Dementia at Duke University Medical Center, Durham, North Carolina.

In a new report that Dr. Trojanowski called "the most exhaustive and thoroughly done [epidemiologic] study I've seen," Dr. Plassman and colleagues performed telephone screening of more than 2,000 World War II veterans who had been hospitalized for head injury, pneumonia, or puncture wounds in 1944 or 1945. Subjects who screened positive for possible dementia underwent a three-hour exam that included neuropsychologic testing, neurologic examination, and DNA collection.

From 1940s armed forces hospital records, the researchers were able to estimate the severity of each subject's head injury, based on the occurrence of amnesia or skull fracture and the duration of unconsciousness. The findings revealed that "the more severe the injury, the greater the risk of Alzheimer's disease and dementia"; the relative risks (compared with controls) ranged from about 2 for moderate head injury to 4 for severe injury. The findings are consistent with those from most other positive epidemiologic studies, Dr. Plassman said. "It's rather striking that all of these studies used different samples, methods, and criteria for head injury, yet all have odds ratios that are pretty close." The relative risk of Alzheimer's disease after head injury is roughly similar to that reported for subjects heterozygous for the apolipoprotein E, (apoE) E4 allele, she added.

431

The study, which was reported, in part, at the February 1999 meeting of the International Neuropsychological Society, was published in the October 24. 1999 issue of *Neurology* with an expanded sample size and the inclusion of new genetic data.

The Genetic Connection

The role of genetic vulnerability is suggested by the fact that only a subset of brain injury patients develop amyloid pathology. Many investigators believe apoE genotype is the key culprit. "There is a clear relationship between having an apoE*E4 allele and your likelihood of developing plaques after a head injury," Dr. Roberts said. "So in a sense the apoE/head injury story gives you the first genetic-environmental interaction in a neurologic disease." This relationship is consistent with apoE's proposed role in the maintenance and repair of neuronal membranes, synaptogenesis, and other processes. Indeed, researchers at the University of Glasgow reported earlier this year that the densities of the ß-amyloid peptides Aß-42 and Aß-40 in head injury patients were related in a dose-dependent manner to apoE*E4 endowment.

However, it is possible that in many cases head injury doesn't induce Alzheimer's disease-like pathology so much as accelerate its arrival. A 1989 retrospective study found that a history of head injury was associated with earlier onset of Alzheimer's disease. And in 1999, a report from the Mayo Clinic suggested that Alzheimer's disease rates were not elevated among subjects with a history of head trauma, but that the head injury hastened the time to Alzheimer's disease onset by about eight years.

Future Interventions

Can prompt, appropriate treatment after brain injury reduce or prevent the development of Alzheimer's disease-like pathology? While the mouse model for Alzheimer's disease that Dr. Trojanowski and others have been using has yielded interesting findings, the rodents' lack of tau pathology and "quirky" behavior did not allow for ideal testing of therapeutic interventions. However, recent work by Dr. Trojanowski and his colleagues, Tracy McIntosh, PhD, and Virginia Lee, PhD, may change that. "I think we may be moving closer to a meaningful model of how to understand the effects of head trauma on amyloid," he said.

At present, "aside from telling football players and soccer players to either not play or to wear a helmet, there's not much in the way of interventions," Dr. Trojanowski noted. However, as researchers gain a better understanding of the relationship between trauma, risk factors, and genetic vulnerability, medical advice could theoretically be targeted to a patient's profile: "If you're apoE*E4 homozygous, you should really think twice about playing football. If you're heterozygous for apoE*E4, you'd better wear a helmet and take vitamin E and aspirin for the rest of your life."

Moreover, the inflammatory model of Alzheimer's disease pathogenesis offers obvious potential for intervention. Epidemiologic studies have found a reduced rate of Alzheimer's disease among people who regularly used nonsteroidal anti-inflammatory drugs. And a study in the August 1, 1999 *Journal of Neuroscience* found that ibuprofen reduced not only inflammation, but Aß plaque burden in a transgenic mouse model for Alzheimer's disease.

Nonetheless, crucial questions remain unanswered. "One of the things that needs fitting together is the link in the biology between the presenilins and APP. [We don't know] how they interact, what the normal function [of presenilins is], and the relationship between that function and the inflammatory process," Dr. Roberts said. Answering these questions, he noted, "would open up clear avenues for drug discovery."

Chapter 63

Hormone Replacement Therapy and Alzheimer's Disease

Estrogen replacement therapy (ERT) does not improve the memory or function of hysterectomized women with mild to moderate Alzheimer's disease, according to a new research report. The findings, from the largest and longest clinical trial to date examining the effects of estrogen therapy on AD, suggest that estrogen should not be used to treat the dementia once the disease is established in women who have had a hysterectomy.

Scientists involved in the study emphasize, however, that estrogen therapy may still play an important role in fighting AD in women at an earlier point in the disease process. A number of epidemiological studies have indicated that estrogen therapy might prevent AD or delay its onset. Clinical trials to validate the usefulness of estrogen to prevent or delay AD are now underway.

This study on estrogen therapy for women with mild to moderate dementia appears in the February 23, 2000, issue of the *Journal of the American Medical Association*. The research was conducted by Ruth Mulnard, R.N., D.N.Sc., University of California, Irvine, and colleagues from 32 Alzheimer's Disease Cooperative Study (ADCS)

This chapter includes "Estrogen Replacement Therapy Not Effective for Alzheimer's Disease," Alzheimer's Disease Education and Referral (ADEAR) Center, National Institute on Aging (NIA), February 23, 2000; "Rates of Dementia Increase Among Older Women on Combination Hormone Therapy," NIH News Release, National Institutes of Health, May 27, 2003; and "Questions and Answers about the Women's Health Initiative Memory Study," National Institute on Aging (NIA), May 22, 2003.

sites across the U.S. The National Institute on Aging (NIA) supports the ADCS, a consortium of academic medical centers and others involved in AD clinical trials.

"A negative finding, particularly one from a study of this size and scope, is critically important in our search for treatments," says Neil Buckholtz, Ph.D., who directs NIA's Dementias of Aging program. "We need to determine where estrogens may or may not be effective for people with AD. This study clearly turns our attention to how estrogens may help protect women who, at the start of therapy, are cognitively healthy. It is also not clear at this time whether estrogen therapy may be effective in women with AD who have an intact uterus."

The 120 hysterectomized women age 60 and above involved in the study had mild to moderate AD. They were divided into three groups of women taking 0.625 mg (milligrams) per day of estrogen, 1.25 mg of estrogen, or placebo pills that looked like the estrogen medication. The women were followed for 15 months (12 months on estrogen therapy with 3 months of additional follow-up); researchers tested for cognitive or functional changes at 2, 6, 12, and 15 months. Primarily, the scientists were examining the overall rate of change the women may have experienced on a scale developed by the ADCS for pinpointing clinical changes in patients with the disease. In addition, they looked for specific effects on mood; certain cognitive functions such as memory, attention, and language; motor function; and standard measures of activities of daily living.

At the end of the study, no significant differences were seen in any of the areas studied, indicating that the ERT had no effect. Estrogen did not, as it has in smaller studies, improve cognitive function, nor did it delay progression of the disease by any of the measures used by Mulnard's group.

Mulnard said that the positive effects of ERT seen in smaller and shorter studies might have been due to short-term effects that estrogen might have had on neurotransmitters in the brain, as seen in animal studies. But, according to Mulnard, the short-term effects could not be sustained over a longer period of time.

Basic research on the etiology of AD may help explain ERT's failure to make a difference in women who already have AD, Mulnard said. Studies on the mechanisms of the disease have indicated that AD may have at least two phases, one called an "initiation" phase and the another a "propagation" phase when the disease has been set in motion. Cell culture studies show that the actions of estrogen may only be effective against some of the mechanisms of the disease, effectively countering those that occur earlier in the disease process. Estrogen receptors, for example are concentrated in the regions of the brain affected first by AD, and ERT may work best before these brain regions are compromised. Mulnard also points to research indicating that estrogen is a relatively weak antioxidant when compared with vitamin E, which has been shown to have some effect at later stages of the disease.

"Research on the basic mechanisms of AD and a range of diseases shows that certain things happen at certain stages," Mulnard notes. "We may find that some therapies, possibly estrogens, may only work during selective phases of the disease process."

The NIA, the National Institute of Neurological Disorders and Stroke (NINDS), National Institute of Mental Health (NIMH), and the National Institute of Nursing Research (NINR) within the National Institutes of Health (NIH), support the AD Prevention Initiative, which funds much of the ongoing clinical research on AD, including additional studies of the preventive possibilities of estrogens. In addition, Wyeth-Ayerst Laboratories is sponsoring a memory study component of NIH's national Women's Health Initiative to test the use of estrogens for preventing AD.

For more information on federally funded AD research and the possibility of participating in a study, contact the NIA's Alzheimer Disease Education and Referral (ADEAR) Center at 800-438-4380, or adear@alzheimers.org. You can view information on AD and on clinical trials specifically on the ADEAR website at http://www.alzheimers.org.

Rates of Dementia Increase Among Older Women on Combination Hormone Therapy

Older women taking combination hormone therapy had twice the rate of dementia, including Alzheimer's disease (AD), compared with women who did not take the medication, according to new findings from a memory substudy of the Women's Health Initiative (WHI). The research, part of the Women's Health Initiative Memory Study (WHIMS) and reported in the May 28, 2003, *Journal of the American Medical Association* (*JAMA*), found the heightened risk of developing dementia in a study of women 65 and older taking Prempro™, a particular form of estrogen plus progestin hormone therapy.

The study also found that the combination therapy did not protect against the development of Mild Cognitive Impairment, or MCI, a form of cognitive decline less severe than dementia.

"Because of possible harm in some areas and lack of a demonstrated benefit in others, we have concluded that combination hormone therapy should not be prescribed at this time for older, postmenopausal women to maintain or improve cognitive function," says Judith A. Salerno, M.D., M.S., Deputy Director of the National Institute on Aging (NIA) at the National Institutes of Health (NIH), U.S. Department of Health and Human Services.

The findings were reported by WHIMS Principal Investigator Sally A. Shumaker, Ph.D., Wake Forest University School of Medicine, Winston-Salem, NC, and colleagues at the 39 sites involved in the study.

The memory substudy WHIMS was funded by Wyeth Pharmaceuticals, which manufactures Prempro™, which it provided for use in the WHI trials. The larger WHI trials are supported by the National Heart, Lung, and Blood Institute (NHLBI) of the NIH. The NIA has been involved in reviewing the current findings as the NIH's lead institute on age-related memory change and dementia.

Importantly, the women in the combined estrogen plus progestin arm of the WHI and substudies such as WHIMS are no longer taking the combination therapy as part of the research trials. In July 2002, all combination therapy components of the WHI were halted when it was found that increased risk of breast cancer, heart disease, stroke, and blood clots among participating women on combined estrogen plus progestin therapy outweighed benefits for hip fractures and colorectal cancer.

As they did in the July 2002 report on increased risk of breast cancer, heart disease, and stroke, researchers stress that the data should be viewed in perspective. While the increased risk of dementia is significant when calculated over a large population of women, the risk to any individual older woman is actually relatively small. (For a detailed discussion of relative versus absolute risk, see the NIA Fact Sheet Understanding Risk: What Do All Those Headlines Mean? online at http://www.nia.nih.gov/health/pubs/understanding-risk/index.htm.)

The current findings address combined estrogen plus progestin therapy, specifically Prempro™, among women 65 years of age and older. For younger women, the cognitive risks and benefits of this combination therapy are unknown. Short-term hormone therapy in younger women for some symptoms of menopause has been approved by the U.S. Food and Drug Administration and the new findings do not directly address decisions about such treatment. Researchers and officials at the NIH suggest that women of any age consult with a physician about their individual risks and benefits.

The memory study findings on women 65 and older showed that over a 5-year period:

- The risk for dementia among women taking estrogen and progestin was twice that of women taking placebo pills. This represents an increase per year from 22 women per 10,000 at risk of dementia in the placebo group to 45 women per 10,000 in the combination therapy group, an additional 23 cases per 10,000 per year among women taking combination therapy. Sixty-one cases of dementia were diagnosed among the 4,500 women participating in the study; 66 percent of those cases occurred among women on combination therapy while 34 percent occurred in women taking placebo.

- Most of the dementia found among women participating in the study was classified as probable Alzheimer's disease, with vascular dementia ranking second. There were 20 cases of Alzheimer's disease among the 40 dementia cases in women in the combination therapy group (50 percent of the cases); in women on placebo, 12 of the 21 cases (57 percent) of dementia were deemed Alzheimer's disease.

- There was no significant difference in the risk of being diagnosed with MCI alone when the placebo and combination therapy groups were compared.

About 4,500 women participated in the WHIMS substudy of women 65 and older. Once the women met the criteria for participation, including screening tests to make sure they did not have dementia at the study's start, they were randomly assigned to take estrogen plus progestin therapy (one pill per day of conjugated equine estrogen (CEE), 0.625 mg, plus medroxyprogesterone acetate (MPA), 2.5 mg—brand name Prempro™) or a look-alike placebo. Cognitive status was evaluated annually, and women who showed signs of decline were examined in greater depth to further characterize their cognitive status.

The researchers looked at several other factors that might influence cognitive status, including socioeconomic status, educational attainment, prior estrogen or progestin use history, and use of cholesterol lowering medications or aspirin or other non-steroidal anti-inflammatory drugs. These factors were not significantly different between the therapy group and the placebo group and did not account for the differences in rates of cognitive decline, the researchers said.

A second report in the same issue of *JAMA* showed general cognitive status to be adversely affected by the combination therapy in older women. WHIMS investigator Stephen Rapp, Ph.D., Wake Forest University School of Medicine, and colleagues at the other sites examined the participants' performance on an often-used test, the Modified Mini-Mental State Exam (3MS). All participants' average performance on the cognitive tests actually improved over time, which researchers suggest may be due to a "practice effect" as a result of taking the same tests every year. However, the rate of increase in the performance of women on the 3MS was somewhat lower for women in the combination therapy group when compared with women receiving the placebo.

About 3,000 women are continuing to participate in a second arm of the WHIMS research, a study of the effects on cognition of estrogen-only therapy in women who have had a hysterectomy. A Data Safety Monitoring Board will continue to monitor the risks and benefits for that part of the study.

The NIH is considering implications of the dementia findings for other clinical studies involving estrogen and progestin.

Questions and Answers about the Women's Health Initiative Memory Study

What do the study results mean?

This finding means that older women should know that:

- Using Prempro™ does not keep you from getting dementia. It doesn't slow the start of the symptoms of dementia. In this study, in fact, it increased the risk for dementia. It also does not stop problems with remembering, paying attention, following directions, or using words correctly.

- Older women should not take this form of estrogen plus progestin to prevent dementia or to keep an alert mind.

- There was no difference between the two groups of women in their chance of having symptoms of mild cognitive impairment (MCI).

What treatment did the women receive in the WHI and WHIMS?

Women were chosen by chance to receive hormones or a placebo. The placebo looks like the hormone pills, but has no hormone in it.

There were two groups that received hormones. The first group took Prempro™ every day. This contained 0.625 mg (milligram) of conjugated equine estrogens and 2.5 mg of medroxyprogesterone acetate, a progestin. The second group took Premarin™ daily. This had just 0.625 mg of conjugated equine estrogens, without the progestin.

These drugs were chosen because at the time the study started they were the ones most often prescribed by doctors in the United States for menopausal hormone therapy. More than six million women used Prempro™ at the time of the study, and around eight million took Premarin™.

What are estrogen and progestin?

Estrogen and progesterone are two hormones that are made by a woman's body before menopause. Progestin is a man-made progesterone. When estrogen alone is given to a woman with a uterus, she often has a thickening of the lining of the uterus. This can cause irregular bleeding. Rarely this thickening can lead to cancer of the lining of the uterus. So, Prempro™ is given to a woman who has a uterus to protect her from changes in the lining of the uterus. Premarin™ is only given to a woman whose uterus has been removed.

What risks and benefits did the WHI scientists find?

An increase in risk and decrease in risk (benefit) can be described in two ways. One, relative risk, compares the chance that a woman using estrogen plus progestin will have a health problem like a heart attack to the chance that a woman not using any menopausal hormone therapy will have the same problem. The other, absolute risk, gives the actual number of health problems that happened or are prevented because of this estrogen plus progestin. An explanation of relative and absolute risk is available at http://www.nia.nih.gov/health/pubs/understanding-risk.

The relative risks and absolute risks found in the WHI and WHIMS studies involving estrogen plus progestin are show in Table 63.1.

Which hormone—estrogen or progestin—causes this dementia? Or is it the combination?

That is not clear from the results of this study. The other part of WHI and WHIMS, using estrogen alone, is continuing with careful monitoring for safety by the National Institutes of Health. When those trials end and scientists are able to compare the results of the studies, they may be able to answer this question.

Do other estrogens and progestins also cause dementia?

Since the WHI was first planned, more types of estrogens and progestins have become available. These include some that are almost identical to the hormones made by a woman's body. Researchers would have to do similar types of large trials with these other types of hormones to know whether they are safer than the ones used in the WHI and WHIMS. The same is true for other forms of hormones—skin patches or creams, for example, rather than pills.

What about the new low-dose versions of Premarin™ and Prempro™?

In spring 2003, the Food and Drug Administration (FDA) approved low-dose Premarin (0.45 mg of conjugated equine estrogens) and Prempro (0.45 mg of conjugated equine estrogens and 1.5 mg of

Table 63.1. Relative and Absolute Risks Found in Studies Involving Estrogen Plus Progestin

Risk or Benefit	Relative Risk	Absolute Risk Each Year
Heart attacks	1.29 or a 29% increase	7 more cases in 10,000 women
Breast cancer	1.26 or a 26% increase	8 more cases in 10,000 women
Strokes	1.41 or a 41% increase	8 more cases in 10,000 women
Blood clots	2.11 or a 111% increase	18 more cases in 10,000 women
Hip fractures	0.66 or a 33% decrease	5 fewer cases in 10,000 women
Colon cancer	0.63 or a 37% decrease	6 fewer cases in 10,000 women
Dementia	2.05 or a 105% increase	23 more cases in 10,000 women over age 65

medroxyprogesterone acetate). These may be used for treating meno-pausal symptoms (hot flashes, night sweats, and vaginal dryness). FDA continues to remind consumers that estrogens and estrogens with progestins should be used at the lowest doses for the shortest length of time needed to reach treatment goals.

What happened in women taking estrogen alone?

At present, this trial is continuing. The safety of the women in this study is reviewed regularly. These women and the scientists will be given any new information that might affect their continued involve-ment in the trial.

I want to use menopausal hormone therapy to relieve my hot flashes. What does this new information mean for me?

Using menopausal hormone therapy for just a short time is still approved by the Food and Drug Administration to control the symp-toms of menopause and to protect women from bone loss that could lead to osteoporosis. However, remember three things. First, in the WHI estrogen plus progestin trial, the increase in breast cancer did not happen until after 4 years of use. Second, in the same trial, the increase in heart disease, stroke, and blood clots began within the first 2 years after starting estrogen plus progestin. Third, in the WHIMS estrogen plus progestin trial, the mental changes also occurred very quickly in these women, who were age 65 and older. That is why it is important to talk to your health care provider about your entire health picture.

Are more findings expected from the WHI?

When the estrogen-only trial of the WHI ends, the scientists will be able to compare the results of that trial with those from the estro-gen plus progestin study and publish the findings. Before then, more details about the estrogen and progestin studies may be published from time to time. Also, scientists in other parts of the WHI, separate from the hormone therapy trial, will be reporting in the future.

Where can I get more details about this study?

The scientific report of the study findings is published in the May 28, 2003, issue of the *Journal of the American Medical Association* (JAMA). You can learn more about menopausal hormone therapy and the Women's Health Initiative by going to the NIH home page, www.nih.gov, and clicking on the link to "Menopausal Hormone Therapy." The WHI Memory Study website is http://www.wfubmc.edu/ whims. Information on memory and Alzheimer's disease can be found at www.alzheimers.org. That's the National Institute on Aging (NIA)'s Alzheimer's Disease Education and Referral (ADEAR) Center. You may also call the ADEAR Center toll free at 800-438-4380 for information and publications. General information on menopause and aging is on the NIA website, www.nia.nih.gov, in "Health Information," and you can order publications by calling the NIA Information Center toll free at 800-222-2225.

Chapter 64

Antioxidant Vitamins May Help Protect against Alzheimer's Disease

Supplementing diets with antioxidant vitamins C and E may boost mental ability in later life and could protect against vascular and some other forms of dementia, according to a study published in the March 28, 2000 issue of *Neurology*, the American Academy of Neurology's scientific journal.

"We believe antioxidants like vitamin E and C may protect against vascular dementia by limiting the amount of brain damage that persists after a stroke," said study author Kamal Masaki, MD, of the University of Hawaii in Honolulu. "The supplements may also play a role in providing protection against brain cell and membrane injury involved in many aging-related diseases, thus resulting in significantly higher scores on mental performance tests in later life."

The study investigated 3,385 Japanese-American men, aged 71–93, participating in the Honolulu Heart Program, a prospective study of heart disease and stroke initiated in 1965. The men were interviewed or surveyed in 1982 and 1988, and were assessed for dementia and mental abilities during exams in 1991 to 1993. Of the participants, 47 were diagnosed with Alzheimer's disease, 35 with vascular dementia, 50 with other or mixed types of dementia, 254 had low cognitive test scores without diagnosed dementia, and 2,999 men showed no cognitive difficulties.

"Vitamins C and E: Protection Against Mental Decline," American Academy of Neurology, March 27, 2000. © 2000 American Academy of Neurology. Reprinted with permission. For additional information about brain diseases, including links to further resources, visit www.thebrainmatters.org.

Participants taking both vitamin E and C supplements regularly (at least once a week) in 1988, were 88 percent less likely to have vascular dementia four years later and 69 percent less likely to have forms of dementia other than vascular or Alzheimer's related dementia or mixed forms of dementia. There was no significant reduction in the occurrence of Alzheimer's disease four years later.

Participants without dementia were evaluated for mental performance and function. Those who reported taking vitamin E and C supplements in 1988 had an approximately 20 percent greater chance of having better cognitive function during the 1991–93 examination than those who did not. However, men taking the supplements in both 1982 and 1988 had an approximately 75 percent greater chance of better mental performance. This suggests that long-term use could significantly improve cognitive function in late life.

"We originally thought that the beneficial impact antioxidant vitamin supplements had against vascular dementia was the prevention of stroke," commented Masaki. "However, to our surprise we found there was not a significant association between vitamin supplement use and clinically recognized stroke."

Previous reports have shown that antioxidants may slow the progression of Alzheimer's disease and the researchers were also surprised when they did not find a protective effect against Alzheimer's.

"It is critically important for patients to practice preventive efforts shown to lower stroke risk and to have broad ranging beneficial effects," said Masaki. "More effective strategies for prevention also must be found. Therefore, a prevention trial of both vitamin E and C to further examine the potential protective effects on both vascular dementia and Alzheimer's disease is needed."

Vascular dementia is the second most common cause of dementia in the United States (following Alzheimer's disease) and the most common cause of dementia in Japan. Those with vascular dementia face the physical impairment related to stroke, such as paralysis, and speech, language and visual disturbances, in addition to mental impairment.

The American Academy of Neurology, an association of more than 16,500 neurologists and neuroscience professionals, is dedicated to improving patient care through education and research. For more information about the American Academy of Neurology, visit its Website at www.aan.com.

Chapter 65

B Vitamins May Be Vital to the Brain

Elevated levels of homocysteine may cause brain atrophy and vascular disease and therefore may be related to the development of dementia and possibly Alzheimer's disease, according to two studies in the May 28, 2002, *Neurology*. About 5% to 7% of the population has mildly elevated levels of homocysteine.

"This is exciting information, because homocysteine levels can be reduced by taking the vitamins B_6, B_{12}, and folic acid," said James F. Toole, MD, Professor of Neurology at Wake Forest University School of Medicine in Winston-Salem, North Carolina, and author of an accompanying editorial. He is currently leading a study to examine if vitamin supplementation to lower homocysteine levels can reduce the risk of stroke. Taking vitamins to lower homocysteine levels may also reduce the risk of Alzheimer's disease and other dementia, he believes.

Brain Atrophy Association Found

The relationship between high homocysteine levels and brain atrophy was examined in 36 healthy community volunteers (mean age, 71.6; range, 59 to 85 years; 18 men and 18 women) with a mean

This chapter includes text from "B Vitamins May Be Vital to the Brain," by Heidi W. Moore, in *Neurology Reviews*, Vol. 10, No. 7, July 2002. Reprinted with permission of Clinicians Group—A Jobson Company. Text beginning with "Folic Acid May Be Important," is from "Folic Acid Possibly a Key Factor in Alzheimer's Disease Prevention," Is from "NIA News: Alzheimer's Disease Research Update," National Institute on Aging (NIA), March 1, 2002.

education level of 12 years and no history of cerebrovascular disease. The researchers hypothesized that "the high homocysteine levels, combined with the increased risk for cerebrovascular disease and possibly neurodegeneration, should manifest in the brains of otherwise healthy elderly individuals in the form of brain atrophy and small vessel disease detectable on MRI [magnetic resonance imaging]." Indeed, the study found that elderly people who had greater brain atrophy were twice as likely to have high homocysteine levels as were those with less atrophy, according to lead author Perminder Sachdev, MD, PhD, Professor of Neuropsychiatry, University of New South Wales in Sydney, Australia.

At the time of assessment, subjects were not taking folate, vitamin B_{12}, or vitamin B_6; they underwent a battery of neuropsychological tests and MRI. It was determined that mean total homocysteine level was not significantly correlated with folate levels but was correlated with creatinine levels. Also, homocysteine levels did have a significant relationship with anterior and midsection ventricle-brain ratios, although not with cortical atrophy.

Significant Correlation in a Small Sample

The authors acknowledged that the sample size was small but noted that the significant correlation between homocysteine levels and an index of brain atrophy in a healthy elderly population is intriguing. The fact that ventricular dilatation and not cortical atrophy was best correlated with homocysteine levels suggested that the measure possibly reflected loss of white matter.

Although the researchers wrote that they "cannot conclude that high homocysteine levels caused brain atrophy," they did speculate on possible mechanisms. While the lack of association between homocysteine levels and white matter hyperintensities makes it unlikely that MRI-visible microangiopathy was a mediating factor, the authors "cannot rule out the possibility that MRI-invisible microangiopathy was related to ventricular dilatation seen in [their] subjects." They allowed that it is possible that homocysteine has a neurotoxic effect or, conversely, may promote neuronal apoptosis. "The association of hyperhomocysteinemia with cerebral atrophy is a possible explanation for its proposal as a risk factor for Alzheimer's disease," they concluded.

Vascular Disease Also Seen

People with hyperhomocysteinemia were also 10 times more likely to have vascular disease, a study from the University of California,

Davis, School of Medicine in Sacramento revealed. The finding was based on a study of 43 people with Alzheimer's disease who were recruited during outpatient visits to the university's Alzheimer's Disease Center and 37 healthy controls who were studied for homocysteine level and B vitamin status.

The patients with Alzheimer's disease underwent testing to exclude other causes of dementia as well as brain imaging (CT or MRI) to determine the presence or absence of cerebral infarction. Of the 43 study participants with a diagnosis of possible or probable Alzheimer's disease, 11 had a coexisting vascular disease such as stroke, myocardial infarction, angina, congestive heart failure, coronary artery disease, transient ischemic attack, or evidence of lacunar or cortical brain infarcts. Of the 37 control subjects without a diagnosis of Alzheimer's disease, 15 had evidence of vascular disease.

Mean plasma homocysteine concentration was higher in the subjects with vascular disease—whether in the Alzheimer's disease group or the control group—than in the subjects without vascular disease, it was reported. No significant effect of Alzheimer's disease on plasma homocysteine concentration was observed.

High Homocysteine Related to Vascular Disease?

"The study didn't find a relationship between high homocysteine levels and Alzheimer's disease per se—as has been reported previously—but rather suggests that in studies that did demonstrate this association, the effect may be mediated by vascular diseases," said lead author Joshua W. Miller, PhD, Assistant Adjunct Professor in the Department of Pathology. The patients with Alzheimer's disease were also found to be 12 times more likely to have low levels of vitamin B_6 than the controls.

The primary conclusion to be drawn from the findings, the authors wrote, is that elevated homocysteine in Alzheimer's disease is not the direct cause or result of Alzheimer's disease pathology or its consequences, either physiologic or behavioral. Instead, they believe, it is related to the well-documented association with vascular disease. It remains to be determined if hyperhomocysteinemia contributes to or is associated with more severe dementia or an accelerated rate of cognitive decline in patients with Alzheimer's disease, they said.

The most effective means for lowering plasma homocysteine is B vitamin supplementation (a combination of folate, vitamin B_{12}, and vitamin B_6), the researchers maintain. Based on previous findings as well as their own, Dr. Miller's group believes that a therapeutic effect of vitamin B$_6$ supplementation may be postulated for patients with Alzheimer's disease.

—Section by Heidi W. Moore

Suggested Reading

Miller JW, Green R, Mungas DM, et al. Homocysteine, vitamin B$_6$, and vascular disease in AD patients. *Neurology*. 2002;58:1471-1475.

Sachdev PS, Valenzuela M, Wang XL, et al. Relationship between plasma homocysteine levels and brain atrophy in healthy elderly individuals. *Neurology*. 2002;58:1539-1541.

Toole JF, Jack CR. Food (and vitamins) for thought. *Neurology*. 2002;58:1449-1450.

Folic Acid May Be Important

Mouse experiments suggest that folic acid could play an essential role in protecting the brain against the ravages of Alzheimer's disease and other neurodegenerative disorders, according to scientists at the National Institute on Aging. This animal study* could help researchers unravel the underlying biochemical mechanisms involved in another recent finding that concluded people with high blood levels of homocysteine have nearly twice the risk of developing the disease.**

In the study, published in the March 1, 2002 issue of the *Journal of Neuroscience*, the investigators fed one group of mice with Alzheimer's-like plaques in their brains a diet that included normal amounts of folate, while a second group was fed a diet deficient in this vitamin. These mice are transgenic, meaning they were bred with mutant genes that cause AD in people. They develop AD-like plaques in their brains that kill neurons.

The NIA team counted neurons in the hippocampus, a brain region critical for learning and memory that is destroyed as plaques accumulate during Alzheimer's disease. The investigators found a decreased number of neurons in the mice fed the folic acid deficient diet.

The scientists also discovered that mice with low amounts of dietary folic acid had elevated levels of homocysteine, an amino acid, in the blood and brain. They suspect that increased levels of homocysteine in the brain caused damage to the DNA of nerve cells in the hippocampus. In transgenic mice fed an adequate amount of folate, nerve cells in this brain region were able to repair damage to their DNA. But in the transgenic mice fed a folate-deficient diet, nerve cells were unable to repair this DNA damage.

"These new findings establish a possible cause-effect relationship between elevated homocysteine levels and degeneration of nerve cells involved in learning and memory in a mouse model of Alzheimer's disease," said Mark Mattson, Ph.D., chief of the NIA's Laboratory of Neurosciences and the study's principal investigator.

People who have Alzheimer's disease often have low levels of folic acid in their blood, but it is not clear whether this is a result of the disease or if they are simply malnourished due to their illness. But based on emerging research, Dr. Mattson speculates consuming adequate amounts of folic acid—either in the diet or by supplementation—could be beneficial to the aging brain and help protect it against Alzheimer's and other neurodegenerative diseases.

Green leafy vegetables, citrus fruits and juices, whole wheat bread, and dry beans are good sources of the vitamin. Since 1998, the Food and Drug Administration has required the addition of folic acid to enriched breads, cereals, flours, corn meals, pastas, rice, and other grain products. However, because it can take a long time for the symptoms of Alzheimer's disease to surface, researchers speculate it will be many years before folate supplementation in food could affect the incidence of dementia in the United States. A human clinical trial is being planned.

In AD, plaques develop first in areas of the brain used for memory and other cognitive functions. They consist of largely insoluble deposits of a protein called beta-amyloid. Although researchers still do not know whether amyloid plaques themselves cause AD or whether they are by-products of the AD process, there is evidence that amyloid deposition may be a central process in the disease. But unlike human brain cells, the brain cells in laboratory mice are not killed by the progressive accumulation of beta amyloid. This finding led Dr. Mattson and his research team to suspect folic acid or some other component of the mouse diet might help these nerve cells resist beta amyloid damage. In earlier work, Dr. Mattson found evidence suggesting folic acid deficiency can increase the brain's susceptibility to Parkinson's disease.

The NIA leads the federal effort to support and conduct basic, clinical, and social and behavioral studies on aging and AD. It supports the Alzheimer's Disease Education and Referral (ADEAR) Center, which provides information on AD research, including clinical trials, to the public, health professionals, and the media. ADEAR can be contacted toll free at 800-438-4380 weekdays or by visiting the website www.alzheimers.org. Press releases, fact sheets, and other materials about aging and aging research can be viewed at the NIA's general information website, www.nia.nih.gov.

Notes

*I. Kruman, T.S. Kumaravel, A. Lohani, W. Pedersen, R.G. Cutler, Y. Kruman, N. Haughey, J. Lee, M. Evans, and M.P. Mattson, "Folic Acid Deficiency and Homocysteine Impair DNA Repair in Hippocampal Neurons and Sensitize Them to Amyloid Toxicity in Experimental Models of Alzheimer's Disease," *Journal of Neuroscience*, 22:5, pp. 1752-1762.

**S. Sesdradri, A. Beiser, J. Selhub, et al., "Plasma Homocysteine as a Risk Factor for Dementia and Alzheimer's Disease," *N Eng J Med*, 346:7, pp. 476-483.

Chapter 66

Developing New Diagnostic Techniques for Alzheimer's Disease

In the past 25 years, scientists have studied Alzheimer's disease (AD) from many angles. They've looked at populations to see how many cases of AD occur and whether there might be links between the disease and lifestyles or genetic backgrounds. They've conducted clinical studies with healthy older people and those at various stages of AD. They've examined individual nerve cells to see how beta-amyloid and other molecules affect the ability of cells to function normally.

These studies have led to better diagnostic tests, new ways to manage behavioral aspects of AD, and a growing number of possible drug treatments. Findings from current research are pointing scientists in promising directions for the future. They are also helping researchers ask better questions about the issues that are still unclear.

Then and Now:
The Fast Pace of Development in AD Research

What We Didn't Know Then

15 years ago: We didn't know any of the genes that could cause AD. We had no idea of the biological pathways that were involved in the development of damage to the brain in AD.

From "Alzheimer's Disease Research: Finding New Answers and Asking Better Questions," excerpted from "Alzheimer's Disease: Unraveling the Mystery," Alzheimer's Disease Education and Referral (ADEAR) Center, a service of the National Institute on Aging, NIH Pub. No. 02-3782, October 2002. The full text of this document is available online at www.alzheimers.org/unraveling/index.htm.

10 years ago: We couldn't model the disease in animals.

5 years ago: NIH did not fund any prevention clinical trials. We had no way to identify people at high risk of developing AD.

1 year ago: We didn't understand anything about how plaques and tangles relate to each other.

What We Know Now (2002)

- We know the 3 major genes for early-onset AD and 1 of the major risk factor genes for late-onset AD.

- We know a lot about the pathways that lead to the development of beta-amyloid plaques in the brain—one of the main features of AD.

- Scientists have developed special kinds of mice that produce beta-amyloid plaques.

- NIH is funding clinical trials that are looking at possible ways to prevent AD.

- We can identify individuals at high risk through imaging, neuropsychological tests, and structured interviews.

- By developing another kind of mice that have both plaques and tangles, we now know that plaques can influence the development of tangles.

Current Tools for Diagnosing AD

A definitive diagnosis of Alzheimer's disease is still only possible after death, during an autopsy, when the plaques and tangles can actually be seen. But with the tools now available, experienced physicians can be pretty confident about making an accurate diagnosis in a living person. Here's how they do it.

They take a detailed patient history, including:

- A description of how and when symptoms developed

- A description of the patient's and his or her family's overall medical condition and history

- An assessment of the patient's emotional state and living environment

They get information from family members or close friends:

- People close to the patient can provide valuable insights into how behavior and personality have changed; many times, family and friends know something is wrong even before changes are evident on tests.

They conduct physical and neurological examinations and laboratory tests:

- Blood and other medical tests help determine neurological functioning and identify possible non-AD causes of dementia.

They do a computerized tomography (CT) scan or a magnetic resonance imaging (MRI) test:

- Brain scans like these can detect strokes or tumors or can reveal changes in the brain's structure and function that indicate early AD.

They conduct neuropsychological testing:

- Question and answer tests or other tasks that measure memory, language skills, ability to do arithmetic, and other abilities related to brain functioning help indicate what kind of cognitive changes are occurring.

Criteria for "Probable" Alzheimer's Disease

Because no simple and reliable biological test for AD is available, the National Institute of Neurological and Communicative Disorders and Stroke and the Alzheimer's Association together established criteria to help physicians diagnose AD. These criteria also help physicians distinguish between AD and other forms of dementia. "Probable" Alzheimer's disease is determined when a person has:

- Dementia confirmed by clinical and neuropsychological examination
- Progressive worsening of memory and other mental functioning
- No disturbances of consciousness (no "blacking out")
- Symptoms beginning between ages 40 and 90
- No other disorders that might account for the dementia

As they get older, some people develop a memory deficit greater than that expected for their age. However, other aspects of cognition are not affected, so these people do not meet all the accepted criteria for AD. Thus, they are said to have "mild cognitive impairment" (MCI). About 40 percent of these individuals will develop AD within 3 years. Others, however, do not seem to progress to AD, at least in the time frame studied thus far (up to approximately 6 years). Understanding more about the characteristics and development of MCI is essential in helping clinicians diagnose early stages of AD.

New Techniques Help in Diagnosing AD

A healthy man in his early 60s begins to notice that his memory isn't as good as it used to be. More and more often, a word will be on the tip of his tongue but he just can't remember it. He forgets appointments, makes mistakes when paying his bills, and finds that he's often confused or anxious about the normal hustle and bustle of life around him. One evening, he suddenly finds himself walking in a neighborhood a couple of miles from his house. He has no idea how he got there.

Not so long ago, this man's condition would have been swept into a broad catch-all category called "senile dementia" or "senility." Today, the picture is very different. We now know that Alzheimer's and other illnesses with dementia are distinct diseases. Armed with this knowledge, we have rapidly improved our ability to accurately diagnose AD. We are still some distance from the ultimate goal—a reliable, valid, inexpensive, and early diagnostic marker—but experienced physicians now can diagnose AD with up to 90 percent accuracy.

Early diagnosis has several advantages. For example, many conditions cause symptoms that mimic those of Alzheimer's disease. Finding out early that the problem isn't AD but is something else can spur people into getting treatment for the real condition. For the small percentage of dementias that are treatable or even reversible, early diagnosis increases the chances of successful treatment.

Even when the cause of the dementia turns out to be Alzheimer's disease, it's good to find out sooner rather than later. One benefit is medical. The drugs now available to treat AD can help some people maintain their mental abilities for months to years, though they do not change the underlying course of the disease .

Other benefits are practical. The sooner the person with AD and family know, the more time they have to make future living arrangements, handle financial matters, establish a durable power of attorney, deal with other legal issues, create a support network, or even make plans to join a research study. Being able to participate for as long as possible in making decisions about the present and future is important to many people with AD.

Finally, scientists also see advantages to early diagnosis. Developing tests that can reveal what is happening in the brain in the early stages of Alzheimer's disease will help them understand more about the cause and development of the disease. It will also help scientists learn when and how to start drugs and other treatments so that they can be most effective.

Scientists are now exploring ways to help physicians diagnose AD earlier and more accurately. For example, some studies are focusing on changes in personality and mental functioning. These changes can be measured through memory and recall tests. Tests that measure a person's abilities in areas such as abstract thinking, planning, and language can also help pinpoint changes in function. Researchers are working hard to improve these standardized tests so that they can better track the changes that might point to early AD or predict which individuals are at higher risk of developing AD in the future.

Other studies are examining the relationship between early damage to brain tissue and outward clinical signs. Still others are looking for changes in blood chemistry that might indicate the progression of Alzheimer's disease.

One of the most exciting areas of ongoing research in this area is neuroimaging. Over the last decade, scientists have developed several highly sophisticated imaging systems that have been used in many areas of medicine, including Alzheimer's disease. Positron emission tomography (PET), single photon emission computed tomography (SPECT), and magnetic resonance imaging (MRI) are all examples. These "windows" on the living brain can help scientists measure the earliest changes in brain function or structure in order to identify those people who are at the very first stages of the disease—even before they develop signs and symptoms.

These types of scans are still primarily research tools, but one day, neuroimaging might be used more commonly to help physicians diagnose AD early. These tools may even be used someday to monitor the progress of the disease and assess patient responses to drug treatment.

Chapter 67

Brain Imaging to Detect Alzheimer's Disease

Even when people have no symptoms, their brains already may be dotted with the plaques and tangles that characterize Alzheimer's disease. As treatments to halt the progress of Alzheimer's disease appear on the horizon, scientists are looking for new ways to identify Alzheimer's-associated changes in the brain before cognitive decline begins.

That's why neuroscientists at the Silvio Conte Center for Neuroscience Research and the Alzheimer's Disease Research Center at Washington University in St. Louis have been working with state-of-the-art imagining techniques to see whether they can identify the presence of Alzheimer's disease in its earliest, pre-clinical stages. At a recent meeting of the Society for Neuroscience, they presented preliminary findings that suggest brain images may help predict future Alzheimer's disease symptoms.

"We screen for diabetes and hypertension," says John G. Csernansky, M.D., the Gregory B. Couch Professor of Psychiatry and director of the Silvio Conte Center for Neuroscience Research. "We don't wait for them to have a stroke or a heart attack. But with Alzheimer's disease, we're in the position where we can't detect the disease until after a person gets sick. By then, it's already too late to prevent much of the damage."

From "Detecting Alzheimer's Disease before Symptoms Begin," *News and Information*, Office of Public Affairs, Washington University in St. Louis. © 2002 Washington University in St. Louis. All rights reserved. Reprinted with permission.

Part of the problem is that the brain is well protected in the skull, preventing easy access. But, with help from modern imaging and computer technology, Csernansky and colleagues believe they are making progress. They are combining magnetic resonance imaging (MRI) scans with complex computer algorithms to locate and identify very small changes in the brain.

"If we compare looking at the brain to looking at a car, past brain imaging techniques required that the car have a big dent in the fender before we could see it," Csernansky explains. "But the continuing evolution of computer assistance allows us to detect the equivalent of hail damage or chips in the paint."

The difference is that these "chips in the paint" do more than affect appearance. Eventually, they have devastating effects on cognitive function.

Because learning and memory are greatly affected by Alzheimer's disease, Csernansky's team has focused on a brain structure known to be important in learning and memory: the hippocampus, a seahorse-shaped structure deep inside the brain.

"We thought this would be a key brain area for changes that may identify the presence of pre-clinical Alzheimer's disease," says Lei Wang, Ph.D., research associate in psychiatry and the lead investigator of the imaging study of patients with and without Alzheimer's disease. "Our preliminary data indicate that there are indeed hippocampal changes in patients who have Alzheimer's disease."

In past imaging studies, Wang and Csernansky found that the hippocampus tends to be slightly smaller in people with Alzheimer's disease than in those without the disorder. They also noted that even healthy older adults had some atrophy and malformations in the hippocampus when compared to younger adults. Because people's brains have individual variations in size and shape, Wang and Csernansky believe that it will be more informative to study how brain structures change over time in order to distinguish normal changes from atrophy that might be associated with disease early on.

To distinguish the differences, they conducted initial MRI scans on 18 patients with mild dementia from Alzheimer's disease and 26 healthy individuals of about the same age. Then, they conducted another MRI two years later.

"In people who didn't have Alzheimer's disease, the volume decrease in the hippocampus was about 4 to 5 percent over those two years," Wang says. "But in people with mild dementia, the volume reduction was closer to 8 to 10 percent. They also showed a shape change that was different than nondemented people, and that pattern of change corresponds well with other post-mortem studies."

Because the rate of atrophy over time is so much slower in healthy adults than in those with Alzheimer's disease, it may be possible to diagnose the presence of pre-clinical Alzheimer's disease by conducting several scans and tracking the rate of volume loss and shape change in key brain structures such as the hippocampus.

"The disease is present in the brain for several years before dementia symptoms are apparent," Csernansky says. "One can logically assume that if you had a sensitive enough measurement, you might be able to detect the illness in people before they become clinically demented. This difference we found in the rate of atrophy is a very powerful discriminator of patients with and without dementia."

MRI scans don't actually show plaques and tangles in the brain. But interestingly, other researchers have shown that plaques often occur in a part of the hippocampus called the CA1 region. In this study, there was a great deal of volume loss in that particular area of the hippocampus.

"It is speculative to assume that this atrophy is being caused by the formation of plaques," Wang says. "But we may be seeing changes as plaques form and the connections between neurons disappear. Eventually, those cells die, and that would certainly cause a reduction in volume But we're not at a point where we're ready to say that's what we've seen in these imaging studies."

Reference

Wang L, Swank JS, Miller MI, Morris JC, Csernansky JG. Progressive hippocampal atrophy distinguishes DAT and healthy aging program no. 228.3 2002 Abstract Viewer/Itinerary Planner. Washington, DC: Society for Neuroscience, 2002. Online.

Note

Funding from the National Institutes of Health and the Gregory B. Couch Endowment at Washington University supported this research.

Chapter 68

Searching for New Alzheimer's Disease Treatments

Research over the last two decades has revealed many pieces of the Alzheimer's disease (AD) puzzle. Using recent advances in genetics and molecular biology, scientists have begun to put these pieces into place. In doing so, they've vastly increased our understanding of AD and opened many avenues that could lead to effective treatments.

It has become clear that there probably isn't a "magic bullet" that will, by itself, prevent or cure AD. However, scientists may be able to identify a number of interventions that can be used to reduce risk and treat the disease. Today, it is estimated that the National Institute on Aging, other NIH Institutes, and private industry are conducting clinical trials (studies involving humans that rigorously test how well an intervention works) on around 30 compounds that may be active against AD. These studies focus on three main areas:

- Helping people with AD maintain their mental functioning

- Slowing the progress of AD, delaying its onset, or preventing it

- Managing symptoms

From "The Search for New Treatments," excerpted from "Alzheimer's Disease: Unraveling the Mystery," Alzheimer's Disease Education and Referral (ADEAR) Center, a service of the National Institute on Aging, NIH Pub. No. 02-3782, October 2002. The full text of this document is available online at www.alzheimers.org/unraveling/index.htm.

Helping People with AD Maintain Their Mental Functioning

In the mid-1970s, scientists discovered that levels of a neurotransmitter called acetylcholine fell sharply in people with Alzheimer's disease. This discovery was one of the first that linked AD with biochemical changes in the brain.

Since then, scientists have conducted hundreds of studies on acetylcholine. They have found that acetylcholine is important for several reasons. It is a critical player in the process of forming memories. It is also commonly used by neurons in the hippocampus and cerebral cortex—two regions devastated by AD. These findings led naturally to the idea that increasing levels of acetylcholine, replacing it, or slowing its breakdown could stop the disease.

The Food and Drug Administration (FDA) has approved four medications for the treatment of mild to moderate AD symptoms. The first, tacrine (Cognex), has been replaced by three newer drugs—donepezil (Aricept), rivastigmine (Exelon), and galantamine (Reminyl). All act by stopping or slowing the action of acetylcholinesterase, an enzyme that normally breaks down acetylcholine. These drugs improve some patients' ability to carry out activities of daily living, such as eating and dressing. The drugs also help with behavioral symptoms, such as delusions and agitation, and can also improve thinking, memory, and speaking skills. However, these medications will not stop or reverse AD and appear to help patients only for months to a few years.

Helping people with AD carry out their daily lives and maintain their mental abilities is one of the most important goals of AD treatment research. Many investigators are working to develop new and better drugs that can preserve this critical function for as long as possible.

Slowing, Delaying, or Preventing Alzheimer's Disease

Understanding all the steps involved in the development of AD—from beginning to end—is important in and of itself. It also can have a big payoff down the road, for if we have this knowledge we might be able to develop drugs that slow, delay, or even prevent the disease process. That's the thinking behind this area of AD treatment research.

Investigators are looking at several possibilities. For example, inflammation of tissue in the brain and overproduction of free radicals are two processes that are thought to be a feature of AD. The NIA is now supporting clinical trials in both of these areas to see whether specific anti-inflammatory agents and agents that protect against oxidative damage can slow or prevent the development of AD.

Scientists are also conducting clinical trials to see whether substances already used to reduce cardiovascular risk factors also help reduce AD risk. The NIA has several ongoing and planned clinical trials to test whether supplementation with folic acid and vitamins B_6 and B_{12} can slow the rate of cognitive decline in cognitively normal men and women, women at increased risk of developing dementia, and in people diagnosed with AD. The Institute will also conduct a study of statins, the most common type of cholesterol-lowering drug, to see whether these drugs can slow the rate of disease progression in AD patients.

Another area of work involves nerve growth factor (NGF). NGF is one of several growth factors in the body that maintain the health of neurons. NGF also promotes the growth of axons and dendrites, the neuron branches that connect with other neurons and that are essential in nerve cells' ability to communicate. Studies have turned up a number of clues that link NGF to the neurons that use acetylcholine as a neurotransmitter, so researchers have been eager to see what happens when NGF is added to aging brain tissue. In animal studies, researchers have been able to reverse most of the age-related neuronal shrinkage and loss of ability to make acetylcholine. This success has led to a small-scale, privately funded gene therapy trial that is testing whether this procedure can be done safely in humans and whether it might lessen symptoms of Alzheimer's disease.

Finally, a number of clinical trials are focusing on the earliest stages of the disease process. For example, scientists are developing drugs that prevent enzymes from clipping beta-amyloid out from APP. Others are working on ways to stop beta-amyloid from clumping together into plaques. Teams of investigators are also studying certain enzymes that seem to be able to break beta-amyloid into pieces after it is released from cells but before it has a chance to form into plaques. Still other scientists are exploring the role of neurotransmitter systems other than acetylcholine, such as glutamate. One especially active area of research involves the possibility that a vaccine might be able to stimulate the immune system into getting rid of plaques once they have formed, stopping beta-amyloid and plaque buildup, or even getting rid of plaques once they have formed.

465

Science on the Cutting Edge

Immunizing Against AD: Just a Neat Idea Or a Real Possibility?

Getting vaccinated against measles, tetanus, polio, and other diseases is common practice these days. A person is injected with a weakened form of a disease-causing bacterium or virus. His or her immune system mobilizes to fight against it, and this protects the person against getting the disease. One scientist wondered whether this approach could work for Alzheimer's disease as well.

Researchers have developed special kinds of mice (called transgenic mice) that gradually develop AD beta-amyloid plaques in the brain. These mice are invaluable tools to test how plaques can be stopped from forming. Over the course of several studies, scientists tested the effects of injections of a vaccine composed of beta-amyloid and a substance known to stimulate the immune system. They found that long-term immunization resulted in much less beta-amyloid being deposited in the brains of the mice. Similar transgenic mice that had been immunized also performed far better on memory tests than did a group of these mice that had not been immunized.

These exciting developments led to preliminary studies in humans to test the safety and effectiveness of the vaccine. Based on positive results, a further study was designed to measure the immune response in participants with AD who received immunizations with the beta-amyloid vaccine. In this study, which began in the fall of 2001, inflammation unexpectedly developed in the brains of some of the participants. As a result of this complication, the pharmaceutical companies that were conducting the research stopped the trial and are continuing to closely monitor the health of the participants.

Despite their disappointment with this development, the scientists and funders involved in this research emphasize that a tremendous amount of valuable information has been gained from this work so far. It is not unusual for such a revolutionary concept to have setbacks, and they are moving forward with other possible strategies.

Managing Symptoms

As Alzheimer's disease makes inroads into memory and mental abilities, it also begins to change a person's emotions and behaviors. Between 70 to 90 percent of people with Alzheimer's disease eventually develop one or more behavioral symptoms. These include sleeplessness, wandering and pacing, aggression, agitation, anger, depression, and hallucinations and delusions. Some of these symptoms may become worse in the evening, a phenomenon called "sundowning," or during daily routines, especially bathing.

Unlike a stroke, in which damage to part of the brain occurs all at once, the damage of Alzheimer's disease spreads slowly over time and affects many different parts of the brain. Even small tasks require the brain to engage in a complex process that can involve more than one region of the brain. If this process is disrupted, the person may not be able to do the task or may act in a strange or inappropriate way.

In light of our growing understanding about the effects of AD on the brain, behavior that may seem bizarre suddenly makes sense:

- For a man who can no longer distinguish between past and present, the anguish caused by the death of his parent may be as real today as it was many years before.

- An unknown young man suddenly appearing in her room may be threatening and terrifying to a woman who does not recognize her grandson.

- Feelings of responsibility toward a long-ago night job resurface and compel a woman to get up in the night to go to work.

- Sitting down to a family meal may produce intense anxiety when a person has no idea what to do with the knife and fork in front of him and all the conversation and activity feel overwhelming.

Behavioral symptoms are one of the hardest aspects of the disease for families and other caregivers to deal with. They are emotional and upsetting. They are also a visible sign of the terrible change that has taken place in the person with AD. Researchers are slowly learning more about why they occur, and they are studying new treatments—both drug and non-drug—to deal with them.

A number of ongoing and planned clinical trials are looking at ways to treat agitation. These trials include participants who are living in nursing homes or at home. They involve the study of a variety of drugs, including a beta-blocker, an anti-seizure medication, a cholinesterase inhibitor, and an antipsychotic.

Chapter 69

Attacking Alzheimer's Disease on Multiple Fronts

Researchers have identified several possible targets for the treatment of Alzheimer's disease. On the forefront of approaches to treat and prevent this disease are inhibitors of amyloid-based ß- and γ–secretase enzymes and an immune-based vaccine that has been found to reduce the burden of plaque in transgenic animal models of Alzheimer's disease.

"Despite decades of intensive study, the precise etiology of Alzheimer's disease remains a mystery," said Ivan Lieberburg, MD, PhD, at the 125th Annual Meeting of the American Neurological Association. "Nevertheless, an overwhelming amount of circumstantial evidence points to the role of ß-amyloid as the causal agent." Dr. Lieberburg is Chief Scientific and Medical Officer, Elan Corporation, South San Francisco, California; and Clinical Professor in the Department of Internal Medicine, University of California, San Francisco.

Production Versus Clearance

"It was always my view that the problem in amyloidosis was really a question of production versus clearance," much like atherosclerosis and hypercholesterolemia, Dr. Lieberburg said. In type 2 hypercholesterolemia, for example, most patients have modestly elevated levels of cholesterol but cannot clear it. Drugs such as the HMG-CoA

"Attacking Alzheimer's Disease on Multiple Fronts," by Debra Hughes, in *Neurology Reviews*, Vol. 9, No. 1, January 2001. Reprinted with permission of Clinicians Group—A Jobson Company.

reductase inhibitors (statins) reduce ongoing production of cholesterol so that clearance mechanisms can operate optimally.

Similarly, therapy being developed for Alzheimer's disease has as its basic premise the question of clearance. "And how do we enhance clearance? We can do it either by decreasing production and allowing endogenous clearance to take place or by enhancing it through some other mechanism." For Alzheimer's disease, this involves three major approaches: inhibiting the 1) ß-secretase and 2) γ–secretase enzyme activity involved to allow endogenous clearance and, alternatively, 3) immunization, which enhances ongoing clearance through an immune-mediated approach.

Secretase Inhibition

Most of the work done over the past several years has centered on γ-secretase. Last year, two groups independently found evidence that the aspartate residues in the presenilin molecule are the sites responsible for γ-secretase activity. Dr. Lieberburg said one problem that has emerged with γ-secretase as a target for therapy is that "presenilin is crucial to the cleavage of Notch," which is a signaling protein important to normal development of the embryo and rapidly dividing cells. "If you inhibit Notch cleavage, you actually can accelerate the differentiation scheme in the adult animal and cause a dramatic phenotype," he said.

The γ-secretase inhibitors under development are orally bioavailable and extremely potent. "They are central nervous system permeant; they are novel compounds; and they have been tested on animals extensively over the past several years. They are capable of dramatically reducing ß-peptide formation in a chronic fashion," said Dr. Lieberburg. He added that in subchronic studies with these inhibitors, "we've achieved as much as 70% reduction of ß-amyloid in the brains of these animals. Now, how that's going to relate to the human situation remains to be seen. But what's important about this is that all the attendant pathology is also reduced," including gliosis and neuritic pathology.

The challenge is to develop not only "a safe drug that's capable of delivering not only this kind of result" but one "with a reasonable therapeutic index that patients can tolerate," Dr. Lieberburg said. While compounds with a therapeutic index of greater than 100 are generally preferred, γ-secretase inhibitors currently under study have indexes that range from 20 to 40. "We understand that this is a very serious disease, but we also understand that we don't want to expose patients to any undue toxicity."

"Part of the reason for the excitement [about] ß-secretase…is because its inhibition may not have many of the attendant therapeutic index issues that are associated with γ-secretase." The ß-secretase enzyme makes only one cleavage at a specific site between two amino acids on amyloid precursor protein (APP). It is an aspartyl protease, few of which are found naturally in humans, allowing for specificity as well as selectivity in drug development. He said that ß-secretase would probably require about 25% inhibition to produce a therapeutic benefit, compared with nearly 99% inhibition for HIV protease. Also, unlike γ-secretase, ß-secretase is relatively selective to the central nervous system.

Inhibition

"The work in this area is not quite as far along as it is with γ-secretase," Dr. Lieberburg said. However, "we're not that far away from getting something that could move into the clinic," he added.

Some of the drawbacks to developing inhibitors include the ubiquitous nature of γ-secretase, the difficulty of working with proteases as targets, and the inhibitors' difficulty in permeating the blood-brain barrier. He said that simulating amyloid clearance mechanisms is much easier than inhibiting the enzymes that promote the production of amyloid. Dr. Lieberburg and his colleagues thus explored whether "we could enhance clearance by activating the immune system and get amyloid to clear from the brain. And in fact you can, rather remarkably."

Or Immunization?

In a prophylaxis study, transgenic animals immunized with ß-amyloid developed almost no amyloid formation in 12 months; the attendant neuritic dystrophy or astrocytosis typically seen was also not present, he said. Given these results, "we were curious to know what would happen if we treated these animals once they developed disease." Treatment begun at 11 months resulted in a "dramatic reduction in pathology," including correction of loss of synapse formation and reduction in neuritic burden and astrocytosis. In reviewing these results, published in *Nature Medicine* in August 2000, the investigators concluded that "antibodies against amyloid ß-peptide triggered microglial cells to clear plaques through Fc receptor-mediated phagocytosis and subsequent peptide degradation. These results indicate that antibodies can cross the blood-brain barrier to act directly

471

in the central nervous system and should be considered as a therapeutic approach for the treatment of Alzheimer's disease and other neurologic disorders."

An immunization based on this approach is currently in phase 1 clinical trials. No data are yet available, other than that it is well tolerated, (including a lack of glomerular nephritis or autoimmune encephalomyelitis). Dr. Lieberburg said that other drugs being tested for safety in animal models prior to their entry into clinical trials include "at least six backup adjuvant-antigen combinations," fusion antigens, and monoclonal antibodies.

Suggested Reading

Bard F, Cannon C, Barbour R, et al. Peripherally administered antibodies against amyloid ß-peptide enter the central nervous system and reduce pathology in a mouse model of Alzheimer disease. *Nat Med*. 2000; 6:916-919.

Chapter 70

Researching Beta Amyloid Plaques, Tau, and Neurofibrillary Tangles

The Latest Research on Stopping Beta Amyloid and Plaques

Beta amyloid, often abbreviated as A-beta, is a protein that builds up in the brains of persons with Alzheimer's disease, collecting in clumps called plaques or senile plaques. While some researchers question whether beta amyloid is the cause of the dementia, most agree that it is involved in the disruption of thinking that is a hallmark of the disease. Efforts at finding medications that would reduce the size or number of plaques are ongoing at research centers throughout the world. In the last several years, a number of approaches have shown promise for inhibiting beta amyloid plaques.

In some cases of familial Alzheimer's disease, mutations in genes for the proteins called the presenilins lead to increased production of amyloid. Researchers at Ludwig-Maximilians University in Munich and other scientists at Harvard have been looking at how presenilin-1 in particular contributes to the excess buildup of beta amyloid. Both groups have concluded that presenilin-1 acts to increase the activity of gamma-secretase, an enzyme that changes a normal protein (amyloid precursor protein or APP) into beta amyloid itself. Further, both

This chapter includes "The Latest Research on Stopping Beta Amyloid and Plaques," "The Latest Research on Tau and Neurofibrillary Tangles," and "The Latest Research on Metals and Alzheimer's Disease," © 2001 American Federation for Aging Research. Reprinted with permission from the American Federation for Aging Research. For further information, please visit www.infoaging.org.

groups have speculated that presenilin-1 might be gamma-secretase. They conclude that drugs that would target the activity of presenilin-1/gamma-secretase may slow the production of beta amyloid and prove to be a useful therapy for Alzheimer's disease.

Chronic inflammation of the brain is a component of Alzheimer's disease. Epidemiological or population studies have shown a lower risk of developing Alzheimer's disease among people who regularly take pain relievers in the category nonsteroidal anti-inflammatory drugs (NSAIDs), such as ibuprofen. A study at UCLA looked at the effects of ibuprofen on the brains of laboratory mice bred to carry the mouse variant of Alzheimer's disease. Those mice fed mouse chow with very high doses of ibuprofen for six months had far fewer beta amyloid deposits in their brains than the mice fed plain mouse chow, showing that at least in mice, an anti-inflammatory medication can at least delay the development of the harmful amyloid plaques.

Some studies have suggested that zinc, a metal necessary in trace amounts for normal growth and development, can be toxic to the brain at high levels, and indeed, beta amyloid collects in plaques at a faster rate in the presence of high levels of zinc. A study at the Sanders-Brown Center on Aging in Louisville, Kentucky, found that at low levels, zinc provided protection against the formation of amyloid plaques, while confirming that at high levels, it promotes their formation, leading the researchers to compare zinc to a double-edged sword.

Many of the dangerous effects of beta amyloid appear to arise from oxidative damage. Our bodies use oxygen to generate energy, and this process produces toxic byproducts called reactive oxygen species, a kind of free radical molecule. Naturally occurring substances called antioxidants (some of which our bodies make and some of which we get in foods) mop up these free radicals, reducing their toxicity. A number of researchers are looking at the effects of antioxidants at reducing the damage caused by amyloid plaques. In vitro (test tube or laboratory) studies done at the University of Kentucky—Lexington, for example, have shown that the antioxidant vitamin E can reduce the amount of damage amyloid can do to brain cells.

Investigators at the University of South Alabama have looked at melatonin, a hormone produced by the pineal gland within the brain, which is known to have antioxidant properties. Their research consistently showed that, at least in tissue culture, melatonin can prevent brain cell death and damage caused by amyloid. The researchers point out that this hormone is presumed by many to play a role in the aging process, since its levels decline with age and decline even more in those with Alzheimer's disease.

474

Gingko biloba is a plant extract reported to have benefits in the treatment of Alzheimer's disease. Scientists at McGill University in Quebec have demonstrated in tissue culture that one form of gingko biloba can prevent the oxidative damage induced by beta amyloid. These same scientists have also looked at the beneficial effects of naturally occurring proteins called insulin-like growth factors (IGFs) at protecting brain cells in culture dishes from the toxic effects of amyloid. IGFs offered the additional benefit of being able to "rescue" brain cells exposed to and damaged by amyloid for up to four days in the tissue cultures.

Researchers from the Massachusetts General Hospital have recently published research that offers a unique and exciting way to reverse the damage caused by amyloid plaques. They created anti-plaque antibodies and injected them directly into the brains of mice with amyloid plaque. Approximately 70% of the plaques were cleared within 3 to 8 days. The researchers speculate that plaque could be formed and removed by the body's own immune system in a similar fashion.

Though all of these approaches offer potential benefits, they have to date been studied extensively only in tissue culture or animal models. Results from ongoing human trials will show which treatments are the best at reducing the toxicity of beta amyloid.

The Latest Research on Tau and Neurofibrillary Tangles

Among the abnormalities found in the brains of people with Alzheimer's disease are neurofibrillary tangles. These are knots composed of the remains of microtubules, tiny structures within cells that assist in the transport of substances into and out of brain cells. Microtubules are composed largely of a protein called tau. If the structure of tau is rendered abnormal, the microtubule structure collapses, and the tau protein collects in neurofibrillary tangles.

Whether tau and the tangles develop before or after beta amyloid plaques has been a source of controversy. Recent evidence seems to suggest that the tangles arise after amyloid has done damage, which implies that preventing the formation of amyloid plaques should also prevent the formation of neurofibrillary tangles. This conclusion, however, still must be demonstrated definitively.

Tau and neurofibrillary tangles are features of aging and Alzheimer's-like diseases in other animal species. Mice bred to develop the mouse form of Alzheimer's disease do develop tangles in the cortex, hippocampus and basal ganglia of their brains. Veterinary researchers have found evidence that other mammals—including dogs, polar bears, and wolverines—develop neurofibrillary tangles as they age. Investigators in Germany have studied baboons and found that they have tangles and abnormal tau proteins, providing a model for studying these abnormalities in a nonhuman primate, a much closer relative of ours than the mouse or the wolverine.

The development of abnormalities in tau appears to be at least a two-step process. First, damaged tau gathers in more diffuse tangles, then later coalesces in denser tangles. The diffuse tangles are found more often in the brains of people with the earlier stages of Alzheimer's disease. The denser, fibrillary tangles are found in those whose disease is more advanced.

The mechanism by which tau is damaged seems to involve the addition of excess phosphate groups to the protein, technically called hyperphosphorylation. Researchers in Kalamazoo, Michigan, have shown that this hyperphosphorylated tau with its excess number of attached phosphates cannot form proper microtubules in tissue culture. They have also offered evidence that adding extra phosphate groups to tau already in microtubules causes those tubules to break down.

Researchers at the University of Pennsylvania have studied tau extensively in "transgenic" mice, which have been bred to have the brain changes of Alzheimer's disease. They have found excess tau gene mutations associated with a number of different brain diseases in these mice. Among the diseases from which the mice suffer are those that resemble human amyotrophic lateral sclerosis (Lou Gehrig's disease) and Parkinson's disease. The researchers are optimistic that learning more about these mouse diseases they call "tauopathies" will lead to a far greater understanding of human tauopathies, including Alzheimer's disease.

The Latest Research on Metals and Alzheimer's Disease

Among the brain abnormalities found in Alzheimer's disease is a buildup of the protein called beta amyloid. Recent studies have shown that beta amyloid is a metalloprotein, housing atoms of zinc, copper and iron deep within its folds. Researchers speculate that those bits of metal might be the key to the damage of Alzheimer's disease—and perhaps to its treatment.

Copper, zinc and iron can all react with oxygen. Oxygen is a critical component in our body's production of energy, but that energy is generated with a price. The by-products of energy production, called free radicals, are toxic, damaging DNA and proteins. Copper can promote the production of these free radicals, while zinc has antioxidant properties, protecting against free radical damage. And free radical damage appears to be a significant component of Alzheimer's disease and the formation of amyloid plaques.

Research teams at Harvard Medical School, the University of Melbourne, and Prana Biotechnology Ltd in Australia are working collaboratively on giving Alzheimer's-prone mice copper chelators, substances that sop up metals and eliminate them from the body. These new metal-binding drugs effectively "melted" the amyloid plaques in living mice in as little as nine weeks, and are now in clinical trials with Alzheimer's patients. Results of the first of these drugs, clioquinol, should be known within 12 months, and further trials of this approach are currently in preparation.

Zinc's role in amyloid plaque is complex. Beta amyloid produces hydrogen peroxide, a toxic free radical. Zinc can squelch the formation of hydrogen peroxide and render beta amyloid itself less toxic. But at the same time, evidence exists that suggests that abnormal zinc levels contribute to the formation of amyloid plaques. Some researchers in this area believe that zinc plays a dual role in Alzheimer's disease, initiating the formation of plaque and then reducing the oxidative damage it causes. So whether taking zinc supplements promotes the disease or treats it is still not clear. However, these researchers suggest, the ideal drug for clearing amyloid should attack copper much more than zinc.

Chapter 71

Is There a Link between Statins and a Decrease in Alzheimer's Disease Risk?

What are statins?

Statins is the common name for a class of drugs formally known as 3-hydroxy-3-methylglutaryl coenzyme A (HMG CoA) reductase inhibitors. These drugs lower levels of low-density lipoprotein (LDL) cholesterol—the type most strongly linked with coronary artery disease and stroke—by blocking a liver enzyme essential for cholesterol production. The U.S. Food and Drug Administration (FDA) approved the first statin in 1987. Statins now marketed in the United States include atorvastatin (Lipitor®), fluvastatin (Lescol®), lovastatin (Mevacor®), pravastatin (Pravachol®), simvastatin (Zocor®), and a number of other formulations.

Why are statins of interest in Alzheimer's disease?

Epidemiological studies have found a link between taking statins to reduce cholesterol levels and a decreased occurrence of Alzheimer's disease. Researchers explored the possibility of such a relationship because several previous studies suggested that people with cardiovascular risk factors have an increased Alzheimer risk. Other studies have shown that in the brain, the cholesterol-carrying protein apolipoprotein E (apoE) promotes aggregation of the protein fragment beta-amyloid into the amyloid plaques that are a hallmark Alzheimer pathology. Further, individuals who have apoE-e4—one of the three common variations of the gene that codes production of ApoE—have an increased likelihood of developing the common, late-onset form of Alzheimer's. These lines of evidence suggest that cholesterol levels and differences in the body's cholesterol-processing pathways may influence Alzheimer risk.

A small study involving 44 participants with normal cholesterol levels and a diagnosis of Alzheimer's has also found preliminary evidence that simvastatin may be of some benefit to individuals with Alzheimer's disease.

Gathering stronger evidence about the effectiveness of statins as a prevention or a treatment will require clinical trials comparing the occurrence of Alzheimer's in a large group of participants assigned to take statins to its frequency in a group similar in all important respects except not taking statins. The trials will need to include participants with normal cholesterol levels, because the effects of statins in this group have not been adequately studied. Additional work is also needed to determine the molecular mechanisms by which statins may modify pathological processes in Alzheimer's.

The Alzheimer's Association and most scientific experts believe that no one should take statins specifically to lower their risk of Alzheimer's until further research clarifies the possible relationship between statins and dementia. However, most physicians do advocate keeping one's cholesterol within levels recommended by the National Cholesterol Education Program of the National Heart, Lung, and Blood Institute, a division of the U.S. National Institutes of Health. The latest guidelines are summarized in: "Executive Summary of the Third Report of the National Cholesterol Education Program (NCEP) Expert Panel on Detection, Evaluation, and Treatment of High Blood Cholesterol in Adults (Adult Treatment Panel III)," published in the May 16, 2001 issue of the *Journal of the American Medical Association* on pages 2486–2497. The guidelines are also posted on the website of the National Heart, Lung, and Blood Institute at http://www.nhlbi.nih.gov/guidelines/cholesterol/index.htm.

Where can I get more information?

You can find the preliminary studies mentioned in this chapter in these sources:

- Haley, Robert W. "Is There a Connection Between the Concentration of Cholesterol Circulating in Plasma and the Rate of Neuritic Plaque Formation in Alzheimer Disease?" (Editorial). *Archives of Neurology*, October 2000: pp. 1410–1412.

- Jick, H., et al. "Statins and the Risk of Dementia." *The Lancet*, November 11, 2000: pp. 1627–1631.

- Simons, M.; Schwartzler, F.; Lutjohann, D.; von Bergmann, K.; Beyreuther, K.; Dichgans, J.; Wormstall, H.; Hartmann, T.; Schultz, J.B. "Treatment with Simvastatin in Normocholesterolemic Patients with Alzheimer's Disease: A 26-Week, Randomized, Placebo-Controlled, Double-Blind Trial." *Annals of Neurology* September 2002; 52 (3): 346–350.

- Wolozin, Benjamin, et al. "Decreased Prevalence of Alzheimer Disease Associated with 3-Hydroxy-3-Methyglutaryl Coenzyme A Reductase Inhibitors." *Archives of Neurology*, October 2000: pp. 1439-1443.

- Yaffe, Kristine, et al. "Serum Lipoprotein Levels, Statin Use, and Cognitive Function in Older Women." *Archives of Neurology*, March 2002: pp. 378–382.

Additional information about heart health and managing your cholesterol is available on the website of the American Heart Association at www.americanheart.org.

For answers to your other questions about Alzheimer's disease, please call the Alzheimer's Association's Contact Center at 800-272-3900 or visit our website at www.alz.org.

Chapter 72

Training Improves Cognitive Abilities of Older Adults

Training sessions for 2 hours a week for 5 weeks improved the memory, concentration, and problem solving skills of healthy independent adults 65 years and older who participated in the nation's largest study of cognitive training. The training not only improved participants' cognitive abilities, but the improvement persisted for 2 years after the training, according to initial findings from the multisite trial of Advanced Cognitive Training for Independent and Vital Elderly, or ACTIVE.[1]

"The trial was highly successful in showing that we can, at least in the laboratory, improve certain thinking and reasoning abilities in older people," says Richard M. Suzman, Ph.D., Associate Director for the Behavioral and Social Research Program at the National Institute on Aging (NIA). "The findings here were powerful and very specific. Although they did not appear to make any real change in the actual, daily activities of the participants, I think we can build on these results to see how training ultimately might be applied to tasks that older people do everyday, such as using medication or handling finances. This intervention research, aimed at helping healthy older people maintain cognitive status as they age, is an increasingly high priority."

The study, published in the November 13, 2002, issue of the *Journal of the American Medical Association*, was funded by the NIA and the National Institute of Nursing Research (NINR), two components

"Training Improves Cognitive Abilities of Older Adults," National Institute on Aging (NIA) News: Alzheimer's Disease Research Update, November 12, 2002.

of the National Institutes of Health at the Department of Health and Human Services.

According to Dr. Patricia A. Grady, Director of the NINR, "The ACTIVE trial provides encouraging preliminary findings that we may be able to conserve or improve some cognitive abilities in older adults not currently having problems in these areas. How this training may affect those who later experience cognitive deficits is a tantalizing question waiting to be answered."

The study looked at several types of cognitive training and then assessed, in the laboratory and in "real world" measures, whether the training was effective. At the outset, certified trainers conducted 10 sessions of 60 to 75 minutes over a 5- to 6-week period. The 2,802 participants were divided into four groups—three groups that received either memory training, reasoning training, or speed of processing training, and a fourth group that received no training. The three types of training were chosen because they showed the most promise in small laboratory studies and were related to tasks of daily living such as telephone use, shopping, food preparation, housekeeping, laundry, transportation, medication use, and personal finances. For all three groups, the training focused on developing strategies as well as providing exercises using these new strategies. All participants were assessed prior to training, immediately after training, and again 1 and 2 years later.

Those in the memory-training group were taught strategies for remembering word lists and sequences of items, text material, and main ideas and details of stories. Participants in the reasoning group were taught how to solve problems that follow patterns. Such strategies can be used in tasks such as reading a bus schedule or filling out an order sheet. Speed of processing training focused on the ability to identify and locate visual information quickly for use in tasks such as looking up a phone number, finding information on medicine bottles, and responding appropriately to traffic signs.

Immediately following the 5-week training period, 87 percent of participants in speed training, 74 percent of participants in reasoning training, and 26 percent of participants in memory training demonstrated reliable improvement on their respective cognitive ability. The training effects continued through 24 months, particularly for the participants who received "booster" training. "The improvements in memory, problem solving, and concentration following training were sizable," noted Karlene Ball, Ph.D., of the University of Alabama at Birmingham, the study's corresponding author. "These roughly counteract the degree of cognitive decline that we would expect to see over a 7- to 14-year period among older people without dementia."

The analysis did not find, however, that participants' improvements in thinking and reasoning also improved their ability to perform everyday tasks like preparing food or handling medications. "Since all participants were living independently, and most were functioning quite well at the outset of the study, it will be interesting to see if those who received training experience less decline in their daily living skills over time," Ball said.

The NIA leads the Federal effort supporting and conducting biomedical, clinical, social, and behavioral research on aging. This effort includes research into the causes and treatment of memory declines and other cognitive problems associated with age. Press releases, fact sheets, and other materials about aging and aging research can be viewed at the NIA's general information website, www.nia.nih.gov.

Note

1. The Advanced Cognitive Training for Independent and Vital Elderly (ACTIVE), a single-blind clinical trial, tested the effectiveness and durability of three techniques to improve the ability of older people to think and reason. ACTIVE investigators included Karlene Ball, Ph.D., Department of Psychology, University of Alabama at Birmingham and Daniel B. Berch, Ph.D., National Institute on Aging, (Current address NICHD.) Karin F. Helmers, Ph.D., National Institute of Nursing Research; Jared B. Jobe, Ph.D., National Heart, Lung and Blood Institute; Mary D. Leveck, Ph.D., National Institute of Nursing Research; Michael Marsiske, Ph.D., Institute on Aging and Departments of Health Policy and Epidemiology and Clinical and Health Psychology, University of Florida; John N. Morris, Ph.D., Hebrew Rehabilitation Center for the Aged; George W. Rebok, Ph.D., Department of Mental Hygiene, Johns Hopkins University; David M. Smith M.D., Department of Medicine, Indiana University School of Medicine; Sharon L. Tennstedt, Ph.D., New England Research Institutes; Frederick W. Unverzagt, Ph.D. Department of Psychiatry, Indiana University School of Medicine; Sherry L. Willis, Ph.D., Department of Human Development and Family Studies, Pennsylvania State University; the ACTIVE Study Group.

Chapter 73

Clinical Trials: What People with Alzheimer's Disease and Their Caregivers Should Know

Participating in a Clinical Trial

Rapid advances in our knowledge about Alzheimer's disease (AD) have led to the development of many new drugs and treatment strategies. However, before these new strategies can be adopted, they must be shown to work in patients. This means that clinical trials—studies in people to rigorously test how well a treatment works—have become an increasingly important part of AD research. Advances in treatment are only possible through the participation of patients and family members in clinical trials.

Clinical trials are the primary way that researchers find out if a promising treatment is safe and effective for patients. Clinical trials also tell researchers which treatments are more effective than others. Trials take place at private research facilities, teaching hospitals, specialized AD research centers, and doctors' offices.

Participating in a clinical trial is a big step for people with AD and their caregivers. That's why physicians and clinical trials staff spend lots of time talking with participants about what it's like to be in a trial and the pros and cons of participating. Here are some things that potential participants might want to know about clinical trials.

From "The Human Side of AD Research," excerpted from "Alzheimer's Disease: Unraveling the Mystery," Alzheimer's Disease Education and Referral (ADEAR) Center, a service of the National Institute on Aging, NIH Pub. No. 02-3782, October 2002. The full text of this document is available online at www.alzheimers.org/unraveling/index.htm.

What kind of trials are there?

- Treatment trials with existing drugs assess whether an already approved drug or compound is useful for other purposes. For example, one current trial is testing whether anti-inflammatory drugs already used to treat arthritis might help to prevent AD.

- Treatment trials with experimental drugs or strategies find out whether a brand new drug or treatment strategy can help improve cognitive function or lessen symptoms in people with AD, slow the progression to AD, or prevent it. Potential drugs tested in these trials are developed from knowledge about the mechanisms involved in the AD disease process. These compounds are rigorously tested in tissue culture and in animals for their action. Safety and effectiveness studies are also conducted in animals before the compounds are tested in humans.

What are the phases of clinical trials?

- During Phase I trials, a study team gives the treatment to a small number of volunteers and examines its action in the body, its safety, and its effects at various doses. Phase I trials generally last only a few months.

- If results show that the treatment appears safe, it will be tested in Phase II and Phase III clinical trials. These trials involve larger numbers of people over longer periods of time. In these trials, the study team wants to know whether the treatment is safe and effective and what side effects it might have.

After these phases are complete and investigators are satisfied that the treatment is safe and effective, the study team may submit its data to the Food and Drug Administration (FDA) for approval. The FDA reviews the data and decides whether to approve the drug or treatment for use in patients.

What happens when a person signs up for a clinical trial?

First it is important to learn about the study. Study staff explain the trial in detail to potential research participants and describe possible risks and benefits. Staff also talk about the participants' rights as research volunteers, including their right to leave the study at any time. Participants and their family members are entitled to have this information repeated and explained until they feel they understand the nature of the study and any potential risks.

Once all questions have been answered and if there is still interest in being a part of the study, a patient participant is asked to sign an informed consent form. Laws and regulations regarding informed consent differ across states and research institutions, but all are intended to ensure that patient participants are protected and well cared for.

In some cases, a patient participant may no longer be able to provide informed consent because of problems with memory and confusion. In such cases, it is still possible for an authorized representative (usually a family member) to give permission for the patient to participate. For example, the patient participant may have previously included research participation as part of his or her durable power of attorney. The person (proxy) exercising the durable power of attorney can decide to let the patient participate in a trial if they are convinced that the patient would have wanted to consent if able to do so. Even so, it is still important that patients assent to be in the study, even if they can no longer formally consent to it. Different states have different laws about who is a legal representative. These laws are in a state of flux as researchers and the public grapple with the ethical issues of proxy consent.

Next, patients go through a screening process to see if they qualify to participate in the study. If they qualify and can safely participate, they can proceed with the other parts of the study.

What happens during a trial?

If participants agree to join the study and the screening process shows they're a good match, they have a "baseline" visit with the study staff. This visit generally involves a full physical exam and extensive cognitive and physical tests. This give the study team information against which to measure future mental and physical changes. Participants also receive the test drug or treatment. As the study progresses, participating patients and family members usually must follow strict medication or treatment instructions and keep detailed records of symptoms. Every so often, participants visit the clinic or research center to have physical and cognitive exams, give blood and urine samples, and talk with study staff. These visits allow the investigators to assess the effects of the test drug or treatment, see how the disease is progressing, and see how the participant and the caregiver are doing.

In most clinical trials, participants are randomly assigned to a study group. One group, the test group, receives the experimental drug. Other groups may receive a different drug or a placebo (an inactive substance that looks like the study drug). Having the different groups is important because only by comparing them can researchers be confident that changes in the test group are the result of the experimental treatment and not some other factor. In many trials, no one—not even the study team—knows who is getting the experimental drug and who is getting the placebo or other drug. This is called "masking" meaning that the patient/family member and the staff are "blind" to the treatment being received.

What should people consider before participating in a clinical trial?

Expectations and motivations. Clinical trials generally don't have miraculous results. The test drug or treatment may relieve a symptom, change a clinical measurement, or reduce the risk of death. With a complex disease like AD, it is unlikely that one drug will cure or prevent the disease. Some people choose not to participate or drop out of a study because this reality doesn't meet their expectations. Others participate because they realize that even if the benefit to them may be slight, they are making a valuable contribution to knowledge that will help future patients.

Uncertainty. Some families have a hard time with the uncertainties of participation—not knowing whether the person is on the test drug or the placebo, not being able to choose which study group to be in, not knowing for a long time whether the study was successful or not. Ongoing and open communication with study staff can help to counter this frustration.

Finding the right clinical trial. Some clinical trials want participants who are cognitively healthy or have only mild symptoms because they are testing a drug that might delay the decline in cognitive function. Other trials are interested in working with participants who have more advanced AD because they are testing a drug that might lessen behavioral symptoms, or they are testing new strategies to help caregivers. Even though a participant may not be eligible for one trial, another trial may be just right.

The biggest benefit of all. Many families find that the biggest benefit of participating in a clinical trial is the regular contact with the study team. These visits provide an opportunity to get state-of-the-art AD care and also to talk on an ongoing basis with experts in AD who have lots of practical experience and a broad perspective on the disease. The study team understands and can provide advice on the emotional and physical aspects of the person with AD and the caregivers' experience. They can suggest ways to cope with the present and give insights into what to expect in the future. They also can share information about support groups and other helpful resources.

Additional Information about Clinical Trials

For more information about AD clinical trials, visit the NIA's Alzheimer's Disease Education and Referral (ADEAR) Center's Clinical Trials Database website (www.alzheimers.org/trials/index.html). This website includes a list of clinical trials on Alzheimer's disease and dementia currently in progress at centers throughout the U.S. It also provides information on the phases of clinical trials and how to participate, and explains the drug development process. The site also provides links to other useful websites with related information. For additional information, visit the clinical trials websites of the Alzheimer's Association www.alz.org/ResourceCenter/ByTopic/Research.htm and the National Institutes of Health www.clinicaltrials.gov.

Chapter 74

Alzheimer's Disease:
Current Clinical Trials

CX516 (Ampalex)

What is CX516?

CX516 (Ampalex) is a drug under investigation as a potential treatment for the cognitive symptoms of Alzheimer's disease. It belongs to a new class of drugs called ampakines, which are being developed by researchers at Cortex Pharmaceuticals, Inc.

How is CX516 designed to treat Alzheimer's?

CX516 may benefit Alzheimer symptoms by enhancing the activity of AMPA receptors, one type of "docking site" that attaches the specialized messenger chemical glutamate. At normal concentrations, glutamate attachment to AMPA receptors plays a key role in learning and memory. Subnormal glutamate levels interfere with learning and memory, while excess glutamate "overstimulates" the cell, leading to cell death. Alzheimer's disease may involve both excesses and deficiencies of glutamate at different times and under different circumstances. CX516 may compensate for decreased

"Fact Sheet: CX516 (Ampalex)," "Fact Sheet: Leteprinim Potassium," "Fact Sheet: Memantine," (revised June 2003) and "Fact Sheet: COGNIShunt™," (revised April 2003) are reprinted with permission of the Alzheimer's Association. For additional information, call the Alzheimer's Association national toll-free number, 800-272-3900, or visit their website at www.alz.org. © 2002–2003 Alzheimer's Association. All rights reserved.

glutamate by enhancing the ability of AMPA receptors to respond to available levels.

What progress has been made in CX516 research?

In Phase I clinical trials, CX516 appeared to be well tolerated and was observed to enhance learning and memory in small groups of healthy young and elderly adults. In current Phase II clinical trials, CX516 is being tested again for safety and for effectiveness in improving cognitive skills in people with Alzheimer's disease.

You can find details about the design and purpose of this trial, criteria for participation, and a list of enrollment centers at ClinicalTrials.gov (http://www.clinicaltrials.gov).

Leteprinim Potassium

What is leteprinim potassium (Neotrofin®)?

Leteprinim potassium (Neotrofin®) is a drug under development by NeoTherapeutics of Irvine, California, to repair and regenerate nerve cells damaged by spinal cord injury, Parkinson's disease, the effects of some chemotherapy drugs, and, until recently, Alzheimer's disease. In preclinical studies, leteprinim showed promise in restoring nerve function in animal models of aging, memory decline, and brain and spinal cord injury. Phase I trials enrolling small numbers of people offered preliminary evidence that leteprinim is safe and well tolerated in human recipients.

NeoTherapeutics then advanced leteprinim to Phase II trials to assess effectiveness, determine optimal dosage, and gain further safety data. In April 2001, the company began recruiting participants for a large U.S. Phase II study enrolling 500 people with mild to moderate Alzheimer's at 52 locations nationwide. On April 30, 2002, the company announced that preliminary analysis of study data revealed that some individuals taking leteprinim showed improvement on tests of mental status and general functioning. However, overall, leteprinim did not perform well enough compared to a placebo (inactive treatment) to meet U.S. Food and Drug Administration (FDA) standards for approving a drug as an Alzheimer's disease treatment.

As a result, the company says that it will suspend all further tests of leteprinim in people with Alzheimer's until it can find a partner to help underwrite such studies. Alvin J. Glasky, PhD, chairman and chief executive officer of NeoTherapeutics, expressed optimism that future trials involving different doses of medication or timing of doses might document a more robust effect of leteprinim as an Alzheimer treatment. In the meantime, NeoTherapeutics will continue studies exploring leteprinim as a treatment for Parkinson's disease, spinal cord injury, and chemotherapy-induced nerve damage.

How does leteprinim work?

Nerve cells produce nerve growth factors, proteins that regulate cell maturation during prenatal development and also play an important role in cell survival, repair, and regeneration during adult life. Because of their significance in cell maintenance and repair, these factors have attracted attention as potential treatments in Alzheimer's disease, stroke, spinal cord injury, and other neurodegenerative conditions. However, nerve growth factors are too large to cross the blood-brain barrier, a protective shield that restricts passage of molecules to the brain. Scientists seek to overcome this difficulty by designing small molecules that cross the blood-brain barrier and mimic the effects of nerve growth factors when they are taken by mouth or injected. The active ingredient in leteprinim is one such small molecule that successfully crosses the blood-brain barrier, where it activates genes that produce nerve growth factors.

What drugs are available now to treat symptoms of Alzheimer's?

The FDA currently approves four drugs specifically to treat symptoms of Alzheimer's disease-tacrine (Cognex®), donepezil (Aricept®), rivastigmine (Exelon®), and galantamine (Reminyl®). All of these drugs are cholinesterase inhibitors that work by increasing the brain's supply of acetylcholine, a specialized chemical messenger produced and secreted by nerve cells that are deficient in people with Alzheimer's disease. There are also several other experimental Alzheimer drugs under investigation. To obtain a fact sheet about cholinesterase inhibitors or trials currently enrolling participants, please call the Alzheimer's Association Contact Center at 1-800-272-3900, or visit the website at www.alz.org.

How can you learn more about the leteprinim (Neotrofin®) trial?

For further information about the trial or to be considered for participation please call the NeoTherapeutics clinical trials hotline at 949-788-6700, extension 300. You may also request details on-line at http://www.neotherapeutics.com. A list of study centers and contacts will help you identify research sites near you.

Memantine

Memantine is a drug developed by the German company Merz + Co. for treatment of symptoms of dementia. The drug has been approved in Germany for more than 10 years, where it is marketed by Merz under the trade name Axura®. In May 2002, the European Union's Committee for Proprietary Medicinal Products approved memantine for treatment of moderately severe to severe Alzheimer's throughout the European Union, where it is marketed by Lundbeck as Ebixa®.

Memantine appears to regulate the activity of glutamate, one of the brain's specialized messenger chemicals that affects the activity of several different types of receptors (cell-surface "docking sites"), including AMPA and NMDA receptors. At normal concentrations, glutamate plays an essential role in learning and memory by attaching to AMPA receptors. This attachment triggers NMDA receptors to allow a certain amount of calcium to flow into a cell.

Subnormal glutamate levels may interfere with learning and memory by leading to insufficient AMPA receptor activity. Excess glutamate, on the other hand, overstimulates AMPA receptors, which in turn leads NMDA receptors to allow excess calcium to flow into cells. Excess calcium causes cell disruption and cell death. Alzheimer's disease may involve both excesses and deficiencies of glutamate at different times and under different circumstances. Memantine may protect against excess glutamate by blocking NMDA receptors, preventing calcium from flowing into cells. It also may increase the activity of AMPA receptors when glutamate levels are low, supporting learning and memory.

Memantine's action in the glutamate system differs from the activity of the cholinesterase inhibitors that are currently approved in the United States for treatment of Alzheimer's. Cholinesterase inhibitors temporarily boost levels of acetylcholine, another messenger chemical that becomes deficient in the Alzheimer brain. These differing modes of action raise the possibility that individuals may be able to take memantine either as stand-alone therapy or in combination with cholinesterase inhibitors.

Where is memantine in the drug development process?

Memantine is now under development by Forest Laboratories, Inc., for marketing in the United States. Three recent trials of memantine have already been completed—one in Latvia, one U.S. Phase III trial testing memantine as a stand-alone treatment, and another Phase III trial testing memantine in combination with donepezil (Aricept®), a cholinesterase inhibitor marketed by Eisai, Inc., and Pfizer, Inc. In the single-therapy trial, participants with moderate to severe Alzheimer's who received 10 milligrams of memantine twice a day during the six months of the study showed significantly less decline in thinking skills and ability to perform daily self-care activities than enrollees who received a placebo (a similar but inactive treatment).

Data from the combination therapy trial, which enrolled more than 400 participants with moderate to severe Alzheimer's disease at 37 U.S. study centers, suggest that individuals who received both memantine and donepezil fared better in terms of their thinking skills and ability to perform daily activities than those who took donepezil and a placebo. These results have been presented at a professional psychopharmacology conference and at the April 2003 meeting of the American Academy of Neurology, but still need to undergo peer review and be published in a scientific journal before they attain the stature of the stand-alone studies.

In June 2003, Forest reported preliminary results from another combination therapy trial enrolling participants with mild to moderate Alzheimer's who were also taking any of three commonly prescribed cholinesterase inhibitors-donepezil (Aricept®), galantamine (Reminyl®), or rivastigmine (Exelon®). According to the company, participants receiving memantine in combination with a cholinesterase inhibitor did not experience any greater benefit in cognition or overall function than those who received a cholinesterase inhibitor and a placebo. These preliminary results suggest that memantine may not be as effective in mild to moderate Alzheimer's as was previously demonstrated in more severely ill individuals. This data has not been peer reviewed or presented in a professional forum.

Two additional nationwide Phase III trials of treatment with memantine alone remain ongoing, one involving individuals with mild to moderate Alzheimer's and one enrolling participants in moderate to severe stages. In December 2002, Forest submitted its new drug application (NDA) to the U.S. Food and Drug Administration (FDA). The NDA, which is the formal request for approval in treating moderate to severe Alzheimer's disease, presents for the FDA's review all of the company's data gathered so far during the drug development process. According to Forest, the FDA "accepted the NDA for filing" on January 30, 2003. The FDA now has 10 months from January 30 to approve memantine or issue a letter finding the drug "not approvable" or "approvable." A "not approvable" letter details defects in the data or the submission that are too serious to fix. An "approvable" determination finds that the drug can ultimately be approved, pending corrections to the submission.

COGNIShunt™

What is COGNIShunt?

COGNIShunt® is a device under investigation as a possible treatment of Alzheimer's disease. It is designed to drain cerebrospinal fluid (CSF) from the skull and into the abdominal cavity. CSF is the protective fluid that fills the empty spaces around the brain and spinal cord. COGNIShunt is similar to the shunt used to treat hydrocephalus, a condition in which an accumulation of CSF results in enlargement of the skull and pressure on the brain.

COGNIShunt is not commercially available for sale or distribution. It is being evaluated per an Investigational Device Exemption (IDE) granted by the U.S. Food and Drug Administration. An IDE permits a device to be shipped in interstate commerce for clinical investigation to determine its medical safety and effectiveness.

What is the premise of a shunt treatment?

CSF is naturally produced and absorbed, but the cycle of "refreshing" declines with age. The researchers investigating the shunt procedure have hypothesized that toxic factors may accumulate in the CSF of an individual with Alzheimer's, contributing to brain cell damage. These factors may include beta-amyloid protein fragments and abnormally altered tau proteins. The shunt treatment is expected to drain off toxic elements and allow the CSF to be replenished.

What research results have been reported to date?

Results of a Phase I/II pilot trial were published in *Neurology* in October 2002 ("Assessment of low-flow CSF drainage as a treatment for AD: Results of a randomized pilot study." *Neurology* 2002, 59:1139–1145). In this study, 15 participants were randomly selected to receive the shunt implantation, and 14 people received no investigational treatment. All participants had been diagnosed with mild to moderate Alzheimer's disease. Subjects were followed for one year.

The primary objective of the pilot study was to assess the safety of the shunt procedure. Side effects among the 15 people receiving the surgical treatment included seizures (2 participants), shunt infection (1), small injury in the abdomen during surgery (1), severe postoperative headache (1), postoperative pain (8), nausea (7), headache (5), abdominal pain (5), and blockage in a shunt (3).

Cognitive assessment tests were done every three months. The researchers noted a trend that symptoms were stabilized in people who received the treatment and a decline in people who did not receive treatment. The assessment of effectiveness included 11 people who received the shunt and 12 people who did not. This sample is too small to make definitive statements about the benefits of the treatment.

What additional research is needed?

Eunoe, Inc., the maker of COGNIShunt, is conducting additional clinical trials to assess the safety and effectiveness of the treatment and to test the hypothesis that the toxic factors in CSF contribute to the destruction of brain cells in Alzheimer's disease.

Additional research is needed to determine if surgery is a viable option for individuals with dementia. Any surgical procedure involves risks, which can be further complicated when an individual may have difficulty understanding those risks. Also, the risks of surgery need to be weighed against the potential long-term benefit of a procedure.

It is important for both the individual with Alzheimer's and family members to understand the conditions of an informed consent for participating in a clinical trial involving surgery.

Update Note

The Alzheimer's Association provides updates as the testing and review processes move forward. The latest version is always available on the Alzheimer's Association's website at http://www.alz.org/ResourceCenter or by calling 800-272-3900. Information about Memantine can be obtained by calling Forest Laboratories directly at 800-678-1605 and asking for the Professional Affairs Division.

Chapter 75

Clinical Antipsychotic Trials of Intervention Effectiveness (CATIE)

About the CATIE Trial for Psychiatric Alzheimer Symptoms

What is the CATIE Alzheimer trial?

CATIE (Clinical Antipsychotic Trials of Intervention Effectiveness) is a nationwide multicenter trial sponsored by the U.S. National Institute of Mental Health (NIMH). The goal of the CATIE Alzheimer's disease trial is to compare the effectiveness of four different medications in treating delusions, agitation, aggression, hallucinations, and other serious disruptions in thinking and behavior that may occur in Alzheimer's disease. The four study medications are already approved by the U.S. Food and Drug Administration (FDA) to treat symptoms of major mental illnesses characterized by serious disruptions in individuals' ability to perceive and interpret the world around them.

Although symptoms of these mental illnesses are in some ways similar to behavioral and psychiatric symptoms of Alzheimer's disease, few clinical studies have tested whether drugs used to treat these conditions are helpful for treating Alzheimer symptoms. Even fewer studies have directly compared the effectiveness of one of these drugs to the benefits of another.

The four drugs involved in this trial are olanzapine (Zyprexa), quetiapine (Seroquel), risperidone (Risperdal), and citalopram (Celexa). The study is designed so enrollees can try each medication until they find the one that may be most helpful for them. Participants will initially be assigned to take one of the study drugs or a placebo (inactive treatment). After two weeks, those assigned to the placebo group will be assigned to one of the active treatments if they have not improved, and enrollees who have not improved on one of the active drugs may switch to another. As the trial progresses, participants who improve on a study medication may stay on it, and those who do not benefit will be offered another active treatment.

Study medications and related medical care will be provided free, and transportation reimbursement is available. In addition, the study team will coordinate care with the participant's regular health care professional. Participants and their caregivers will also receive basic counseling, psychological support, advice on managing challenging behavior, education, and skill development.

Who may participate in this trial?

Individuals with Alzheimer's disease may be eligible to participate if they are experiencing one or more of the following symptoms:

- Delusions or irrational ideas, such as believing that "someone is out to get them" or that their caregivers are not who they say they are

- Agitation—being restless or easily upset

- Physically or verbally aggressive behavior

- Hallucinations—seeing or hearing things that are not actually there

Participants must also have a family member or caregiver available to accompany them to approximately 12 clinic visits over nine months. With some exceptions, enrollees will be allowed to continue taking medications for Alzheimer's disease and other health conditions. There are study sites in Alabama, California, Connecticut, Florida, Georgia, Hawaii, Illinois, Iowa, Louisiana, Maryland, Missouri, New Jersey, New York, North Carolina, Ohio, Pennsylvania, South Carolina, and Texas.

Where can I get more information?

To find a site near you or to request an information sheet prepared by CATIE, please call the Alzheimer's Association Contact Center at 800-272-3900 or visit the CATIE Website at http://www.catie.unc.edu/home.htm. Information about the trial, including a complete list of sites, can also be accessed through the Clinical Trials section of the Alzheimer's Association website at www.alz.org.

Chapter 76

Alzheimer's Disease Cooperative Study (ADCS)

As part of intensifying efforts to expand and expedite the search for Alzheimer's disease (AD) treatments, the National Institute on Aging (NIA) has awarded $54 million to support the Alzheimer's Disease Cooperative Study (ADCS), a national consortium of medical research centers and clinics. The network of 83 sites in the U.S. and Canada, coordinated by the University of California, San Diego (UCSD), will develop improved diagnostic tools and test a variety of drugs to slow down the progression of AD or prevent the disease altogether.

The consortium was first organized in 1991 under a cooperative agreement between NIA, part of the National Institutes of Health, and UCSD. During its first decade, thc ADCS put in place an infrastructure of leading researchers to carry out clinical trials for promising new therapies for AD, developed new and more reliable ways to evaluate patients enrolled in these and other studies, and initiated a number of clinical trials. This next 5-year award will allow that work to continue and will move AD treatment research in new directions, including the study of a cholesterol-lowering statin drug, an antioxidant, and a high-dose vitamin regimen. The ADCS will also develop evaluation tools for AD prevention research.

"Basic and epidemiological studies over just the past few years have given us important clues about compounds that might prove more

"Alzheimer's Disease Clinical Trials Expanded, Expedited," *NIA News: Alzheimer's Disease Research Update*, National Institute on Aging (NIH), September 20, 2001.

effective against AD," says Neil Buckholtz, Ph.D., chief of the Dementias of Aging Branch at the NIA and project officer for the ADCS. "This award will help us test out a number of these possibilities quickly and reliably so that we can give clinicians, patients, and families new weapons in the fight against Alzheimer's disease." A degenerative disorder of the brain, AD is a devastating disease that robs its victims of memory and causes cognitive failure, leading to total dependence and, ultimately, death. It is estimated that as many as 4 million Americans suffer from AD.

Leon Thal, M.D., chair of the Department of Neurosciences at the UCSD School of Medicine and principal investigator of the ADCS, notes that some 2,500 people have participated in 13 ADCS research studies over the past decade. Their contribution, he says, has greatly informed medical practice, as ADCS findings over the past few years have suggested what may—and what may not—work against the disease. Previous ADCS studies have looked at the use of vitamin E, the anti-Parkinson's disease drug selegiline, and estrogen, among other drugs.

Several studies are continuing or are being initiated in the 5-year effort. These include:

- Vitamin E and donepezil—This ongoing prevention trial, begun in 1999, examines whether vitamin E, an antioxidant, or donepezil, an agent that slows the breakdown of the neurotransmitter acetylcholine, may keep patients with Mild Cognitive Impairment from "converting" to AD. Some 700 patients are participating.

- Statins—This new study will test evidence from population and animal research that cholesterol might play a role in AD development. Patients with mild or moderate AD taking a cholesterol-lowering statin drug will be compared with AD patients of similar age and stage after 1 year to see if the use of the drug slowed down the progression of clinical signs of AD.

- High-dose folate/B_6/B_{12} supplements—Research has shown that blood levels of homocysteine may be elevated in AD patients. This study is an 18-month clinical trial designed to test whether reducing homocysteine levels with the high-dose vitamin supplements can slow the rate of cognitive decline in people with AD.

- Valproate—Psychiatric symptoms associated with AD include agitation and psychosis, especially in later stages of the disease. In this 2-year trial, scientists will study whether low-dose valproate, an anti-convulsant drug, can help delay the emergence of agitation and psychosis. They will look at whether valproate may delay clinical progression of AD as well, in light of new studies suggesting that the drug may also be neuroprotective.

- Indole-3-Propionic Acid (IPA)—IPA, a highly potent, naturally occurring anti-oxidant, has been shown to interfere with the action of enzymes contributing to amyloid plaque formation, a hallmark of AD. This preliminary study will look at the safety and tolerability of IPA in patients with AD.

- Improved Assessment Measures—ADCS researchers will continue their work developing new or improved measures for evaluating the clinical effectiveness of drugs being tested for prevention or treatment of AD.

The NIA leads the Federal effort to support and conduct basic, clinical, and social and behavioral studies on AD. It also supports the Alzheimer's Disease Education and Referral (ADEAR) Center, which provides information on clinical trials and other research to the public, health professionals, and media. ADEAR can be contacted toll free at 1-800-438-4380 weekdays during business hours or by viewing www.alzheimers.org. As these clinical trials move forward and begin recruiting patients, the public will be able to find out more about participation through the ADEAR Center's Clinical Trials Database.

A directory of Alzheimer's Disease Centers can be found in Chapter 82.

Chapter 77

Brain Autopsy:
The Gift of Knowledge

The word "autopsy" stems from the Greek word autopsia, meaning to see with one's own eyes. Researchers have made significant progress in developing accurate tests to detect AD in living patients, and as a result, a diagnosis of "probable" AD now can be made with up to 90 percent certainty in specialized research facilities. However, the disease can be diagnosed conclusively only by examining the brain after death in an autopsy to see for sure the characteristic plaques and tangles that define AD. Autopsy provides valuable information that can educate and enlighten families, physicians, and researchers, who are working to discover more reliable tests for AD. Information gained from autopsies is a vital part of the research conducted at the Alzheimer's Disease Centers (ADCs) supported by the National Institute on Aging (NIA). The autopsy results of AD patients who have been followed over time at an ADC are especially valuable. For these patients, doctors usually have substantial treatment and care history which can give them insights into the disease course and provide information essential to the search for effective treatments and an eventual cure for AD. In the past, brain tissue samples were essential for AD research because no animal model for AD existed. According to University of Pennsylvania ADC Director John Q. Trojanowski, M.D., Ph.D. "Autopsy may be even more important today than in the past. The animal models we now have for AD provide a good "caricature"

"Brain Autopsy: The Gift of Knowledge," *Connections*, Vol. 9(1), Winter 2001. *Connections* is a publication of the Alzheimer's Disease Education and Referral Center (ADEAR), a service of the National Institute on Aging.

of the disease, but it is essential that we be able to compare them to actual diseased human brain tissue obtained through autopsy." Marcelle Morrison-Bogorad, Ph.D., Associate Director of Neuroscience and Neuropsychology of Aging Program, NIA agrees with Dr. Trojanowski and adds, "Ultimately, this research will uncover the chain of events that leads to AD and related dementias. Many families of dementia patients make the commitment in order to help further AD research by agreeing to donate the brain for research. It is vitally important that people without brain disorders also make tissue donations, so that we can understand how healthy brains work."

Benefits of Autopsy

To Families: Advancing medical knowledge often is cited as the most important benefit of autopsy. Family members also may feel a sense of relief once they know the exact cause of death and that their loved one was given appropriate care during his or her illness. Findings from an autopsy can help family members understand genetic risk factors that can be associated with AD and related dementias, and provide an opportunity for genetic counseling. Participation in brain autopsy can help family members attach meaning and purpose to the suffering that occurs with AD and related dementias. Autopsy can provide family members and loved ones with a sense of closure to facilitate the grieving process.

To Researchers and the Medical Community: Autopsy provides an important quality control tool by confirming the diagnosis. In AD clinical trials, autopsy results help researchers confirm that the people in the trial actually had AD and not some other dementia. Autopsy results can help researchers develop and test better, more accurate diagnostic tools. Autopsies of non-demented persons and those in the early stages of AD can help scientists pinpoint the earliest signs of age-related brain changes and how they differ from brain changes in early AD. Research of this type may lead to interventions that might help in the earliest stages.

To Society: Autopsies provide more accurate disease rates of dementia, including vital statistics for State and national registries. Accurate diagnostic data from autopsy can provide information to those who advocate for laws and funding in support of AD patients and their families. As a result, society as a whole may benefit by additional services designed to ease the burden caused by AD and related dementias.

Planning for an Autopsy

The time immediately after the death of a family member is stressful and is not the best time to start making decisions about an autopsy. Planning ahead allows family members time to reach a decision and prepare the needed paperwork. Putting things in place before the person's death helps ensure that brain tissue can be removed promptly. A variety of professionals can help make the process of donating tissue through an autopsy service easier. Social workers, nurses, and other support staff at the ADCs are available to answer questions about the donation in advance. This may ease the decision-making process for the family. Often, ADCs have designated an autopsy coordinator who helps people through the entire process. Once a decision to donate brain tissue is made, paperwork giving consent can start. If the patient is in a nursing home or other long-term care facility, staff there should be notified in advance of the family's wishes. Next, a funeral home is selected and notified of the arrangement. Usually, within several weeks of the autopsy, a written report is presented to the family. The physician or support staff at the autopsy service often are available to discuss the findings. For more information about planning for an autopsy or becoming involved in a research study, families may contact any ADC. Each of the ADCs provides autopsy services to patients who have participated in their research programs. Some of the ADCs offer broader autopsy services to patients who have been seen and followed by an ADC physician. In some cases, they will provide autopsy services to others by request. Many of the ADCs refer patients from outside their programs to the pathology departments of their institutions. Typically, this is a fee-for-service arrangement. Other ADCs refer families to local Alzheimer's Association chapters, area brain banks, and State medical examiners.

Frequently Asked Questions about Brain Autopsy

Who should get an autopsy?

AD patients and research volunteers without dementia.

When should the autopsy be performed?

As soon as possible after death. The family should contact the autopsy coordinator immediately—day or night and send them the signed consent form.

511

Will the autopsy procedure disfigure the body and delay the funeral?

No. The physician, a pathologist, removes the brain through an incision in the back of the head. The face is never touched or scarred during the procedure. An open casket is still an option. The examination will not delay preparation of the body for burial.

Hasn't the patient suffered enough?

The person who has died suffered a great deal during his or her illness, but it is important to remember that he or she is no longer suffering and that the autopsy will provide valuable information to those who survive.

Are there religious objections to brain donations?

Often, there are cultural or religious concerns that practitioners need to address in order to help the family feel more at ease with the decision. Most religions and cultural traditions agree that organ donation is valuable. Your own religious advisor is the best person to guide you. You are encouraged to talk with your own minister, priest, or rabbi.

Who may grant permission for an autopsy?

The consent for an autopsy is legally binding only when it is signed after death by the legal next-of-kin. Check with your lawyer or the facility performing the autopsy since these laws differ for each State. The following is an example of persons, in order of priority, who may provide such consent:

- Spouse
- Adult son or daughter
- Either parent
- Adult brother or sister
- Guardian of the deceased at the time of death
- Any other person authorized or under obligation to dispose of the body

What can the family expect to learn from the autopsy report?

The report will explain the final diagnosis and any major changes found in the brain. It will say whether or not the diagnosis of Alzheimer's disease was confirmed and if there were any other conditions affecting the brain. The primary, attending physician, or pathologist can interpret the report.

How much will the brain autopsy cost the family?

Costs usually range from $500 to $1,500 (can be higher) for the autopsy, which does not include transportation costs. Research programs at medical institutions like the ADCs offer free services to those who qualify.

Autopsy Resources

Dementia Postmortem Network, Websites, and ADC Autopsy Program Directory

The Michigan Dementia Postmortem Network helps families of people in Michigan who are affected by dementing diseases. It was established to help people to obtain an autopsy. The network includes four types of medical professionals and volunteers: referral liaisons, autopsy liaisons, pathologists, and neuropathologists. Each is trained to help families by providing a specific service. Referral liaisons—usually social workers, nurses, or Alzheimer's Association chapter volunteers—provide general information about brain autopsy in Michigan and help the family complete enrollment. Autopsy liaisons—often pathology assistants or funeral directors—help coordinate arrangements for the autopsy. Services include obtaining patient medical information and consent for autopsy, and helping the family arrange transportation for the body. At autopsy, pathologists (doctors specializing in the study of tissue) remove the brain. Neuropathologists (doctors with additional training in studying brain tissue) examine the brain cells, make a diagnosis, and complete an autopsy report for the patient's physician and family. The Michigan Dementia Postmortem Network serves Michigan residents, but it has an informative website available to families and professionals across the country. The Website, http://www.mdpn.msu.edu/ includes information about the value of autopsy, answers frequently asked questions and offers guidance on how to talk to other family members about whether to have an autopsy performed. On the website, network advisors emphasize the importance of deciding in advance whether to request a brain autopsy and include a checklist for family members considering autopsy. The Network's website also provides information, referrals, a list of publications, and recommendations from the Michigan Postmortem Examination Workgroup. All of the information on the site is free to the public. The following is a sample of other websites that offer information about brain autopsy.

List of Websites

Alzheimer's Association List of Local Chapters
http://www.alz.org/findchapter.asp

Alzheimer's Association San Diego Chapter
http://www.sanalz.org/support_services/services7.html

The Diagnostic Center for Alzheimer's Disease and Neuropathology Laboratory at the University of Oklahoma Health Sciences Center in Oklahoma City Autopsy Network
http://w3.ouhsc.edu/pathology/deptlabs/
diagnostic_center_for_alzheimer.htm#Autopsy Assistance Network

Tulane University Medical Center Autopsy Service
http://www.mcl.tulane.edu

Florida Alzheimer's Disease Initiative Brain Bank (affiliated with Suncoast Gerontology Center)
http://www.med.usf.edu/suncoast/alzheimer

University of Virginia Health Services Department of Neurology Brain Research Facility
http://www.med.virginia.edu/medicine/clinical/neurology/facilities/
brain-resource.html

A Checklist for Family Members

- Discuss the autopsy decision with all involved family members, physician(s), your religious leader, and/or people in your support group.

- Identify the patient's legal next-of-kin.

- Obtain a consent form from the facility that will perform the autopsy.

- Keep a copy of the consent form in an accessible place.

514

- Give your family members and physician a copy of the consent form.

- Become familiar with the procedure for signing the consent form at the time of death. Though you will not sign the consent form until after death occurs, it will be helpful to identify the method you will use.

- Request to place an information sheet that explains the procedures to follow at the time of death and an alert sticker in the patient's chart.

- Give your family members a copy of the procedures to be followed at the time of death.

- Find out who you need to call at the time of death and how to reach the appropriate person during the daytime, evening hours, weekends, or holidays.

- Discuss arrangements and costs involved with transportation of the body with the facility performing the autopsy.

- Contact the funeral director and explain that you are planning a brain-only autopsy for your family member.

- Notify the director or administrator, director of nursing, hospice nurse, and social worker of the nursing home or other institution of your plans for autopsy (if applicable).

- Notify the physician who will need to complete required paperwork.

Alzheimer's Disease Centers Autopsy Program Directory

The National Institute on Aging currently funds 30 Alzheimer's Disease Centers (ADC's) at major medical institutions across the Nation. Researchers at these Centers are working to translate research advances into improved care and diagnosis for Alzheimer's Disease (AD) patients while, at the same time, focusing on the program's long-term goal—finding a way to cure and possibly prevent AD.

Areas of investigation range from the basic mechanisms of AD to managing the symptoms and helping families cope with the effects of the disease. Center staff conduct basic, clinical, and behavioral research.

Each of the ADCs provides autopsy services to dementia patients and volunteers without dementia who are enrolled in clinical research studies and trials. Some of the ADCs offer autopsy services to a broader range of people in the community both with and without dementia.

Autopsies of non-demented persons and those in the early stages of AD are helping ADC researchers find the first signs of age-related brain changes and how they may differ from brain changes in early AD. Research of this type may lead to interventions that might help in the first stages of the disease. For patients and families affected by AD, many ADC's offer:

- Opportunities for AD patients and those without dementia to volunteer to participate in drug trials and other clinical research projects.

- Diagnostic and medical management (costs may vary). Many Centers accept Medicare, Medicaid, and private insurance.

- Opportunities for AD patients and their families to participate in support groups and other special programs.

For more information, you may contact any of the Alzheimer's Disease Centers. For the most current listing of the ADCs visit the ADEAR Center's website at: http://alzheimers.org/pubs/adcdir.html.

Part Seven

Additional Help and Information

Chapter 78

Glossary of Terms Related to Alzheimer's Disease and Other Dementias

To help you better understand some of the terminology used to describe aspects of Alzheimer's disease, the Alzheimer's Association has developed this glossary of frequently used terms.

A

abilities: Level at which certain actions and activities can be carried out.

acetylcholine: A neurotransmitter that appears to be involved in learning and memory. Acetylcholine is severely diminished in the brains of persons with Alzheimer's disease.

activities of daily living (ADLs): Personal care activities necessary for everyday living, such as eating, bathing, grooming, dressing, and toileting. People with dementia may not be able to perform necessary functions without assistance. Professionals often assess a person's ADLs to determine what type of care is needed.

adult day services: Programs that provide participants with opportunities to interact with others, usually in a community center or facility. Staff lead various activities such as music programs and support groups. Transportation is often provided.

advance directives: Written documents, completed and signed when a person is legally competent, that explain a person's medical wishes in advance, allowing someone else to make treatment decisions on his or her behalf later in the disease process.

adverse reaction: An unexpected effect of drug treatment that may range from trivial to serious or life-threatening, such as an allergic reaction.

age-matched controls: See controls.

agent: The individual—usually a trusted family member or friend—authorized by a power of attorney to make legal decisions for another individual. In scientific terms, "agent" sometimes refers to a drug as well.

aggression: Hitting, pushing, or threatening behavior that commonly occurs when a caregiver attempts to help an individual with Alzheimer's with daily activities, such as dressing. It is important to control such behavior because aggressive persons can cause injury to themselves and others.

agitation: Vocal or motor behavior (screaming, shouting, complaining, moaning, cursing, pacing, fidgeting, wandering, etc.) that is disruptive, unsafe, or interferes with the delivery of care in a particular environment. An abnormal behavior is considered agitation only if it poses risk or discomfort to the individual with Alzheimer's or his/her caregiver. Agitation can be a nonspecific symptom of one or more physical or psychological problems (e.g., headache, depression).

allele: One of two or more alternative forms of a gene; for example, one allele of the gene for eye color codes for blue eyes, while another allele codes for brown eyes.

Alzheimer's disease: A progressive, neurodegenerative disease characterized by loss of function and death of nerve cells in several areas of the brain, leading to loss of mental functions such as memory and learning. Alzheimer's disease is the most common cause of dementia.

ambulation: The ability to walk and move about freely.

amino acids: The basic building blocks of proteins. Genes contain the code for assembling protein of the 20 amino acids necessary for human growth and function.

amyloid: A protein deposit associated with tissue degeneration; amyloid is found in the brains of individuals with Alzheimer's.

amyloid plaque: Abnormal cluster of dead and dying nerve cells, other brain cells, and amyloid protein fragments. Amyloid plaques are one of the characteristic structural abnormalities found in the brains of individuals with Alzheimer's. Upon autopsy, the presence of amyloid plaques and neurofibrillary tangles is used to positively diagnose Alzheimer's.

amyloid precursor protein (APP): A protein found in the brain, heart, kidneys, lungs, spleen, and intestines. The normal function of APP in the body is unknown. In Alzheimer's disease, APP is abnormally processed and converted to beta amyloid protein. Beta amyloid is the protein deposited in amyloid plaques.

animal models: Normal animals modified mechanically, genetically, or chemically, used to demonstrate all or part of the characteristics of a disease. With models, researchers can study the mechanisms of a disease and test therapies.

antibodies: Specialized proteins produced by the cells of the immune system that counteract a specific foreign substance. The production of antibodies is the first line of defense in the body's immune response.

anti-inflammatory drugs: Drugs that reduce inflammation by modifying the body's immune response.

anxiety: A feeling of apprehension, fear, nervousness, or dread accompanied by restlessness or tension.

apathy: Lack of interest, concern, or emotion.

aphasia: Difficulty understanding the speech of others and/or expressing oneself verbally.

apolipoprotein E: A protein whose main function is to transport cholesterol. The gene for this protein is on chromosome 19 and is referred to as apoE. There are three forms of apoE: e2, e3, and e4. ApoE-e4 is associated with about 60 percent of late-onset Alzheimer's cases and is considered a risk factor for the disease.

apoptosis: Programmed cell death.

APP: See amyloid precursor protein.

art therapy: A form of therapy that allows people with dementia opportunities to express their feelings creatively through art.

assay: The evaluation or testing of a substance for toxicity, impurities, or other variables.

assessment: An evaluation, usually performed by a physician, of a person's mental, emotional, and social capabilities.

assisted living facility: A residential care setting that combines housing, support services, and health care for people typically in the early or middle stages of Alzheimer's disease.

atrophy: Shrinking of size; often used to describe the loss of brain mass seen in Alzheimer's disease during autopsy.

autonomy: A person's ability to make independent choices.

autopsy: Examination of a body organ and tissue after death. Autopsy is often performed (upon request) to confirm a diagnosis of Alzheimer's disease.

axon: The arm of a nerve cell that normally transmits outgoing signals from one cell body to another. Each nerve cell has one axon, which can be relatively short in the brain but can be up to three feet long in other parts of the body.

B

behavioral symptoms: In Alzheimer's disease, symptoms that relate to action or emotion, such as wandering, depression, anxiety, hostility, and sleep disturbances.

beneficiary: An individual named in a will who is designated to receive all or part of an estate upon the death of a will maker.

beta amyloid protein: A specific type of amyloid normally found in humans and animals. In Alzheimer's disease, beta amyloid is abnormally processed by nerve cells and becomes deposited in amyloid plaques in the brains of persons with the disease.

Binswanger's disease: A type of dementia associated with stroke-related changes in the brain.

biomarker: Used to indicate or measure a biological process (for instance, levels of a specific protein in blood or spinal fluid, genetic mutations, or brain abnormalities observed in a PET scan or other imaging test). Detecting biomarkers specific to a disease can aid in the identification, diagnosis, and treatment of affected individuals and people who may be at risk but do not yet exhibit symptoms.

blood-brain barrier: The selective barrier that controls the entry of substances from the blood into the brain.

brain: One of the two components of the central nervous system, the brain is the center of thought and emotion. It is responsible for the coordination and control of bodily activities, and the interpretation of information from the senses (sight, hearing, smell, etc.).

C

calcium: An element taken in through the diet that is essential for a variety of bodily functions, such as neurotransmission, muscle contraction, and proper heart function. Imbalances of calcium can lead to many health problems and can cause nerve cell death.

calcium channel blocker: A drug that blocks the entry of calcium into cells, thereby reducing activities that require calcium, such as neurotransmission. Calcium channel blockers are used primarily in the treatment of certain heart conditions but are being studied as potential treatments for Alzheimer's disease.

caregiver: The primary person in charge of caring for an individual with Alzheimer's disease, usually a family member or a designated health care professional.

care planning: A written action plan containing strategies for delivering care that address an individual's specific needs or problems.

case management: A term used to describe formal services planned by care professionals.

cell: The fundamental unit of all organisms; the smallest structural unit capable of independent functioning.

cell body: In nerve cells, the central portion from which axons and dendrites sprout. The cell body controls the life-sustaining functions of a nerve cell.

cell culture: Cells grown in a test tube or other laboratory device for experimental purposes.

cell membrane: The outer boundary of the cell. The cell membrane helps control what substances enter or exit the cell.

central nervous system (CNS): One of the two major divisions of the nervous system. Composed of the brain and spinal cord, the CNS is the control network for the entire body.

cerebral cortex: The outer layer of the brain, consisting of nerve cells and the pathways that connect them. The cerebral cortex is the part of the brain in which thought processes take place. In Alzheimer's disease, nerve cells in the cerebral cortex degenerate and die.

cerebrospinal fluid (CSF): The fluid that fills the areas surrounding the brain and spinal cord.

choline: A natural substance required by the body that is obtained from various foods, such as eggs; an essential component of acetylcholine.

choline acetyltransferase (CAT): An enzyme that controls the production of acetylcholine; appears to be depleted in the brains of individuals with Alzheimer's disease.

cholinergic system: The system of nerve cells that uses acetylcholine as its neurotransmitter and is damaged in the brains of individuals with Alzheimer's.

cholinesterase: An enzyme that breaks down acetylcholine, into active parts that can be recycled.

chromosome: An H-shaped structure inside the cell nucleus made up of tightly coiled strands of genes. Each chromosome is numbered (in humans, 1-46). Genes on chromosome 1, 14, 19, and 21 are associated with Alzheimer's disease.

clinical trials: Organized studies that test the value of various treatments, such as drugs or surgery, in human beings.

coexisting illness: A medical condition that exists simultaneously with another, such as arthritis and dementia.

cognitive abilities: Mental abilities such as judgment, memory, learning, comprehension, and reasoning.

cognitive symptoms: In Alzheimer's disease, the symptoms that relate to loss of thought processes, such as learning, comprehension, memory, reasoning, and judgment.

combativeness: Incidents of aggression.

competence: A person's ability to make informed choices.

computed tomography (CT scan): A type of imaging scan that shows the internal structure of a person's brain. In diagnosing dementia, CT scans can reveal tumors and small strokes in the brain.

conservator: In some states, the guardian who manages an individual's assets.

continuum of care: Care services available to assist individuals throughout the course of the disease.

controls: A group of people or animals that does not receive a treatment or other intervention or that is not affected with the disease being studied. This group is used as a standard to compare any changes in a group that receives treatment or has the disease. In Alzheimer research patients are often compared with controls of the same age (age-matched) to rule out the effects of age on study results.

Creutzfeldt-Jakob disease: A rare disorder of infectious and genetic origin that typically causes memory failure and behavioral changes.

CT scan: See computed tomography.

cueing: The process of providing cues, prompts, hints, and other meaningful information, direction, or instruction to aid a person who is experiencing memory difficulties.

D

deficits: Physical and/or cognitive skills or abilities that a person has lost, has difficulty with, or can no longer perform due to his or her dementia.

delusion: A false idea typically originating from a misinterpretation but firmly believed and strongly maintained in spite of contradictory proof or evidence.

dementia: The loss of intellectual functions (such as thinking, remembering, and reasoning) of sufficient severity to interfere with a person's daily functioning. Dementia is not a disease itself but rather a group of symptoms that may accompany certain diseases or conditions. Symptoms may also include changes in personality, mood, and behavior. Dementia is irreversible when caused by disease or injury but may be reversible when caused by drugs, alcohol, hormone or vitamin imbalances, or depression.

dementia-capable: Skilled in working with people with dementia and their caregivers, knowledgeable about the kinds of services that may help them, and aware of which agencies and individuals provide such services.

dementia-specific: Services that are provided specifically for people with dementia.

dendrites: Branched extensions of the nerve cell body that receive signals from other nerve cells. Each nerve cell usually has many dendrites.

diagnosis: The process by which a physician determines what disease a patient has by studying the patient's symptoms and medical history and analyzing any tests performed (blood, urine, brain scans, etc.).

disorientation: A cognitive disability in which the senses of time, direction, and recognition become difficult to distinguish.

DNA (deoxyribonucleic acid): A chain of nucleotides (cytosine, guanine, adenine, or thymine) linked with ribose sugar molecules that form the basis of genetic material. Specific patterns of nucleotides represent particular genes.

double-blind, placebo-controlled study: A research procedure in which neither researchers nor patients know who is receiving the experimental substance or treatment and who is receiving a placebo.

Down syndrome: A syndrome that causes slowed growth, abnormal facial features, and mental retardation. Down syndrome is caused by an extra copy of all or part of chromosome 21. Most individuals with Down syndrome develop Alzheimer's disease in adulthood.

durable power of attorney: A legal document that allows an individual (the principal) an opportunity to authorize an agent (usually a trusted family member or friend) to make legal decisions for when the person is no longer able to do so themselves.

durable power of attorney for health care: A legal document that allows an individual to appoint an agent to make all decisions regarding health care, including choices regarding health care providers, medical treatment, and, in the later stages of the disease, end-of-life decisions.

E

early-onset Alzheimer's disease: An unusual form of Alzheimer's in which individuals are diagnosed with Alzheimer's before the age of 65. Less than 10 percent of all Alzheimer patients have early-onset. Early-onset Alzheimer's is associated with mutations in genes located on chromosomes 1, 14, and 21.

early stage: The beginning stages of Alzheimer's disease when an individual experiences very mild to moderate cognitive impairments.

elder law attorney: An attorney who practices in the area of elder law, a specialized area of law focusing on issues that typically affect older adults.

electron microscope: A powerful microscope that employs a stream of electrons to magnify an image.

environment: Physical and interpersonal surroundings that can affect mood and behaviors in people with dementia.

enzyme: A protein produced by living organisms that promotes or otherwise influences chemical reactions.

excitotoxicity: Overstimulation of nerve cells by nerve impulses. Excitotoxicity often leads to cell damage or death.

executor: The individual named in a will who manages the estate of a deceased individual.

F

familial Alzheimer's disease: A form of Alzheimer's disease that runs in families.

fatty acids: Acids within the body derived from the breakdown of fats.

free radicals: Highly reactive molecules capable of causing damage in brain and other tissue. Free radicals are common by-products of normal chemical reactions occurring in cells. The body has several mechanisms to deactivate free radicals.

free-standing, dementia-specific care center: A facility solely dedicated to the care of people with dementia. This building can sometimes be part of a larger campus.

G

gait: A person's manner of walking. People in the later stages of Alzheimer's often have "reduced gait," meaning their ability to lift their feet as they walk has diminished.

gene: The basic unit of heredity; a section of DNA coding for a particular trait.

gene linkage: A group of genes located close together on a chromosome.

gene regulation: The control of the rate or manner in which a gene is expressed.

genetic susceptibility: The state of being more likely than the average person to develop a disease as a result of genetics.

genome: All the genes of an organism.

glucose: A simple sugar that is a major energy source for all cellular and bodily functions. Glucose is obtained through the breakdown, or metabolism, of food in the digestive system.

glutamate: An amino acid neurotransmitter normally involved in learning and memory. Under certain circumstances it can be an excitotoxin and appears to cause nerve cell death in a variety of neurodegenerative disorders.

guardian: An individual appointed by the courts who is authorized to make legal and financial decisions for another individual.

H

hallucination: A sensory experience in which a person can see, hear, smell, taste, or feel something that isn't there.

hippocampus: A part of the brain that is important for learning and memory.

hoarding: Collecting and putting things away in a guarded manner.

hospice: Philosophy and approach to providing comfort and care at life's end rather than heroic lifesaving measures.

Huntington's disease: An inherited, degenerative brain disease affecting the mind and body, characterized by intellectual decline and involuntary movement of limbs.

I

immune system: A system of cells that protect a person from bacteria, viruses, toxins, and other foreign substances that enter the body.

incontinence: Loss of bladder and/or bowel control.

inflammatory response: The immune system's normal response to tissue injury or abnormal stimulation caused by a physical, chemical, or biological substance. Immune system cells, if abnormally stimulated, can often cause further tissue damage while responding to the injured site.

instrumental activities of daily living (IADLs): Secondary level of activities (different from ADLs, such as eating, dressing, and bathing) important to daily living, such as cooking, writing, and driving.

L

late-onset Alzheimer's disease: The most common form of Alzheimer's disease, usually occurring after age 65. Late-onset Alzheimer's strikes almost half of all people over the age of 85 and may or may not be hereditary.

late stage: Designation given when dementia symptoms have progressed to the extent that a person has little capacity for self-care.

layering: Behavior that involves inappropriately changing or layering clothing, wearing some on top of others.

Lewy body dementia: A dementing illness associated with protein deposits called Lewy bodies, found in the cortex of the brain.

living trust: A legal document that allows an individual (the grantor or trustor) to create a trust and appoint someone else as trustee (usually a trusted individual or bank) to carefully invest and manage his or her assets.

living will: A legal document that expresses an individual's decision on the use of artificial life support systems.

M

magnetic resonance imaging (MRI): A brain scanning technique that generates cross-sectional images of a human brain by detecting small molecular changes. MRI scans reveal a contrast between normal and abnormal tissues. The image produced is similar to those generated by CT scans. There are no side effects or risks associated with MRI scans, although MRI can affect electrical devices like pacemakers and hearing aids.

Medicaid: A program sponsored by the federal government and administered by states that is intended to provide health care and health-related services to low-income individuals.

Medicare: A federal health insurance program for people age 65 and older and for individuals with disabilities.

memory: The ability to process information that requires attention, storage, and retrieval.

metabolism: The complex chemical and physical processes of living organisms that promote growth, sustain life, and enable all other bodily functions to take place.

microglia (microglial cells): A type of immune cell found in the brain. Microglia are scavengers, engulfing dead cells and other debris. In Alzheimer's disease, microglia are found associated with dying nerve cells and amyloid plaques.

MID: See multi-infarct dementia.

Mini-Mental State Examination (MMSE): A standard mental status exam routinely used to measure a person's basic cognitive skills, such as short-term memory, long-term memory, orientation, writing, and language.

mitochondria: Components found in cells that serve as primary energy sources for all cellular functions.

model system: A system used to study processes that take place in humans or other living organisms.

monoamine oxidase B (MAO-B): An enzyme that breaks down certain neurotransmitters, including dopamine, serotonin, and noradrenaline.

monoamine oxidase inhibitor (MAOI): A drug that interferes with the action of monoamine oxidase, slowing the breakdown of certain neurotransmitters. Used in the treatment of depression.

MRI: See magnetic resonance imaging.

multi-infarct dementia (MID): A form of dementia, also known as vascular dementia, caused by a number of strokes in the brain. These strokes can affect some intellectual abilities, impair motor and walking skills, and cause an individual to experience hallucinations, delusions, or depression. The onset of MID is usually abrupt and often progresses in a stepwise fashion. Individuals with MID are likely to have risk factors for strokes, such as high blood pressure, heart disease, or diabetes. MID cannot be treated; once the nerve cells die, they cannot be replaced. However, risk factors can be treated, which may help prevent further damage.

music therapy: Use of music to improve physical, psychological, cognitive, and social functioning.

N

nerve cell (neuron): The basic working unit of the nervous system. The nerve cell is typically composed of a cell body containing the nucleus, several short branches (dendrites), and one long arm (the axon) with short branches along its length and at its end. Nerve cells send signals that control the actions of other cells in the body, such as other nerve cells and muscle cells.

nerve cell line: A group of nerve cells derived from a cell culture that can be used for experimental purposes.

nerve cell transplantation: An experimental procedure in which normal brain cells are implanted into diseased areas of the brain to replace dying or damaged cells.

nerve growth factor (NGF): A protein that promotes nerve cell growth and may protect some types of nerve cells from damage.

neuritic plaque: See amyloid plaque.

neurodegenerative disease: A type of neurological disorder marked by the loss of nerve cells. See Alzheimer's disease, Parkinson's disease.

neurofibrillary tangle: Accumulation of twisted protein fragments inside nerve cells. Neurofibrillary tangles are one of the characteristic structural abnormalities found in the brains of Alzheimer patients. Upon autopsy, the presence of amyloid plaques and neurofibrillary tangles is used to positively diagnose Alzheimer's.

531

neurological disorder: Disturbance in structure or function of the nervous system resulting from developmental abnormality, disease, injury, or toxin.

neurologist: A physician who diagnoses and treats disorders of the nervous system.

neuron: See nerve cell.

neuropathology: Changes in the brain produced by a disease.

neurotransmission: Passage of signals from one nerve cell to another via chemical substances or electrical signals.

neurotransmitter: Specialized chemical messenger (e.g., acetylcholine, dopamine, norepinephrine, serotonin) that sends a message from one nerve cell to another. Most neurotransmitters play different roles throughout the body, many of which are not yet known.

neurotrophic factor: A protein, such as nerve growth factor, that promotes nerve cell growth and survival.

nucleus: The central component of a cell; contains all genetic material.

O, P

onset: Defines time of life when Alzheimer's disease begins (e.g., early-onset, late-onset).

pacing: Aimless wandering, often triggered by an internal stimulus (e.g., pain, hunger, or boredom) or some distraction in the environment (e.g., noise, smell, temperature).

paranoia: Suspicion of others that is not based on fact.

Parkinson's disease: A progressive, neurodegenerative disease characterized by the death of nerve cells in a specific area of the brain; the cause of nerve cell death is unknown. Parkinson patients lack the neurotransmitter dopamine and have such symptoms as tremors, speech impediments, movement difficulties, and often dementia later in the course of the disease.

peripheral nervous system (PNS): One of the two major divisions of the nervous system. Nerves in the PNS connect the central nervous system with sensory organs, other organs, muscles, blood vessels, and glands.

perseveration: Persistent repetition of an activity, word, phrase, or movement, such as tapping, wiping, and picking.

personal care: See activities of daily living.

PET scan: See positron emission tomography scan.

pharmacology: The study of drugs, including their composition, production, uses, and effects in the body.

phosphorylation: The chemical addition of a phosphate group (phosphate and oxygen) to a protein or another compound.

Pick's disease: Type of dementia in which degeneration of nerve cells causes dramatic alterations in personality and social behavior but typically does not affect memory until later in the disease.

pillaging: Taking things that belong to someone else. A person with dementia may think something belongs to her, even when it clearly does not.

placebo: An inactive material in the same form as an active drug—for example, a sugar pill. See double-blind, placebo-controlled study.

plaques and tangles: See amyloid plaque and neurofibrillary tangle.

positron emission tomography scan (PET scan): An imaging scan that measures the activity or functional level of the brain by measuring its use of glucose.

presenilins: Proteins that may be linked to early-onset Alzheimer's disease. Genes that code for presenilin 1 and presenilin 2 have been found on chromosomes 14 and 1, respectively, and are linked to early-onset familial Alzheimer's disease.

principal: The individual signing the power of attorney to authorize another individual to legally make decisions for him or her.

prions: Protein segments that may cause infection that may lead to some forms of dementia.

proteases: Enzymes that aid in the breakdown of proteins in the body.

protein metabolism: The breakdown of proteins into amino acids, a process essential to human growth and metabolism.

psychosis: A general term for a state of mind in which thinking becomes irrational and/or disturbed. It refers primarily to delusions, hallucinations, and other severe thought disturbances.

Q, R

quality care: Term used to describe care and services that allow recipients to attain and maintain their highest level of mental, physical, and psychological function, in a dignified and caring way.

reassurance: Encouragement intended to relieve tension, fear, and confusion that can result from dementing illnesses.

receptor: A site on a nerve cell that receives a specific neurotransmitter; the message receiver.

receptor agonist: A substance that mimics a specific neurotransmitter, is able to attach to that neurotransmitter's receptor, and thereby produces the same action that the neurotransmitter usually produces. Drugs are often designed as receptor agonists to treat a variety of diseases and disorders in which the original chemical substance is missing or depleted.

recombinant DNA technology: Artificial rearrangement of DNA; segments of DNA from one organism can be incorporated into the genetic makeup of another organism. Using these techniques, researchers can study the characteristics and actions of specific genes. Many modern genetic research methods are based on recombinant DNA technology.

reinforcement: Employment of praise, repetition, and stimulation of the senses to preserve a person's memory, capabilities, and level of self-assurance.

reminiscence: Life review activity aimed at surfacing and reviewing positive memories and experiences.

repetitive behaviors: Repeated questions, stories, and outbursts or specific activities done over and over again, common in people with dementia.

respite: A short break or time away.

respite care: Services that provide people with temporary relief from tasks associated with caregiving (e.g., in-home assistance, short nursing home stays, adult day care).

restraints: Devices used to ensure safety by restricting and controlling a person's movement. Many facilities are "restraint free" or use alternative methods to help modify behavior.

risk factors: Factors that have been shown to increase one's odds of developing a disease. In Alzheimer's disease, the only established risk factors are age, family history, and genetics.

S

Safe Return: The Alzheimer's Association's nationwide identification, support, and registration program that assists in the safe return of individuals with Alzheimer's or related dementia who wander and become lost.

senile plaque: See amyloid plaque.

senility: Term meaning "old," once used to describe elderly diagnosed with dementia. Today, we know dementia is caused by various diseases (e.g., Alzheimer's) and is not a normal part of aging.

sequencing: In human behavior, doing things in a logical, predictable order.

shadowing: Following, mimicking, and interrupting behaviors that people with dementia may experience.

side effect: An undesired effect of a drug treatment that may range in severity from barely noticeable, to uncomfortable, to dangerous. Side effects are usually predictable.

skilled nursing care: Level of care that includes ongoing medical or nursing services.

special care unit: Designated area of a residential care facility or nursing home that cares specifically for the needs of people with Alzheimer's.

spinal cord: One of the two components of the central nervous system. The spinal cord is the main relay for signals between the brain and the rest of the body.

stages: Course of disease progression defined by levels or periods of severity: early, mild, moderate, moderately severe, severe.

sundowning: Unsettled behavior evident in the late afternoon or early evening.

support group: Facilitated gathering of caregivers, family, friends, or others affected by a disease or condition for the purpose of discussing issues related to the disease.

suspiciousness: A mistrust common in Alzheimer patients as their memory becomes progressively worse. A common example is when patients believe their glasses or other belongings have been stolen because they forgot where they left them.

synapse: The junction where a signal is transmitted from one nerve cell to another, usually by a neurotransmitter.

synaptic vesicles: Small sacs located at the ends of nerve cell axons that contain neurotransmitters. During activity the vesicles release their contents at the synapse, and the neurotransmitter stimulates receptors on other cells.

T, U, V

tangles: See neurofibrillary tangles.

tau protein: The major protein that makes up neurofibrillary tangles found in degenerating nerve cells. Tau is normally involved in maintaining the internal structure of the nerve cell. In Alzheimer's disease, tau protein is abnormally processed.

tissue: A group of similar cells that act together in the performance of a particular function.

toxin: A substance that can cause illness, injury, or death. Toxins are produced by living organisms.

trigger: An environmental or personal stimulus that sets off particular and sometimes challenging behavior.

trustee: The individual or bank managing the assets of the living trust.

vesicle: A small pouch or pouch-like structure (sac). Vesicles in nerve cell axons contain neurotransmitters.

vitamins: Various substances found in plants and animals that are required for life-sustaining processes.

W, X, Y, X

wandering: Common behavior that causes people with dementia to stray and become lost in familiar surroundings.

will: A legal document created by an individual that names an executor (the person who will manage the estate) and beneficiaries (persons who will receive the estate at the time of death).

zinc: A metal that is essential for proper nutrition. It is unknown if zinc plays a role in the development of Alzheimer's disease.

Chapter 79

Additional Reading about Alzheimer's Disease and Other Dementias

To make topics easier to identify, resources in this chapter are listed alphabetically by title under the following headings:

- Books
- Booklets, Brochures, and Fact Sheets
- Video and Multimedia Resources

For price and availability, please contact the source indicated. Some books may also be available from your local library or bookstore.

Books

Decoding Darkness: The Search for the Genetic Causes of Alzheimer's Disease
By R.E. Tanzi and A.B. Parson, Perseus Publishing, 2000. 281 pages. Available from Perseus Books Group. Customer Service, 5500 Central Avenue, Boulder, CO 80301. 800-386-5656; Website: http://www. perseuspublishing.com.

This chapter includes information excerpted from 2001 and 2002 issues of *Connections*, a newsletter of the Alzheimer's Disease Education and Referral (ADEAR) Center, National Institute on Aging, with updated information from CHID (The Combined Health Information Database), a bibliographic database produced by the health-related agencies of the U.S. government. To search CHID online for additional information, go to http://chid.nih.gov.

Diagnosis and Management of Alzheimer's Disease and Other Dementias

By R. C. Green, Professional Communications, Inc. 2001. 224 pages. Available from Professional Communications Inc., Fulfillment Center, P.O. Box 10, Caddo, OK 74729-0010; 800-337-9838; Website: http://www.pcibooks.com.

The Forgetting. Alzheimer's: Portrait of an Epidemic

By David Shenk. Random House, Inc. 2001. 292 pages. Available from local book stores or Random House, Inc. 1540 Broadway, New York, NY 10036; Website: http://www.randomhouse.com.

Handbook on Dementia Caregiving: Evidence-Based Interventions for Family Caregivers

Edited by R. Schulz, Springer Publishing Company, 2000. 330 pages. Available from Springer Publishing Company, 536 Broadway, New York, NY 10012-3955. 212-431-4370; Website: http://www.springer pub.com.

Handholder's Handbook: A Guide for Caregivers of People with Alzheimer's or Other Dementias

By R. Teitel, Rutgers University Press, 2001. 192 pages. Available from Rutgers University Press, 100 Joyce Kilmer Avenue, Piscataway, NJ 08854. 800-446-9323. Website: http://rutgerspress.rutgers.edu.

Interventions in Dementia Care: Toward Improving Quality of Life

Edited by M.P. Lawton and R.L. Rubinstein, Springer Publishing Company, Inc., 2000. 188 pages. Available from Springer Publishing Company, Inc., 536 Broadway, New York, NY 10012-3955. 212-431-4370; Website: http://www.springerpub.com.

Keep Your Brain Young: The Complete Guide to Physical and Emotional Health and Longevity

By G. McKann and M. Albert. John Wiley and Sons, Inc. 2002. 296 pages. Available from John Wiley and Sons, Inc., 111 River Street, Hoboken, NJ 07030, 201-748-6000, Website: www.wiley.com.

Love Is Ageless: Stories about Alzheimer's Disease. 2nd ed.

Edited by J. Bryan; Lompico Creek Press, 2002. 244 pages. Available from Lompico Creek Press. P.O. Box 1403, Felton, CA 95018-1403.

(831) 335-7696. E-mail: editor@sasquatch.com. Website: www.loveis ageless.com.

Love Never Sleeps: Living at Home with Alzheimer's
By M.S. Rain; Hampton Roads Publishing Company, 2002. 371 pages. Available from Hampton Roads Publishing Company, 1125 Stoney Ridge Road, Charlottsville, VA 22902; 434-296-2772; E-mail: hrpc@ hrpub.com. Website: www.hrpub.com.

Mayo Clinic on Alzheimer's Disease
Edited by R. Petersen; Mayo Clinic Health Information, 2002. 210 pages. Available from: Mayo Clinic Health Management Resources, Centerplace 4, 200 First Street, S.W., Rochester, MN 55905; 800-430-9699.

Moral Challenge of Alzheimer Disease: Ethical Issues from Diagnosis to Dying. Second Edition.
By S.G. Post, The Johns Hopkins University Press, 2000. 162 pages. Available from The Johns Hopkins University Press, 2715 North Charles Street, Baltimore, MD 21218-4363; 800-537-5487; 410-516-6900; Website: http://www.press.jhu.edu.

Planning Care at Home: A Guide for Advocates and Families
Prepared by the National Senior Citizens Law Center, 2000. 127 pages. Available from National Senior Citizens Law Center, 1101 14th Street, NW, Washington, DC 20005; 202-289-6976; Website: http://www. nsclc.org.

Who Cares: A Loving Guide for Caregivers
By D. Marrella; DC Press, 2002. 222 pages. Available from DC Press, 2445 River Tree Circle, Sanford, FL 32771; (866) 602-1476. Website: www.focusonethics.com/whocares.html.

Booklets, Brochures, and Fact Sheets

Alzheimer's Disease: A Guide for Clergy
By the Alzheimer's Association, 2000. 13 pages. Available from the Alzheimer's Association, 919 North Michigan Avenue, Suite 1100, Chicago, IL 60611-1676; 800-272-3900 or 800-223-4405; TDD: 312-335-8882. Website: http://www.alz.org.

Assisted Living and Supportive Housing

Produced by the Family Caregiver Alliance, January 2001. 6 pages. Available from the Family Caregiver Alliance, 425 Bush Street, Suite 500, San Francisco, CA 94108; 415-434-3388; Toll-free calls in California (800) 445-8106; E-mail: info@caregiver.org; Website: www.caregiver.org.

Brain Connections: Your Guide to Information on Brain Diseases and Disorders. Fifth Edition

Produced by the Dana Alliance for Brain Initiatives, 2000. 49 pages. Available from the Dana Alliance for Brain Initiatives, 745 Fifth Avenue, Suite 700, New York, NY 10151. 212-223-4040; Website: http://www.dana.org.

Caregiving at a Glance: Fingertip Help for Families Taking Care of People with Alzheimer's Type Illnesses. 2nd Edition.

By L.E. Noyes, Family Respite Center. 2000. 28 pages. Available from Family Respite Center, 2036 Westmoreland Street, Falls Church, VA 22043; 703-532-8899. Website: http://www.familyrespitecenter.org.

Guide for Alzheimer's Disease and Related Disorders. 3rd ed.

Produced by the Kansas Department on Aging, Topeka, KS, March 2002. 63 pages. Available from the Kansas Department on Aging. New England Building, 503 South Kansas Avenue, Topeka, KS 66603-3404; 800-432-3535; 785-296-4986; TDD 785-291-3167. Website: www.k4s.org/kdoa.

Hospitalization Happens: A Guide to Hospital Visits for Your Loved Ones with Memory Disorders

By the North Carolina Division of Aging, Joseph and Kathleen Bryan Alzheimer's Disease Research Center, Alzheimer's Disease Education and Referral (ADEAR) Center, 2001. 6 pages. Available from Alzheimer's Disease Education and Referral (ADEAR) Center. P.O. Box 8250, Silver Spring, MD 20907-8250; 800-438-4380, 301-495-3311. Website: http://www.alzheimers.org

Managing Nutrition in Dementia Care: A Supportive Approach for Caregivers

By E. H. Weiss, E.H. and others. Alzheimer's Association—Western New York Chapter, 2001. 30 pages. Available from the Alzheimer's Association—Western New York Chapter, 1284 French Road, Depew, NY 14043. 716-656-8448 or 800-273-6737. Website: http://www.alzwny.org.

Male Caregivers' Guidebook: Caring for Your Loved One with Alzheimer's at Home

Produced by the Alzheimer's Association Mid-Iowa Chapter, 1999. 69 pages. Available from the Alzheimer's Association Mid-Iowa Chapter, 700 East University Avenue, Des Moines, IA 50316-2392; 800-738-8071; 515-263-2464.

Moving a Relative with Memory Loss: A Family Caregiver's Guide

By L. White and B. Spencer, Whisp Publications, 2000. 50 pages. Available from Whisp Publications, P.O. Box 5426, Santa Rosa, CA 95402, 707-525-9633.

Pressure Points: Alzheimer's and Anger

By E.L. Ballard, L.P. Gwyther, and T.P. Toal. Duke Family Support Program. 2000. 68 pages. Available from Alzheimer's Disease Education and Referral Center. P.O. Box 8250, Silver Spring, MD 20907-8250; 800-438-4380. Website: http://www.alzheimers.org.

Respite Services: Enhancing the Quality of Daily Life for Caregivers and Persons with Dementia

By D.A. Lund and S.D. Wright, University of Utah. 2001. 12 pages. Available from University of Utah Gerontology Center, 10 South 2000 East Front, Salt Lake City, UT 84112-5880; 801-581-8198; E-mail: geron@nurs.utah.edu; Website: www.nurs.utah.edu/gerontology/respite brochure.pdf.

Steps to Facing Late-Stage Care: Making End-of-Life Decisions

By the Alzheimer's Association, 2000. 15 pages. Available from the Alzheimer's Association, 919 North Michigan Avenue, Suite 1100, Chicago, IL 60611-1676; 800-272-3900, TDD: 312-335-8882.

Steps to Success: Decisions about Help at Home for Alzheimer's Caregivers

By L. Gwyther, E. Ballard, and J. Pavon, AARP Andrus Foundation, 2002. 16 pages. Available from the AARP Andrus Foundation, 601 E. Street, N.W., Washington, DC 20049; 800-775-6776; Website: http://www.andrus.org/caregiving/pdf/alzcare.pdf.

Travelling with a Person Who Has Dementia
A 2-page fact sheet produced by Alzheimer's Association NSW, 2002. Available from Alzheimer's Association NSW, P.O. Box 6042, North Ryde, NSW, 1670 Australia. E-mail: ahall@alznsw.asn.au; Website: www.alznsw.asn.au/library/travel.htm.

Who? What? Where? Resources for Women's Health and Aging
By the Alliance for Aging Research, 2000. 36 pages. Available from the National Institute on Aging Information Center. P.O. Box 8057, Gaithersburg, MD 20898-8057. 800-222-2225; TTY: 800-222-4225; Website: http://www.nia.nih.gov.

Video and Multimedia Resources

Caregiver Survival Kit
A multimedia kit prepared by the National Family Caregivers Association, 2000. Available from the National Family Caregivers Association, 10400 Connecticut Avenue, Suite 500, Kensington, MD 20895-3944; 800-896-3650, Website: www.nfcacares.org.

Communication: How to Communicate with Someone Who Has Alzheimer's Disease or Related Dementia
A videotape produced by Healing Arts Communication, Medford, OR, 2001. Available from Healing Arts Communication, 33 North Central, Suite 211, Medford, OR 97501. 888-846-7008. Website: http://www. homecarecompanion.com.

He's Doing This to Spite Me: Emotional Conflicts in Dementia Care
A video by S. Hartman and D. Kleber, Terra Nova Films. 2000. 22 minutes. Available from Terra Nova Films, 9848 South Winchester Avenue, Chicago, IL 60643; 800-779-8491; 773-881-8491 Website: http://www.terranova.org.

Participating in Research: A Legacy of Hope
A video recording produced by Northwestern Cognitive Neurology and Alzheimer's Disease Center, Chicago, IL, 2001. 13 minutes. Available from Alzheimer's Disease Education and Referral Center, PO Box 8250, Silver Spring, MD 20907-8250. 800-438-4380; Website: http:// www.alzheimers.org.

Chapter 80

The Safe Return Program

Safe Return is a national, government-funded program of the Alzheimer Association that assists in the identification and safe, timely return of individuals with Alzheimer's disease and related dementias who wander off, sometimes far from home, and become lost.

The Alzheimer's Association's Safe Return Program is the only nationwide program of its kind. Since the program began in 1993, more than 93,000 individuals have registered in Safe Return nationwide. The program has helped locate and return more than 7,400 individuals to their families and caregivers.

What Is Wandering?

People with Alzheimer's disease are prone to wander. They can become lost (even in familiar settings), leave a safe environment, or intrude in inappropriate places. Wandering can happen anytime or anyplace and can be life-threatening for the individual.

How Does Safe Return Work?

The Safe Return program helps unite families by working through Alzheimer's Association chapters across the country and trained com-

"Safe Return" is reprinted with permission of the Alzheimer's Association. For additional information, call the Alzheimer's Association national toll-free number, 800-272-3900, or visit their website at www.alz.org. © 2003 Alzheimer's Association. All rights reserved.

munity members like law enforcement officials, emergency medical technicians, and transit operators. The program includes:

- Identification products, including wallet cards, jewelry, clothing labels, lapel pin, bag tags
- A national photo/information database
- A 24-hour toll-free emergency crisis line
- Alzheimer's Association local chapter support
- Wandering behavior education and training for caregivers and families

If the registrant wanders and is found, the person who finds him/her can call the Safe Return toll-free number located on the wanderer's identification wallet card, jewelry, or clothing labels. The Safe Return telephone operator immediately alerts the family members or caregiver listed in the database, so they can be reunited with their loved one.

If a person is reported missing by a family member or caregiver, Safe Return can fax local law enforcement agencies the missing person's information and photograph. Local Alzheimer's Association chapters provide family support and assistance while police conduct the search and rescue.

Registration

To register, a person with dementia or their caregiver fills out a simple form, supplies a photograph, and chooses the type of identification product that the registrant will wear and/or carry. The registration fee is $40, and caregiver jewelry is $5. Check with your local Alzheimer's Association chapter to find out if scholarships are available in your area to cover the cost of registration.

To register by phone using a credit card, call 888-572-8566, Monday through Friday, 8 a.m. to 8 p.m. central time.

Chapter 81

Directory of Alzheimer's Disease Resources

Administration on Aging (AoA)
One Massachusetts Avenue
Washington, DC 20201
Phone: 202-619-0724
Fax: 202-401-7620
Website: www.aoa.gov
E-mail: AoAInfo@aoa.gov

Working in close partnership with its sister agencies in the U.S. Department of Health and Human Services, the AoA is the Federal agency dedicated to policy development, planning and the delivery of supportive home-and community-based services to older persons and their caregivers. The AoA works through the national aging network of State and Area Agencies on Aging, Tribal and Native organizations, and thousands of service providers, adult care centers, caregivers, and volunteers.

Information in this chapter was compiled from "Resource Directory for Older People," National Institute on Aging and the Administration on Aging, NIH Pub. No. 01-738, August 2001; "Alzheimer's Disease: Unraveling the Mystery," National Institute on Aging, NIH Pub. No. 02-3782, October 2002; and the "Directory of Health Organizations (DIRLINE)," a database of the National Library of Medicine (http://dirline.nlm.nih.gov), and other sources deemed accurate. All contact information was verified in July 2003.

Agency for Healthcare Research and Quality (AHRQ)
Publications Clearinghouse
P.O. Box 8547
Silver Spring, MD 20907-8547
Toll-Free: 800-358-9295
Website: http://www.ahrq.gov

AHRQ, part of the federal government, provides an information clearinghouse service that distributes *Evidence-Based Summaries and Reports*, *Clinical Practice Guidelines*, and other medical statistics and information. Call to order copies of guidelines on topics such as cardiac rehabilitation, treatment of pressure sores, or other publications on elder and long-term health care, health insurance, and minority health data. Visit the website to download *Clinical Practice Guidelines* on topics such as urinary incontinence, screening for Alzheimer's disease, and post-stroke rehabilitation.

Alliance for Aging Research
2021 K Street, NW, Suite 305
Washington, DC 20006
Phone: 202-293-2856
Fax: 202-785-8574
Website: http://www.agingresearch.org

The Alliance is a national, citizen advocacy organization offering free publications including *Investing in Older Women's Health*, *Meeting the Medical Needs of the Senior Boom*, *Delaying the Diseases of Aging*, and other aging-related subjects such as menopause, how to age with ease, and health care options under Medicare. The Alliance supports the health and independence of older people through public and private funding of medical research and geriatric education.

Alzheimer Society of Canada
20 Eglinton Avenue W., Suite 1200
Toronto, ON M4R 1K8 Canada
Toll-Free: 800-616-8816 (Canada only)
Phone: 416-488-8772
Fax: 416-488-3778
Website: http://www.alzheimer.ca
E-mail: info@alzheimer.ca

Alzheimer Society of Canada provides information to Alzheimer's disease patients, their families, and physicians. The website includes basic information, current news, and links to resources. Online support is available for caregivers.

Alzheimer's Association
225 North Michigan Avenue
Suite 1700
Chicago, IL 60601-7633
Toll-free: 800-272-3900
Phone: 312-335-8700
Fax: 312-335-1110
TTY: 312-335-8882
Website: http://www.alz.org
E-mail: info@alz.org

The Association is a nonprofit organization offering information and support services to people with Alzheimer's disease (AD) and their families. Contact the 24-hour, toll-free telephone line to link with local chapters and community resources. The Association funds research to find a cure for AD and provides information on caregiving. A free catalog of educational publications is available in English and Spanish.

Alzheimer's Australia NSW
P.O. Box 6042
North Ryde, NSW, Australia
Toll-Free: 800-639-331 (in Australia)
Website: www.alznsw.asn.au

Alzheimer's Australia NSW provides support services to people with Alzheimer's disease and other dementias and their families in New South Wales, Australia. The website includes a wealth of information in the dementia library.

Alzheimer's Disease Cooperative Study
University of California at San Diego (UCSD)-ADCS
8950 Villa La Jolla Dr., Suite C772
La Jolla, CA 92037
Phone: 858-622-5880

The Alzheimer's Disease Cooperative Study at the University of California at San Diego works in cooperation with the National Institute of Aging to conduct research in the development of drug treatments for Alzheimer's disease patients.

Alzheimer's Disease Education and Referral (ADEAR) Center
P.O. Box 8250
Silver Spring, MD 20907-8250
Toll-Free: 800-438-4380 (English, Spanish)
Phone: 301-495-3311
Fax: 301-495-3334
Website: http://www.alzheimers.org
E-mail: adear@alzheimers.org

The ADEAR Center, funded by the National Institute on Aging, distributes information about Alzheimer's disease (AD) to health professionals, patients and their families, and the public. Contact the Center for information about the symptoms, diagnosis, and treatment of AD; recent research; and referrals to State and other national services. The ADEAR website has searchable publications and databases, including the AD Clinical Trials Database of studies accepting volunteers.

Alzheimer's Disease Research Center
Baylor College of Medicine, Department of Neurology
6550 Fannin Street
Smith Tower, #1801
Houston, TX 77030
Phone: 713-798-6660
Website: http://www.bcm.tmc.edu/neurol/struct/adrc/adrc1.html

The Alzheimer's Disease Research Center at Baylor College conducts research designed to help identify better ways to diagnose and treat dementia patients.

American Academy of Neurology
1080 Montreal Avenue
St. Paul, MN 55116
Phone: 651-695-1940
Fax: 651-695-2791
Website: http://www.aan.com

The Academy is an association of doctors specializing in disorders of the brain and central nervous system. Contact AAN for information about neurology. Visit the Academy's website for referrals to accredited neurologists. Publications include the AAN's "Patient Information Guide" on neurological disorders and treatment.

American Association for Geriatric Psychiatry
7910 Woodmont Avenue, Suite 1050
Bethesda, MD 20814-3004
Phone: 301-654-7850
Fax: 301-654-4137
Website: http://www.aagponline.org
E-mail: main@aagponline.org

The Association works to improve the mental health and well-being of older people. Contact AAGP for information on geriatric psychiatry and to receive referrals to specialists. Available publications include "Growing Older, Growing Wiser: Coping with Expectations, Challenges and Changes in Later Years," and brochures on topics such as Alzheimer's disease, depression, and the role of the geriatric psychiatrist.

American Association of Critical-Care Nurses
101 Columbia
Aliso Viejo, CA 92656-4109
Toll-free: 800-899-AACN (2226)
Fax: 949-362-2020
Website: http://www.aacn.org
E-mail: info@aacn.org

AACN is a nonprofit professional association dedicated to meeting the needs of its members who care for acutely and critically ill patients and their families. The Association provides practice and educational resources as well as professional support for its members. Contact AACN for publications and audiovisual materials on critical care.

American Association of Retired Persons (AARP)
601 E Street, NW
Washington, DC 20049
Toll-free: 800-424-3410 (members only)
Phone: 202-434-2277
Website: http://www.aarp.org

AARP is a nonprofit organization that advocates for older Americans' health, rights, and life choices. Local chapters provide information and services on crime prevention, consumer protection, and income tax preparation. Members can join group health, auto, life, and home insurance programs, investment plans, or a discount mail-order pharmacy service. The AgeLine database, available on CD-ROM, contains extensive resources on issues of concern to older people. Publications are available on housing, health, exercise, retirement planning, money management, leisure, and travel.

American Federation for Aging Research
70 West 40th Street, 11th Floor
New York, NY 10018
Toll-Free: 888-582-2327
Phone: 212-703-9977
Fax: 212-997-0030
Website: www.afar.org
E-mail: info@afar.org

AFAR is a nonprofit organization dedicated to supporting basic aging research. AFAR funds a wide variety of cutting-edge research on the aging process and age-related diseases. Visit the website for a list of free publications.

American Geriatrics Society
350 Fifth Avenue
New York, NY 10118
Phone: 212-308-1414
Fax: 212-832-8646
Website: http://www.americangeriatrics.org
E-mail: info.amger@americangeriatrics.org

AGS is a nonprofit organization of physicians and health care professionals supporting the study of geriatrics. Contact AGS for information on geriatrics, long-term care, acute and chronic illnesses, rehabilitation, and nursing home care. Publications include the *AGS Complete Guide to Aging and Health* and the *AGS Medical Reference Guide*.

American Health Assistance Foundation
22512 Gateway Center Dr.
Clarksburg, MD 20871
Toll-Free: 800-437-AHAF (2423)
Phone: 301-948-3244
Fax: 301-258-9454
Website: http://www.ahaf.org

AHAF provides information and supports research on age-related illnesses. The Foundation supports three research programs: Alzheimer's

Disease (AD) Research (along with the Alzheimer's Family Relief Program) offers emergency grants of up to $500 to AD patients in need and their caregivers, National Glaucoma Research, and the National Heart Foundation. Contact AHAF for free publications on AD, glaucoma, heart disease, and stroke.

American Health Care Association
1201 L Street, NW
Washington, DC 20005
Phone: 202-842-4444
Fax: 202-842-3860
Website: http://www.ahca.org

AHCA is an organization representing the interests of nursing homes, assisted living centers, and subacute care facilities. Publications are available about nursing homes, guardianship, assisted living, financing, and long-term care services.

American Medical Association (AMA)
515 North State Street
Chicago, IL 60610
Toll-free: 800-621-8335
Phone: 312-464-5000
Fax: 312-464-5600
Website: http://www.ama-assn.org

AMA is an organization of licensed doctors that distributes scientific information on health and sets standards on medical law and practice. Local AMA associations can provide referrals to qualified doctors. AMA publishes the *Journal of the American Medical Association*, other subscription medical journals, and books for sale, including an encyclopedia of medicine.

American Psychiatric Association
1000 Wilson Blvd., Suite 1825
Arlington, VA 22209-3901
Phone: 703-907-7300
Fax: 703-907-1085
Website: http://www.psych.org
E-mail: apa@psych.org

The American Psychiatric Association is an association of psychiatrists, physicians specializing in diagnosing and treating people with mental and emotional disorders. Its Council on Aging establishes standards for psychiatric care of older people. Contact the APA for information on elder care issues, including medication use by older people, treatment of Alzheimer's disease, and nursing homes. Contact APA for referrals to local psychiatrists.

American Psychological Association

750 First Street, NE
Washington, DC 20002-4242
Toll-Free: 800-374-2721
Phone: 202-336-5500
Website: http://www.apa.org
E-mail: webmaster@apa.org

The American Psychological Association is a professional society of psychologists that provides assistance and information on mental, emotional, and behavioral disorders. Contact the APA for a list of State chapters, information on the psychosocial aspects of aging, and referrals to APA-member psychologists. The APA's section on older people produces publications on topics such as dementia and dementia research. Publications include a quarterly subscription magazine, *Psychology and Aging*.

American Society on Aging

833 Market Street, Suite 511
San Francisco, CA 94103
Toll-Free: 800-537-9728
Phone: 415-974-9600
Fax: 415-974-0300
Website: http://www.asaging.org
E-mail: info@asaging.org

ASA is a nonprofit organization providing information about medical and social practice, research, and policy pertinent to the health of older people. Membership and subscriptions to *Generations*, a quarterly journal, and *Aging Today*, the Society's bimonthly news magazine, are available to the public. A catalog of books for sale and other educational materials is available on the website.

Brookdale Center on Aging (BCOA) of Hunter College

425 E. 25th Street
New York, NY 10010

Brookdale Center on Aging, continued
Phone: 212-481-3780
Fax: 212-481-3791
Website: http://www.brookdale.org
E-mail: info@brookdale.org

BCOA sponsors a variety of programs including the Institute on Law and Rights of Older Adults which fights for grandparent rights. Other programs focus on elder care services, guardianship, caregiving, Medicare, intergenerational activities, and Alzheimer's disease.

Center for Neurologic Study
9850 Genesee, Suite 320
La Jolla, CA 92037
Phone: 858-455-5463
Fax: 858-455-1713
Website: www.cnsonline.org
E-mail: cns@cts.com

A non-profit organization, the Center for Neurologic Study (CNS) conducts neurologic research into the causes and cures of presently untreatable nervous system diseases. CNS offers support and education for neurologic disease patients. Interests of CNS include: nervous system diseases (including multiple sclerosis, amyotrophic lateral sclerosis, Alzheimer's disease); neuropharmacology; growth factors; and patient education. Staff provides information and materials on topics of interest; answers inquiries; offers advisory, reference, and current-awareness services; conducts seminars and workshops; distributes publications; and makes referrals to other sources of information.

Center for the Study of Aging and Human Development
Duke University Medical Center
3502A Busse Building Hospital South
Box 3003
Durham, NC 27710
Phone: 919-660-7500
Fax: 919-684-8569
Website: http://www.geri.duke.edu

The Center is a free-standing, nonprofit organization promoting research, education, and training in the field of aging. IAPAAS is the

Center's membership division. It organizes programs on health, fitness, prevention, and aging. Contact the Center for a list of publications and information about the quarterly newsletter, *Lifelong Health and Fitness.*

Cleveland Clinic Health Information Center
9500 Euclid Avenue
Cleveland, OH 44195
Phone: 216-444-3371
Website: http://www.clevelandclinic.org/health

The Cleveland Clinic Health Information Center, part of the Cleveland Clinic, offers a searchable database of health information on its website.

Cognitive Neurology and Alzheimer's Disease Center at Northwestern University
320 East Superior Street
Chicago, IL 60611-3008
Phone: 312-908-9339
Fax: 312-908-8789
Website: http:// www.brain.nwu.edu

CNADC conducts research to understand the causes of dementia. The Center also works to provide needed information to patients and their caregivers.

Dana Alliance for Brain Initiatives
745 Fifth Avenue
Suite 900
New York, NY 10151
Phone: 212-223-4040
Fax: 212-317-8721
Website: http://www.dana.org
E-mail: dabiinfo@danany.dana.org

The Dana Alliance promotes public education about brain research. The Alliance links the public, press, and policy makers with experts and resources in the field of neuroscience. It also hosts conferences on the brain and brain diseases. Contact the Dana Alliance for publications on brain research and diagnosis and treatment of brain disorders.

Elderweb

1305 Chadwick Drive
Normal, IL 61761
Phone: 309-451-3319
Fax: 866-422-8995
Website: http://www.elderweb.com
E-mail: ksb@elderweb.com

Elderweb is a research website for older people, professionals, and families seeking information on elder care and long-term care. Visit Elderweb for news and information on legal, financial, medical, and housing issues for older people and links to other websites.

Fisher Center for Alzheimer's Research Foundation

One Intrepid Square
West 46th Street & 12th Avenue
New York, NY 10036
Toll-Free: 800-259-4636
Phone: 212-245-5434
Website: http://www.alzinfo.org
E-mail: info@alzinfo.org

The Center's three primary areas of interest are understanding the causes of Alzheimer's disease, improving the care of people with Alzheimer's disease, and searching for a cure.

Gerontological Society of America

1030 15th Street, NW
Suite 250
Washington, DC 20005-1503
Phone: 202-842-1275
Fax: 202-842-1150
Website: http://www.geron.org
E-mail: geron@geron.org

GSA is a professional organization providing information, advocacy, and support for research into the study of aging. GSA has a database of information on biological and social aspects of aging, links to aging information resources, and referrals to researchers and specialists in gerontology. GSA distributes publications on a variety of aging-related topics.

Huntington's Disease Society of America
158 West 29th Street, 7th Floor
New York, NY 10001-5300
Toll-Free: 800-345-HDSA (4372)
Phone: 212-242-1968, ext. 10
Fax: 212-239-3430
Website: http://www.hdsa.org
E-mail: hdsainfo@hdsa.org

The Society is a nonprofit organization providing information, services, and advocacy for people with Huntington's disease (HD) and their families. Contact HDSA for research information on causes, diagnosis, and treatment of HD as well as referrals to testing centers, specialists, self-help groups, and social services. Publications and audiovisual materials on HD are available.

Institute for Advanced Studies in Immunology and Aging
1700 Wisconsin Ave., NW, 1st Floor
Washington, DC 20007
Phone: 202-333-8845
Fax: 202-333-8898
Website: www.iasia.org
E-mail: iasia@iasia.org

The Institute for Advanced Studies in Immunology and Aging (IASIA) is a nonprofit medical research and education organization which, since 1985, has supported research on the body's complex immune system. The Institute is dedicated to defining the linkage between the immune system, the brain, and aging; accelerating the application of research in the diagnosis, prevention, and treatment of AIDS, cancer, and Alzheimer's disease; and educating the medical community and the public on the latest advances in immunology and aging research and treatment.

International Center for the Disabled
340 East 24th St.
New York, NY
Phone: 212-585-6000
Fax: 212-585-6161
Website: http://www.icdrehab.org
E-mail: info@icdrehab.org

A private, nonprofit organization, ICD provides outpatient rehabilitation services, medical and vocational services to patients, conducts research, and administers education programs on the rehabilitation of the disabled. Primary concerns include evaluation and treatment of the disabled in fields of medicine; sensory feedback therapy; speech and hearing therapy; behavioral medicine treatment for the physically disabled; Alzheimer's Disease Program; cognitive rehabilitation of the head injured; programs to help businesses deal with stress, supervision and retention of disabled persons on the job, and returning the disabled to working status; chemical dependency; vocational rehabilitation; advanced rehabilitation research.

John Douglas French Alzheimer's Foundation
11620 Wilshire Boulevard, Suite 270
Los Angeles, CA 90025
Toll-Free: 800-477-2243
Phone: 310-445-4650
Fax: 310-479-0516
Website: http://www.jdfaf.org

The Foundation funds scientific research into the causes and cure for Alzheimer's disease. Contact the Foundation for the free publication "Caring for a Person with Memory Loss and Confusion."

National Academy of Elder Law Attorneys, Inc.
1604 North Country Club Road
Tucson, AZ 85716
Phone: 520-881-4005
Fax: 520-325-7925
Website: http://www.naela.org

NAELA is a nonprofit association assisting lawyers, bar associations, and others who work with older people and their families. Contact NAELA for information on lawyers specializing in issues pertinent to older people, resources to legal information, assistance, and education. A list of publications is available.

National Association of Community Health Centers
7200 Wisconsin Avenue, Suite 210
Bethesda, MD 20814
Phone: 301-347-0400
Fax: 301-347-0459
Website: http://www.nachc.com
E-mail: contact@nachc.com

NACHC is a national association representing community health centers nationwide. Contact NACHC for referrals to local health centers and information on the Association's programs as well as health care regulation and policy updates.

National Association of Nutrition and Aging Service Programs
1101 Vermont Avenue, NW
Washington, DC 20005
Phone: 202-682-6899
Fax: 202-682-3984
Website: http://www.nanasp.org

NANASP, a membership organization, supports a broad range of nutrition and related services for community-dwelling older people by training nutrition providers and advocating for older people. Publications include a "Legislative Action Manual" and *The Washington Bulletin*.

National Association of State Units on Aging
1201 15th St., NW, Suite 350
Washington, DC 20005
Phone: 202-898-2578
Fax: 202-898-2583
Website: http://www.nasua.org
E-mail: info@nasua.org

NASUA is a public-interest organization providing information, assistance, and advocacy on behalf of older people. Contact NASUA for information on rights of older people, health care and social services regulations, and referrals to lawyers specializing in elder law and aging issues. Publications are available on topics such as the Older Americans Act, long-term care, older worker issues, elder abuse, and nutrition programs. The Association cooperates in administering the Eldercare Locator, AoA's toll-free information service.

National Center for Health Statistics
3311 Toledo Road
Hyattsville, MD 20782-2003
Phone: 301-458-4636
Website: http://www.cdc.gov/nchs

NCHS, part of the federal government, is the agency that monitors and compiles information on the Nation's health. NCHS statistical programs on aging collect information on the health of older people, their lifestyles, exposure to unhealthy influences, diagnosis and age of onset for illnesses or disabilities, and patterns of health care service use. Contact NCHS for reports on trends in health and aging.

National Center on Elder Abuse
1201 15th Street, NW, Suite 350
Washington, DC 20005
Phone: 202-898-2586
Fax: 202-898-2583
Website: http://www.elderabusecenter.org
E-mail: NCEA@nasua.org

NCEA is operated jointly by the National Association of State Units on Aging, the National Committee for the Prevention of Elder Abuse, and the University of Delaware to disseminate information about abuse and neglect of older people. NCEA operates the Clearinghouse on Abuse and Neglect of the Elderly and can provide referrals to agencies and specialists. Publications are available on prevention of abuse, neglect, and state regulations.

National Center on Women and Aging
Heller School for Social Policy and Management
Mail Stop 035
Brandeis University
Waltham, MA 02254-9110
Toll-free: 800-929-1995
Phone: 781-736-3866
Fax: 781-736-3865
Website: http://www.brandeis.edu/heller/national
E-mail: natwomctr@brandeis.edu

The Center focuses on older women's issues and provides policy analysis, research, and assistance to the network of Administration on Aging-funded State and Area Agencies on Aging. The Center provides information and publications on women's health, caregiving, income security, and housing as well as prevention of crime and violence toward older women.

National Council on Aging, Inc.
300 D Street, SW, Suite 801
Washington, DC 20024

National Council on Aging, Inc., continued
Phone: 202-479-1200
Fax: 202-479-0735
Website: http://www.ncoa.org
E-mail: info@ncoa.org

NCOA is a private, nonprofit organization providing information, training, technical assistance, advocacy, and leadership in all aspects of aging services and issues. Contact NCOA for information on training programs and in-home services for older people. NCOA publications are available on topics such as lifelong learning, senior center services, adult day care, long-term care, financial issues, senior housing, rural issues, intergenerational programs, and volunteers in aging.

National Gerontological Nursing Association
7794 Grow Drive
Pensacola, FL 32514
Toll-free: 800-723-0560
Fax: 850-484-8762
Website: http://www.ngna.org
E-mail: ngna@puetzamc.com

NGNA, an organization of nurses specializing in care of older adults, informs the public on health issues affecting older people, supports education for nurses and other health care practitioners, and provides a forum to discuss topics such as nutrition in long-term care facilities and elder law for nurses. NGNA offers information on gerontological nursing and conducts nursing research related to older people.

National Health Information Center
P.O. Box 1133
Washington, DC 20013-1133
Toll-free: 800-336-4797
Phone: 301-565-4167
Fax: 301-984-4256
Faxback: 301-468-1204
Website: http://www.health.gov/NHIC
E-mail: nhicinfo@health.org

NHIC, a service of the federal government, links consumers and health professionals with resources and information. The Center provides health information, contacts for federally supported health information centers, lists of national health observances, and toll-free numbers sponsored by the federal government.

National Hispanic Council on Aging
2713 Ontario Road, NW
Washington, DC 20009
Phone: 202-265-1288
Fax: 202-745-2522
Website: http://www.nhcoa.org
E-mail: nhcoa@nhcoa.org

NHCoA is a national organization providing advocacy, education, and information for older Hispanic people. Contact the Council for facts and resources on health, employment, housing, strengthening families, and building communities, as well as referrals to local Council chapters. Publications in English and Spanish are available.

National Indian Council on Aging
10501 Montgomery Boulevard, NE, Suite 210
Albuquerque, NM 87111-3846
Phone: 505-292-2001
Fax: 505-292-1922
Website: http://www.nicoa.org
E-mail: dave@nicoa.org

NICOA provides services, advocacy, and information on aging issues for older American Indian and Alaska Native people. Contact NICOA for information about its resources and support groups serving the national Indian community, and NICOA's clearinghouse for issues affecting older Indian people. Publications are available, including the newsletter *Elder Voices*.

National Institute of Mental Health
6001 Executive Boulevard
Room 8184, MSC 9663
Bethesda, MD 20892-9663
Toll-free: 800-421-4211
Phone: 301-443-4513
Fax: 301-443-4279
TTY: 301-443-8431
Website: www.nimh.nih.gov
E-mail: nimhinfo@nih.gov

NIMH, part of NIH, is the lead agency conducting and supporting mental health research including mental disorders of aging. Contact NIMH for information on mental health and aging, Alzheimer's disease, anxiety disorders, depression, and suicide.

National Institute of Neurological Disorders and Stroke
Bethesda, MD 20892-2540
Toll-Free: 800-352-9424
Phone: 301-496-5751
Fax: 301-402-2186
Website: http://www.ninds.nih.org

NINDS, part of NIH, conducts and supports research on stroke and neurological disorders. NINDS provides information on its research targets, including stroke, head and spinal injuries, tumors of the central nervous system, epilepsy, multiple sclerosis, Huntington's disease, Parkinson's disease, and Alzheimer's disease. A directory of voluntary health agencies is available.

National Institute on Aging (NIA)
P.O. Box 8057
Gaithersburg, MD 20898-8057
Toll-Free: 800-222-2225 (NIA Information Center)
TTY: 800-222-4225
Phone: 301-496-1752
Website: http://www.nia.nih.gov

NIA, part of NIH, conducts and supports biomedical, social, and behavioral research on aging processes, diseases, and the special problems and needs of older people. NIA develops and disseminates publications on topics such as the biology of aging, exercise, doctor/patient communication, and menopause. The Institute produces the *Age Pages*—a series of fact sheets for consumers on a wide range of subjects including nutrition, medications, forgetfulness, sleep, driving, and long-term care. Information, publications, referrals, resource lists, and database searches on Alzheimer's disease are available through the Institute-funded ADEAR Center.

National Mental Health Association (NMHA)
2001 N. Beauregard Street, 12th Floor
Alexandria, VA 22311
Toll-Free: 800-969-NMHA (6642) (Mental Health Resource Center)

National Mental Health Association (NMHA), continued
Phone: 703-684-7722
Fax: 703-684-5968
TTY: 800-433-5959
Website: http://www.nmha.org

The NMHA Information Center provides referrals to mental health specialists, as well as publications such as "Coping with Growing Older, Answers to Your Questions about Clinical Depression."

National Resource Center on Native American Aging
P.O. Box 9037
Grand Forks, ND 58202-9037
Toll-Free: 800-896-7628
Phone: 701-777-3437
Fax: 701-777-6779
Website: http://www.med.und.nodak.edu/depts/rural/nrcnaa

The Resource Center, funded by the Administration on Aging, provides support, advocacy, and information for older Native Americans, including American Indians, Alaska Natives, and Native Hawaiians. Contact the Center for legal information and references, geriatric leadership training, cultural awareness, and a variety of publications.

National Senior Citizens Law Center
1101 14th Street, NW, Suite 400
Washington, DC 20005
Phone: 202-289-6976
Fax: 202-289-7224
Website: http://www.nsclc.org
E-mail: nsclc@nsclc.org

NSCLC offers assistance to Legal Aid Offices and private lawyers working on behalf of low-income older and disabled people. The Center does not accept individual clients but acts as a clearinghouse of information on legal problems such as age discrimination, Social Security, pension plans, Medicaid, Medicare, nursing homes, and protective services.

Older Women's League (OWL)
1750 New York Ave., NW, Suite 350
Washington, DC 20006

Older Women's League (OWL), *continued*
Toll-Free: 800-TAKE-OWL (825-3695)
Phone: 202-783-6686
Fax: 202-628-0458
Website: http://www.owl-national.org
E-mail: owlinfo@owl-national.org

OWL is a national organization advocating for the special concerns of older women. OWL helped develop the Campaign for Women's Health and the Women's Pension Policy Consortium. Contact OWL's 24-hour PowerLine for information about legal and political activity related to health care, access to housing, economic security, individual rights, and violence against women and older people. OWL newsletters are available.

Society for Neuroscience
11 Dupont Circle, NW, Suite 500
Washington, DC 20036
Phone: 202-462-6688
Fax: 202-462-9740
Website: http://www.sfn.org
E-mail: info@sfn.org

The Society is an organization of scientists and physicians interested in the brain, spinal cord, and peripheral nervous system. Members seek to advance an understanding of the nervous system by encouraging research, promoting education in the neurosciences, and informing the public about the results of research. Contact the Society for the fact sheet series called *Brain Briefings*, short newsletters explaining how basic neuroscience research leads to clinical applications.

Stanford/VA Alzheimer's Research Center of California
3801 Miranda Avenue
Palo Alto, CA 94304
Phone: 650-858-3915
Fax: 650-849-0183
Website: http://arcc.stanford.edu

The multi-faceted research conducted at the Stanford/VA Alzheimer's Research Center of California includes work on understanding memory problems and diagnosing Alzheimer's disease. In addition to research, the Center offers diagnostic evaluations, support groups, and community education.

Taub Institute for Research on Alzheimer's Disease and the Aging Brain
College of Physicians and Surgeons, Columbia University
630 West 168th St.
P.O. Box 16
New York, NY 10032
Phone: 212-305-1818
Fax: 212-342-2849
Website: http://www.healthsciences.columbia.edu/dept/taub/index.html

The Taub Institute for Research on Alzheimer's Disease and the Aging Brain sponsors and facilitates research and educational programs relating to Alzheimer's Disease (AD) and other age-related neurodegenerations. Areas of research interest include: the underlying causes of AD; the genetic contribution to AD susceptibility; and improving the diagnosis and treatment of AD. Staff answers inquiries; distributes publications; maintains an Internet site; sponsors seminars and conferences; and makes referrals to other sources of information.

Chapter 82

Alzheimer's Disease Centers (ADCs) Program Directory

About the Alzheimer's Disease Centers (ADC's)

The National Institute on Aging currently funds 29 Alzheimer's Disease Centers (ADC's) at major medical institutions across the nation. In addition, there are three Affiliate Centers. Researchers at these centers are working to translate research advances into improved care and diagnosis for Alzheimer's disease (AD) patients while, at the same time, focusing on the program's long-term goal—finding a way to cure and possibly prevent AD.

Areas of investigation range from the basic mechanisms of AD to managing the symptoms and helping families cope with the effects of the disease. Center staff conduct basic, clinical, and behavioral research, and train scientists and health care providers new to AD research.

Although each center has its own unique area of emphasis, a common goal of the ADC's is to enhance research on AD by providing a network for sharing new ideas as well as research results. Collaborative studies draw upon the expertise of scientists from many different disciplines. The National Alzheimer's Coordinating Center (see listing under Washington State) coordinates data collection and fosters collaborative research among the ADC's.

Many ADC's have satellite facilities, which offer diagnostic and treatment services and collect research data in underserved, rural, and minority communities.

"NIA Alzheimer's Disease Centers (ADC's) Program Directory," National Institute on Aging, 2003. Contact information verified in July 2003.

For patients and families affected by AD, many ADC's offer:

- Diagnosis and medical management (costs may vary—centers may accept Medicare, Medicaid, and private insurance).

- Information about the disease, services, and resources.

- Opportunities for volunteers to participate in drug trials, support groups, clinical research projects, and other special programs for volunteers and their families.

For more information, you may contact any of the centers on the following list. While the addresses and telephone numbers given are for the center directors, you may ask for information about any of the activities described above and about offices and satellite clinics at other locations throughout the country.

Alabama

University of Alabama at Birmingham
Alzheimer's Disease Center
454 Sparks Center
1720 7th Avenue South
Birmingham, AL 35294-0010
Phone: 205-934-3847 (Family Program Information)
Website: http://main.uab.edu/show.asp?durki=11627

Arizona

Sun Health Research Institute/Arizona Consortium
Arizona Alzheimer's Disease Center
10515 W. Santa Fe Drive
Sun City, AZ 85351
Phone: 623-876-5328
Website: http://www.shri.org

Arkansas

University of Arkansas for Medical Sciences
Alzheimer's Disease Center
4301 W. Markham, Slot 811
Little Rock, AR 72205-7199
Toll-Free: 800-942-8267
Phone: 501-603-1294 (Information Line)
Website: http://alzheimer.uams.edu

California

Stanford University
Stanford/VA Alzheimer's Research Center of California
Department of Psychiatry
3801 Miranda Avenue
Palo Alto, CA 94304
Phone: 650-858-3915
Fax: 650-849-0183
Website: http://arcc.stanford.edu

University of California, Davis
Alzheimer's Disease Center
Department of Neurology
4860 Y Street
Suite 3900
Sacramento, CA 95817
Phone: 916-734-5496 (Information Line)
Fax: 916-456-9350
Website: http://alzheimer.ucdavis.edu

University of California, Irvine
Alzheimer's Disease Center
Institute for Brain Aging and Dementia
Gottschalk Medical Plaza 1100
Medical Plaza Drive
University of California
Irvine, CA 92697
Phone: 949-824-2382
Fax: 949-824-3049
Website: http://www.alz.uci.edu

University of California, Los Angeles
Alzheimer's Disease Center
Department of Neurology
710 Westwood Plaza
Room 2238
Los Angeles, CA 90095-1769
Phone: 310-206-5238
Website: http://www.adc.ucla.edu
E-mail: adc@ucla.edu

University of California, San Diego
Alzheimer's Disease Research Center
Department of Neurosciences
UCSD School of Medicine
8950 La Jolla Drive
Suite C129
La Jolla, CA 92093-0624
Phone: 858-622-5800 (Information Line)
E-mail: adrc@ucsd.edu
Website: http://adrc.ucsd.edu

University of Southern California
Ethel Percy Andrus Gerontology Center
3715 McClintock Avenue
Los Angeles, CA 90089-0191
Phone: 213-740-7777 (Information Line for current studies and enrollment only)
Website: http://www.usc.edu/dept/gero/ADRC

Georgia

Emory University*
Emory Alzheimer's Disease Center
1841 Clifton Road, NE
Atlanta, GA 30329
Phone: 404-728-6950 (Information Line)
Fax: 404-728-6955
Website: http://www.emory.edu/WHSC/MED/ADC

*Affiliate Center

Illinois

Northwestern University
Cognitive Neurology and Alzheimer's Disease Center
Northwestern University Medical School
320 East Superior Street
Chicago, IL 60611
Phone: 312-908-9339
Fax: 312-908-8789
Website: http://www.brain.nwu.edu

Rush-Presbyterian-St. Lukes Medical Center
Alzheimer's Disease Center
Rush Institute for Healthy Aging
710 South Paulina Street
Chicago, IL 60612
Phone: 312-942-4463 (Information Line)
Website: http://www.rush.edu/patients/radc

Indiana

Indiana University
Indiana Alzheimer's Disease Center
Indiana University School of Medicine
635 Barnhill Drive
MS-B029
Indianapolis, IN 46202-5120
Phone: 317-278-2030 (Information Line)
E-mail: iadc@iupui.edu

Kentucky

University of Kentucky
Sanders-Brown Research Center on Aging
8100 South Limestone
101 Sanders-Brown Building
Lexington, KY 40536-0230
Phone: 859-323-6040 (Information Line)
Fax: 859-323-2866
Website: http://www.coa.uky.edu

Maryland

Johns Hopkins Medical Institutions
Alzheimer's Disease Research Center
Division of Neuropathology
The Johns Hopkins University School of Medicine
550 N. Broadway
Suite 201
Baltimore, MD 21205-2196
Phone: 443-287-4720
E-mail: troncoso@jhmi.edu
Website: http://www.alzresearch.org

Massachusetts

Boston University
Alzheimer's Disease Center
715 Albany St., E-842
Boston, MA 02118
Toll-Free: 888-458-BUAD (2823)
Phone: 617-638-5426
Fax: 617-414-1197
Website: http://www.bu.edu/alzresearch
E-mail: buad@bu.edu

Harvard Medical School/Massachusetts General Hospital
Massachusetts General Hospital
Department of Neurology
55 Fruit Street
Boston, MA 02114
Phone: 617-726-2000
Fax: 617-726-2353
Website: http://neurowww.mgh.harvard.edu

Michigan

University of Michigan
Alzheimer's Disease Research Center
Department of Neurology
1500 E. Medical Center Drive
1914 Taubman Street
Ann Arbor, MI 48109-0316
Phone: 734-764-2190 (Information Line)
Website: http://www.med.umich.edu/madrc

Minnesota

Mayo Clinic
Department of Neurology
200 First Street, SW
Rochester, MN 55905
Phone: 507-284-1324 (Information Line)
Fax: 507-538-0878
E-mail: mayoADC@mayo.edu
Website: http://www.mayo.edu/research/alzheimers_center

Missouri

Washington University
Alzheimer's Disease Research Center
Memory and Aging Project, Department of Neurology
Washington University Medical Center
4488 Forest Park Avenue, Suite 130
St. Louis, MO 63108-2293
Phone: 314-286-2881
Fax: 314-286-2763
Website: http://alzheimer.wustl.edu/adrc2

New York

Columbia University
Taub Institute for Research on Alzheimer's Disease and the Aging Brain
630 West 168th Street
P&S Box 16
New York, NY 10032
Phone: 212-305-1818 (Information Line)
E-mail: taubinstitute@columbia.edu
Website: http://www.alzheimercenter.org

Mount Sinai School of Medicine/Bronx VA Medical Center
Alzheimer's Disease Research Center
Department of Psychiatry, Box 1230
One Gustave L. Levy Place
New York, NY 10029-6574
Phone: 212-241-8329 (Information Line)
Fax: 212-860-3945
Website: http://www.mssm.edu/psychiatry/adrc.shtml

New York University
Alzheimer's Disease Center
New York University School of Medicine
Silberstein Aging and Dementia Research Center
Alzheimer's Disease Center
550 First Avenue
Room THN 310
New York, NY 10016
Phone: 212-263-5700 (Information Line)
Website: http://aging.med.nyu.edu

University of Rochester*
Alzheimer's Disease Center
Center for Aging and Developmental Biology
University of Rochester Medical Center
601 Elmwood Avenue
Box 645
Rochester, NY 14642
Phone: 585-273-1506
Website: http://www.urmc.rochester.edu/adc/index.html

*Affiliate Center

North Carolina

Duke University
Joseph and Kathleen Bryan Alzheimer's Disease Research Center
2200 West Main Street
Suite A-230
Durham, NC 27705
Phone: 919-416-5380
Website: http://adrc.mc.duke.edu

Ohio

Case Western Reserve University
University Memory and Aging Center
University Hospitals of Cleveland
12200 Fairhill Road
Cleveland, OH 44120-1013
Phone: 800-252-5048
Website: http://www.ohioalzcenter.org

Oregon

Oregon Health Sciences University
Aging and Alzheimer's Disease Center
3181 SW Sam Jackson Park Road
Department of Neurology
CR 131
Portland, OR 97201-3098
Phone: 503-494-6976
Website: http://www.ohsu.edu/som-alzheimers

Pennsylvania

University of Pennsylvania
Alzheimer's Disease Center
Center for Neurodegenerative Disease Research
University of Pennsylvania School of Medicine
3rd Floor Maloney Building
3600 Spruce Street
Philadelphia, PA 19104-4283
Phone: 215-662-4708 (Information Line)
Website: http://www.med.upenn.edu/ADC

University of Pittsburgh
Alzheimer's Disease Research Center
4-West Montefiore University Hospital
200 Lothrop Street
Pittsburgh, PA 15213-2582
Phone: 412-692-2700 (Information Line)
Website: http://www.adrc.pitt.edu

Texas

Baylor College of Medicine*
Alzheimer's Disease Research Center
Department of Neurology
6550 Fannin Street
Smith Tower
Suite 1801
Houston, TX 77030
Phone: 713-798-6660 (Information Line)
Website: http://www.bcm.tmc.edu/neurol/struct/adrc/adrc1.html

*Affiliate Center

University of Texas, Southwestern Medical Center
Alzheimer's Disease Research Center
5323 Harry Hines Boulevard
Dallas, TX 75390-9070
Phone: 214-648-7444 (Information Line)
Fax: 214-648-7460
Website: http://www2.swmed.edu/alzheimer

Washington

University of Washington
Alzheimer's Disease Center
VAPSHCS 116 MIRECC
1660 S. Columbian Way
Seattle, WA 98108
Phone: 206-277-3281 (Information Line)
Patient Recruitment: 800-317-5382
Fax: 206-768-5456
Website: http://depts.washington.edu/adrcweb

National Alzheimer's Coordinating Center (NACC)
4225 NE Roosevelt Way, Suite 301
Seattle, WA 98105
Phone: (206) 543-8637
Fax: (206) 543-8791
E-mail: naccmail@alz.washington.edu
Website: http://www.alz.washington.edu

The NACC coordinates data collection and fosters collaborative research among the ADC's.

Chapter 83

Resources for Discount Medications

Caregivers everywhere are familiar with the high-wire act involved in paying for medications for a loved one in their care. Already working within tight budgets, families find it difficult to absorb recent increases in prescription costs. Carol Thomson, for example, pays $700–800 a month for her mother's medications, and even though a small grant helped cover the cost over the past year, the grant is about to run out. So far, she has made 30 or 40 phone calls in an attempt to find discounted medications. Fortunately, a few generous physicians have helped her with free samples.

Caregiver Lucille Marinko will be forced to give up the attendant care which affords her a little respite time, because she is unable to pay for both the eight medications she needs for her mother and the additional help.

As we know, Medicare does not cover the cost of prescription medicines. For a while, Medicare supplemental policies—in particular the HMO policies—did cover prescriptions to a greater or lesser extent— sometimes with a cap on how much could be spent each year, sometimes with a given amount for co-pay, and sometimes with options for using generic medications.

However, because prescription costs are the largest cause of the increase in the cost of medical care in the United States—rising at twice the rate of inflation—most insurance companies have put limits on their coverage. Congress continues to debate different prescription coverage programs for Medicare recipients. Meanwhile, caregivers continue to scramble to find money to pay for drugs as well as the myriad other expenses involved in caring for someone with a long-term illness.

As the government and insurance companies struggle with this problem, some help is available—although it may take access to a computer and considerable time to find the right program.

Help on the Web

- The easiest way to review the kinds of programs drug companies offer is to visit www.needymeds.com.

- A new drug savings card called Together Rx is now available. It offers a 20–40% discount on the cost of medications. See www.togetherrx.com.

- The Medicine Program, www.themedicineprogram.com, helps people find assistance in obtaining medications, as does the Directory of Prescription Drug Assistance Programs, www.phrma.org.

- AARP has a mail order prescription program that gives discounts on medications. See www.aarppharmacy.com.

- Many people are talking about the "Canadian connection," whereby people can save money on medications by importing them from Canada. Canadian pharmacies include www.canada meds.com, www.realfastdrugstore.com, and www.thecanadian drugstore.com. Medicine Assist in Vermont will also help you access Canadian medications at www.unitedhealthalliance.com.

- The Kaiser Family Foundation has a summary of programs at their web site, www.kff.org.

Other Resources

- Although it is often necessary to apply to each drug company for their particular discount card, the Association of Chain Drug Stores is promoting a Pharmacy Care One Card that links the company cards. Call (703) 837-4244.

- Costco's pharmacy offers some of the lowest prices on medication, and Costco membership is not required.

- Eisai and Pfizer have an Aricept Assistance Program for people with dementia. Call (800) 226-2072.

- Your local Area Agency on Aging, through their HICAP program (Health Insurance Counseling and Advocacy Program) will also have information on drug programs.

- People who qualify for Veteran's benefits can get lower cost prescriptions through the VA—see http://www.va.gov/health_benefits.

Prescription drug discount programs change quickly, and the available options may be different or even eliminated by the time you read this. If you need help finding the right program for you, call your local Area Agency on Aging or HICAP program or Family Caregiver Alliance for assistance, (800) 445-8106.

Chapter 84

Caregiver Resources

Aging Network Services
4400 East-West Highway
Suite 907
Bethesda, MD 20814
Phone: 301-657-4329
Fax: 301-657-3250
Website: www.agingnets.com
E-mail: ans@AgingNetS.com

Aging Network Services (ANS) is a Bethesda, Maryland-based service with a group of 250 Masters-level social workers throughout the United States who provide counseling, referrals, and geriatric services to families and individuals in need of grief and loss counseling and Alzheimer's care. ANS specializes in situations where there is resistance from the person in need to outside intervention.

Information in this chapter was compiled from "Resource Directory for Older People," National Institute on Aging and the Administration on Aging, NIH Pub. No. 01-738, August 2001; "Alzheimer's Disease: Unraveling the Mystery," National Institute on Aging, NIH Pub. No. 02-3782, October 2002; "Caregiver Guide: Tips for Caregivers of People with Alzheimer's Disease," National Institute on Aging, NIH Pub. No. 01-4013, April 2002; the "Directory of Health Organizations (DIRLINE)," a database of the National Library of Medicine (http://dirline.nlm.nih.gov), and other sources deemed accurate. All contact information was verified in July 2003.

Alzheimer's Disease Support Groups
Family Caregivers and Friends Program
c/o Alzheimer's Association
225 North Michigan Avenue, Suite 1700
Chicago, IL 60601-7633
Toll-free: 800-272-3900
Phone: 312-335-8700
Fax: 312-335-1110
TTY: 312-335-8882
Website: www.alz.org/chapter/respite.htm
E-mail: info@alz.org

This nonprofit association supports families and caregivers of patients with Alzheimer's disease. Almost 300 chapters nationwide provide referrals to local resources and services, and sponsor support groups and educational programs. Online and print versions of publications are also available at the website.

American Association of Homes and Services for the Aging
2519 Connecticut Avenue, NW
Washington, DC 20008-1520
Phone: 202-783-2242
Fax: 202-783-2255
Website: http://www.aahsa.org
E-mail: inform@aahsa.org

AAHSA is a national, nonprofit organization providing older people with services and information on housing, health care, and community involvement.

American Health Assistance Foundation
Alzheimer's Family Relief Program
22512 Gateway Center Drive
Clarksburg, MD 20871
Toll-Free: 800-437-AHAF (2423)
Phone: 301-948-3244
Fax: 301-258-9454
Website: http://www.ahaf.org

AHAF provides information and supports research on age-related illnesses. The Foundation supports three research programs: Alzheimer's Disease (AD) Research (along with the Alzheimer's Family Relief Program) offers emergency grants of up to $500 to AD patients in need and their caregivers, National Glaucoma Research, and the National Heart Foundation. Contact AHAF for free publications on AD, glaucoma, heart disease, and stroke.

Assisted Living Federation of America
11200 Waples Mill Road, Suite 150
Fairfax, VA 22030
Phone: 703-691-8100
Fax: 703-691-8106
Website: http://www.alfa.org

ALFA represents for-profit and nonprofit providers of assisted living, continuing care retirement communities, independent living, and other forms of housing and services. The Federation works to advance the assisted living industry and enhance the quality of life for consumers.

Children of Aging Parents
1609 Woodbourne Road, Suite 302A
Levittown, PA 19057
Toll-Free: 800-227-7294
Phone: 215-945-6900
Fax: 215-945-8720
Website: http://www.caps4caregivers.org

This nonprofit group provides information and materials for adult children caring for their older parents. Caregivers of people with Alzheimer's disease also may find this information helpful.

Eldercare Locator
Toll-Free: 800-677-1116
Website: www.eldercare.gov

The Eldercare Locator is a nationwide, directory assistance service helping older people and their caregivers locate local support and resources for older Americans. It is funded by the Administration on Aging (AoA), which also provides a caregiver resource called *Because We Care—A Guide for People Who Care*. The AoA *Alzheimer's Disease Resource Room* contains information for families, caregivers, and professionals about AD, caregiving, working with and providing services to persons with AD, and where you can turn for support and assistance.

Family Caregiver Alliance
690 Market St., Suite 600
San Francisco, CA 94104
Toll-Free: 800-445-8106
Phone: 415-434-3388
Fax: 415-434-3508
Website: www.caregiver.org
E-mail: info@caregiver.org

The Family Caregiver Alliance (FCA), founded in 1977, is a community-based, non-profit organization that addresses the needs of the families and friends who provide long-term care by: developing services (specialized information and assistance; consultation on long-term care planning; service linkage and arrangement; legal and financial consultation; respite services; counseling; and education); advocating for public and private support; conducting research; and educating the public. FCA is a support organization for caregivers, offering specialized information on Alzheimer's disease, stroke, traumatic brain injury, Parkinson's disease, ALS, other disorders, and long-term care concerns. FCA provides practical, hands-on information for caregivers in order to assist them in: care planning; stress relief; and locating and using community resources such as in-home or daycare services. FCA publishes an online Policy Digest covering policy issues related to caregiving and long-term care. FCA offers a wide range of publications. FCA's National Center on Caregiving (NCC) is a central source of information and technical assistance on caregiving and long-term care for policy makers, families, service providers, media, program developers, and funders. The mission of the NCC is to advocate the development of high-quality, cost-effective policies and programs for caregivers in every state in the country.

MedSupport Friends Supporting Friends International
3132 Timberview Drive
Dunedin, FL 34698
Website: www.medsupport.org

MedSupport Friends Supporting Friends International, also known as MedSupport FSF International, founded in 1994, is a nonprofit organization dedicated to educating and assisting persons with disabilities in the community, their caregivers and their families; educating and informing the disabled about the wide range of services available to them through traditional and non-traditional resources;

educating and informing the general population about disabilities and the many facets of being disabled; providing the disabled, their caregivers and families a forum to discuss and interact with similar persons via the Internet, and providing moderated chats allowing for ongoing online support and establishment of relationships with other persons in similar situations; and assisting and enabling the disabled to get online, thereby having a means of contact and socialization as well as support and information.

National Association for Continence
P.O. Box 1019
Charleston, SC 29402
Toll-Free: 800-252-3337
Fax: 843-377-0905
Website: http://www.nafc.org
E-mail: memberservices@nafc.org

NAFC, formerly Help for Incontinent People, is a nonprofit organization providing advocacy, education, and support to people with incontinence and their families. Contact NAFC for referrals to specialists, resources, and information about the causes, prevention, diagnosis, treatments, and management alternatives for incontinence. Publications are available.

National Association for Home Care
228 7th Street, SE
Washington, DC 20003
Phone: 202-547-7424
Fax: 202-547-3540
Website: http://www.nahc.org
E-mail: webmaster@nahc.org

NAHC promotes hospice and home care, sets standards of care, and conducts research on aging, health, and health care policy. Association publications include "How to Choose a Home Care Provider" and other free consumer guides on home and hospice care.

National Association of Area Agencies on Aging (N4A)
15th Street NW, 6th Floor
Washington, DC 20005
Toll-Free: 800-677-1116 (Eldercare Locator)
Phone: 202-296-8130
Website: www.n4a.org

N4A is the umbrella organization for the AoA-funded Area Agencies on Aging. It also represents the interests of Title VI Native American aging programs. The Association administers the AoA-sponsored Eldercare Locator, a toll-free number linking older adults and their family members with local aging resources. N4A publishes the "National Directory for Eldercare Information and Referral."

National Caregiving Foundation
801 North Pitt St.
Suite 116
Alexandria, VA 22314-1765
Toll-Free: 800-930-1357
Phone: 703-299 9300
Website: www.caregivingfoundation.org
E-mail: info@caregivingfoundation.org

The National Caregiving Foundation is a national organization dedicated to assisting persons who provide and care for a friend or loved one on a permanent or impermanent basis. The National Caregiving Foundation helps caregivers identify and access supportive services and professionals who can provide information, counseling, or other support. The primary focus is helping the caregivers of Alzheimer's patients, however, the National Caregiving Foundation will assist anyone who provides emotional and/or hands-on care for a friend or loved one. In addition, the National Caregiving Foundation distributes support and educational materials; provides funding for research; and works for increased public awareness.

National Family Caregivers Association
10400 Connecticut Avenue
#500
Kensington, MD 20895-3944
Toll-Free: 800-896-3650
Fax: 301-942-2302
Website: http://www.nfcacares.org
E-mail: info@nfcacares.org

NFCA is a grass roots organization providing advocacy, support, and information for family members who care for chronically ill, older, or disabled relatives. There is no charge for family members to be on the mailing list and to receive the newsletter, *Take Care!* Contact NFCA for help finding resources.

National Hospice and Palliative Care Organization
1700 Diagonal Road
Suite 625
Alexandria, VA 22314
Toll-Free: 800-658-8898 (Hospice Helpline and Locator)
Toll-Free: 800-646-6460
Phone: 703-837-1500
Fax: 703-837-1233
Website: http://www.nhpco.org
E-mail: info@nhpco.org

NHPCO is a nonprofit, membership organization working to enhance the quality of life for individuals who are terminally ill and advocating for people in the final stage of life. Contact NHPCO for information, resources, and referrals to local hospice services. Publications, fact sheets, and website resources are available on topics including how to find and evaluate hospice services.

National Hospice Foundation
1700 Diagonal Road, Suite 625
Alexandria, VA 22314
Toll-Free: 800-338-8619
Phone: 703-516-4928
Website: http://www.hospiceinfo.org

NHF, a nonprofit, charitable organization affiliated with the National Hospice and Palliative Care Organization, provides support and information about hospice care options. NHF publications include "Hospice Care: A Consumer's Guide to Selecting a Hospice Program," "Communicating Your End-of-Life Wishes," and "Hospice Care and the Medicare Hospice Benefit."

National Information and Referral Support Center
1201 15th Street
Suite 350
Washington, DC 20005-3914
Phone: 202-898-2578
Fax: 202-898-2583
Website: http://www.nasua.org
E-mail: staff@nasua.org

NIRSC provides technical assistance, consultation, and training to State and Area Agencies on Aging and to local information and referral providers funded under the Older Americans Act. Contact the Center for referrals, resources, and information on how to locate services for older people. A list of Center publications is available.

Partnership for Caring, Inc.
1620 Eye Street, NW, Suite 202
Washington, DC 20006
Toll-Free: 800-989-9455
Phone: 202-406-8345 (voice mail)
Fax: 202-296-8352
Website: http://www.partnershipforcaring.org

PFC is a national, nonprofit organization providing advocacy, resources, and information on the reform and enhancement of care for the dying. Contact the Partnership for referrals to resources and support groups, legal assistance, and information on end-of-life issues.

Simon Foundation for Continence
Box 835-F
Wilmette, IL 60091
Toll-Free: 800-237-4666
Website: http://www.simonfoundation.org

The Simon Foundation for Continence helps individuals with incontinence, their families, and the health professionals who provide their care. The Foundation provides books, pamphlets, tapes, self-help groups, and other resources.

Visiting Nurse Associations of America
99 Summer Street, Suite 1700
Boston, MA 02110
Toll-Free: 888-866-8773
Phone: 617-737-3200
Fax: 617-737-1144
Website: http://www.vnaa.org
E-mail: vnaa@vnaa.org

VNAA is an association of nonprofit, community-based home health care providers. Visiting nurses offer quality in-home medical care including physical, speech, and occupational therapy; social services; and nutritional counseling. Local agencies operate adult day-care centers, wellness clinics, hospices, and meals-on-wheels programs. A fact sheet and caregiver's handbook are available.

Well Spouse Foundation
63 West Main Street, Suite H
Freehold, NJ 07728
Toll-Free: 800-838-0879
Website: http://www.wellspouse.org

Well Spouse is a nonprofit membership organization that gives support to wives, husbands, and partners of the chronically ill and/or disabled. Well Spouse publishes the bimonthly newsletter, *Mainstay*.

Chapter 85

If You Suspect Elder Abuse

Elder Abuse Is a Serious Problem

Each year hundreds of thousands of older persons are abused, neglected, and exploited by family members and others. Many victims are people who are older, frail, and vulnerable and cannot help themselves and depend on others to meet their most basic needs.

Legislatures in all 50 states have passed some form of elder abuse prevention laws. Laws and definitions of terms vary considerably from one state to another, but all states have set up reporting systems. Generally, adult protective services (APS) agencies receive and investigate reports of suspected elder abuse.

National Elder Abuse Incidence Study

Reports to APS agencies of domestic elder abuse increased 150 percent between 1986 and 1996. This increase dramatically exceeded the 10 percent increase in the older population over the same period.

A national incidence study conducted in 1996 found the following:

- 551,011 persons, aged 60 and over, experienced abuse, neglect, and/or self-neglect in a one-year period;

"Fact Sheets: Elder Abuse Prevention," U.S. Administration on Aging, U.S. Department of Health and Human Services, January 2003.

- Almost four times as many new incidents of abuse, neglect, and/ or self-neglect were not reported as those that were reported to and substantiated by adult protective services agencies;

- Persons, aged 80 years and older, suffered abuse and neglect two to three times their proportion of the older population; and

- Among known perpetrators of abuse and neglect, the perpetrator was a family member in 90 percent of cases. Two-thirds of the perpetrators were adult children or spouses.

Generally Accepted Definitions

Physical abuse is the willful infliction of physical pain or injury, for example, slapping, bruising, sexually molesting, or restraining.

Sexual abuse is the infliction of non-consensual sexual contact of any kind.

Psychological abuse is the infliction of mental or emotional anguish, for example, humiliating, intimidating, or threatening.

Financial or material exploitation is the improper act or process of an individual, using the resources of an older person, without his/her consent, for someone else's benefit.

Neglect is the failure of a caretaker to provide goods or services necessary to avoid physical harm, mental anguish or mental illness, for example, abandonment, denial of food or health related services.

The Role of the Administration on Aging

The Administration on Aging (AoA) is the only federal agency dedicated to policy development, planning, and the delivery of supportive home and community-based services to our nation's diverse population of older persons and their caregivers. They provide critical information and assistance and programs that protect the rights of vulnerable, at-risk older persons through the national aging network. State elder abuse prevention activities include:

- Professional training, for example, workshops for adult protective services personnel and other professional groups, statewide conferences open to all service providers with an interest in elder abuse, and development of training manuals, videos, and other materials.

- Coordination among state service systems and among service providers, for example, creation of elder abuse hotlines for reporting, formation of statewide coalitions and task forces, and creation of local multi-disciplinary teams, coalitions, and task forces;

- Technical assistance, for example, development of policy manuals and protocols that outline the proper or preferred procedures;

- Public education, for example, development of elder abuse prevention education campaigns for the public, including media public service announcements, posters, flyers, and videos.

AoA funds the National Center on Elder Abuse as a resource for public and private agencies, professionals, service providers, and individuals interested in elder abuse prevention information, training, technical assistance, and research. The website includes a state-by-state listing of statewide toll-free telephone numbers.

The Role of State and Local Adult Protective Service Agencies

State law charges state and local Adult Protective Service (APS) agencies with the responsibility to protect and provide services to vulnerable, incapacitated, or disabled adults. The laws vary in the amount of authority they invest in state APS agencies to oversee local APS programs. Local APS agencies receive and investigate reports of suspected abuse, neglect, and exploitation, and provide follow-up services.

What If You Suspect Abuse?

If you, as a concerned citizen or a service provider, suspect that abuse has occurred or is occurring, report your suspicions to the local APS agency. If the suspected incident involves an older person living in an institutional setting, call the office of the local long-term care (LTC) ombudsman. It is essential to call the office with jurisdiction over the geographical area where the older person lives. If you are unsure which office to call, you can obtain the correct telephone number by calling AoA's Eldercare Locator at 1-800-677-1116

What Happens after You Report?

The APS agency screens calls for potential seriousness. The agency keeps the information it receives confidential. If the agency decides the situation possibly violates state elder abuse laws, the agency assigns a caseworker to conduct an investigation (in cases of an emergency, usually within 24 hours). If the victim needs crisis intervention, services are available. If elder abuse is not substantiated, most APS agencies will work as necessary with other community agencies to obtain any social and health services that the older person needs.

The older person has the right to refuse services offered by APS. The APS agency provides services only if the older person agrees or has been declared incapacitated by the court and a guardian has been appointed. The APS agency only takes such action as a last resort.

If You Have Questions about the APS Services

If you have questions about the services provided to an older person by a local APS agency, call the Director of the local APS agency or the State APS agency. Give them the name and address of the older person and ask them to look into the matter. The AoA does not have oversight responsibility for APS.

For More Information

Working in close partnership with its sister agencies in the U.S. Department of Health and Human Services, the AoA is the official Federal agency dedicated to policy development, planning and the delivery of supportive home and community-based services to older persons and their caregivers. The AoA works through the national aging network of 56 State Units on Aging, 655 Area Agencies on Aging, 236 Tribal and Native organizations representing 300 American Indian and Alaska Native Tribal organizations, and two organizations serving Native Hawaiians, plus thousands of service providers, adult care centers, caregivers, and volunteers. For more information about the AoA, please contact:

U.S. Administration on Aging
Department of Health and Human Services
Washington, DC 20201
Phone: (202) 401-4541; Fax: (202) 357-3560
Website: http://www.aoa.gov; E-mail: aoainfo@aoa.gov
Eldercare Locator: 1-800-677-1116, Monday-Friday, 9 a.m. to 8 p.m. ET

Index

Index

Page numbers followed by 'n' indicate a footnote. Page numbers in *italics* indicate a table or illustration.

A

AAA Foundation for Traffic Safety, contact information 257
AARP *see* American Association of Retired Persons
abilities, defined 519
accessory apartments, described 401
acetaminophen 190
acetylcarnitine 190
acetylcholine
  defined 519
  described 116, 189, 464
acetylcholinesterase inhibitors, described 17, 464
activities of daily living (ADL)
  caregivers 313
  defined 519
  housing options 401–2
  see also instrumental activities of daily living
acupuncture, Alzheimer's disease 199–200
acute confusional state *see* delirium
AD *see* Alzheimer's disease

A.D.A.M., Inc., publications
  Alzheimer's disease diagnosis 181n
  Wernicke-Korsakoff syndrome 159n
ADC *see* AIDS dementia complex
ADCS *see* Alzheimer's Disease Cooperative Study
ADEAR Center *see* Alzheimer's Disease Education and Referral Center
ADL *see* activities of daily living
Administration on Aging (AoA)
  contact information 257, 371, 547, 596
  Eldercare Locator, contact information 225, 257, 310, 585, 595
  publications
    elder abuse prevention 593n
    home care employees 383n
    housing options 395n
    resource directory 547n, 583n
adrenoleukodystrophy 106
"AD Research - Finding New Answers and Asking Better Questions" (ADEAR Center) 409n
adult day care
  caregivers 314, 384
  described 375, 401
adult day services
  Alzheimer's disease 233
  defined 519

599

adult protective services (APS) agencies, elder abuse prevention 593, 595–96
advance directives
  caregivers 280
  defined 520
  described 172, 214–15, 265, 267–70, 404
adverse reaction, defined 520
Advil 190
age factor
  Alzheimer's disease 4, 48–49
  brain 24
  delirium 103–4
  Down syndrome risk factor 59–60
  frontotemporal dementia 122
  genetic testing 133
  hormone replacement therapy 437–40
  Huntington's disease 128
  intimacy issues 363–64
  Pick's disease 149
Ageless Design, Web site address 311
age-matched controls *see* controls
Agency for Healthcare Research and Quality (AHRQ), contact information 548
AgeNet, Inc.
  financial strategies publication 271n
  Solutions for Better Aging program, contact information 271n, 277n
agent, defined 520
"Age-Related Memory Changes" (Alzheimer's Association) 11n
age-related memory loss, overview 11–17
aggression, defined 520
Aging Network Services, contact information 583
agitation
  coping strategies 328–31
  defined 520
AHRQ *see* Agency for Healthcare Research and Quality
AIDS dementia complex (ADC), overview 77–84
"AIDS Dementia Complex" (Project Inform) 77n

akinesia, frontotemporal dementia 121, 123
Alabama, Alzheimer's Disease Center 570
alcohol use
  Alzheimer's disease 421–22
  delirium 101–2, 109
  memory loss 15, 170
  see also Wernicke-Korsakoff syndrome
Aleve (naproxen) 7
alleles
  Alzheimer's disease 49
  defined 52, 520
Alliance for Aging Research, contact information 548
alprazolam 102
ALS *see* amyotrophic lateral sclerosis
Altman, Joseph 25
aluminum
  Alzheimer's disease 423–24, 425–27
  Alzheimer's disease risk factor 44, 55–56, 239
Alzheimer, Alois 3
"Alzheimer Disease and Down Syndrome" (Alzheimer Society of Canada) 59n
"Alzheimer Disease and Risk Factors" (Alzheimer Society of Canada) 41n
Alzheimer's Association
  contact information 225, 232, 308, 324, 549
  publications
    age-related memory loss 11n
    Alzheimer's diagnosis 203n
    caregiving challenges 327n
    clinical trials 493n, 501n
    dementia tests 177n
    glossary 519n
    Safe Return program 545n
    statins 479n
    statistics 3n
Alzheimer's Australia NSW, contact information 549
Alzheimer Scotland - Action on Dementia, vascular dementia publication 151n
"Alzheimer's Disease" (A.D.A.M., Inc.) 181n

600

G

613

Health Reference Series
COMPLETE CATALOG

Adolescent Health Sourcebook

Basic Consumer Health Information about Common Medical, Mental, and Emotional Concerns in Adolescents, Including Facts about Acne, Body Piercing, Mononucleosis, Nutrition, Eating Disorders, Stress, Depression, Behavior Problems, Peer Pressure, Violence, Gangs, Drug Use, Puberty, Sexuality, Pregnancy, Learning Disabilities, and More

Along with a Glossary of Terms and Other Resources for Further Help and Information

Edited by Chad T. Kimball. 658 pages. 2002. 0-7808-0248-9. $78.

"It is written in clear, nontechnical language aimed at general readers. . . . Recommended for public libraries, community colleges, and other agencies serving health care consumers."
— American Reference Books Annual, 2003

"Recommended for school and public libraries. Parents and professionals dealing with teens will appreciate the easy-to-follow format and the clearly written text. This could become a 'must have' for every high school teacher." *— E-Streams, Jan '03*

"A good starting point for information related to common medical, mental, and emotional concerns of adolescents." *— School Library Journal, Nov '02*

"This book provides accurate information in an easy to access format. It addresses topics that parents and caregivers might not be aware of and provides practical, useable information." *— Doody's Health Sciences Book Review Journal, Sep-Oct '02*

"Recommended reference source."
— Booklist, American Library Association, Sep '02

AIDS Sourcebook, 3rd Edition

Basic Consumer Health Information about Acquired Immune Deficiency Syndrome (AIDS) and Human Immunodeficiency Virus (HIV) Infection, Including Facts about Transmission, Prevention, Diagnosis, Treatment, Opportunistic Infections, and Other Complications, with a Section for Women and Children, Including Details about Associated Gynecological Concerns, Pregnancy, and Pediatric Care

Along with Updated Statistical Information, Reports on Current Research Initiatives, a Glossary, and Directories of Internet, Hotline, and Other Resources

Edited by Dawn D. Matthews. 664 pages. 2003. 0-7808-0631-X. $78.

ALSO AVAILABLE: AIDS Sourcebook, 1st Edition. Edited by Karen Bellenir and Peter D. Dresser. 831 pages. 1995. 0-7808-0031-1. $78.

AIDS Sourcebook, 2nd Edition. Edited by Karen Bellenir. 751 pages. 1999. 0-7808-0225-X. $78.

"Highly recommended."
— American Reference Books Annual, 2000

"Excellent sourcebook. This continues to be a highly recommended book. There is no other book that provides as much information as this book provides."
— AIDS Book Review Journal, Dec-Jan 2000

"Recommended reference source."
— Booklist, American Library Association, Dec '99

"A solid text for college-level health libraries."
— The Bookwatch, Aug '99

Cited in *Reference Sources for Small and Medium-Sized Libraries, American Library Association, 1999*

Alcoholism Sourcebook

Basic Consumer Health Information about the Physical and Mental Consequences of Alcohol Abuse, Including Liver Disease, Pancreatitis, Wernicke-Korsakoff Syndrome (Alcoholic Dementia), Fetal Alcohol Syndrome, Heart Disease, Kidney Disorders, Gastrointestinal Problems, and Immune System Compromise and Featuring Facts about Addiction, Detoxification, Alcohol Withdrawal, Recovery, and the Maintenance of Sobriety

Along with a Glossary and Directories of Resources for Further Help and Information

Edited by Karen Bellenir. 613 pages. 2000. 0-7808-0325-6. $78.

"This title is one of the few reference works on alcoholism for general readers. For some readers this will be a welcome complement to the many self-help books on the market. Recommended for collections serving general readers and consumer health collections."
— E-Streams, Mar '01

"This book is an excellent choice for public and academic libraries."
— American Reference Books Annual, 2001

"Recommended reference source."
— Booklist, American Library Association, Dec '00

"Presents a wealth of information on alcohol use and abuse and its effects on the body and mind, treatment, and prevention." *— SciTech Book News, Dec '00*

"Important new health guide which packs in the latest consumer information about the problems of alcoholism." *— Reviewer's Bookwatch, Nov '00*

SEE ALSO Drug Abuse Sourcebook, Substance Abuse Sourcebook

Allergies Sourcebook, 2nd Edition

Basic Consumer Health Information about Allergic Disorders, Triggers, Reactions, and Related Symptoms, Including Anaphylaxis, Rhinitis, Sinusitis, Asthma, Dermatitis, Conjunctivitis, and Multiple Chemical Sensitivity

Along with Tips on Diagnosis, Prevention, and Treatment, Statistical Data, a Glossary, and a Directory of Sources for Further Help and Information

Edited by Annemarie S. Muth. 598 pages. 2002. 0-7808-0376-0. $78.

ALSO AVAILABLE: *Allergies Sourcebook, 1st Edition.* Edited by Allan R. Cook. 611 pages. 1997. 0-7808-0036-2. $78.

"This book brings a great deal of useful material together. . . . This is an excellent addition to public and consumer health collections."
— *American Reference Books Annual, 2003*

"This second edition would be useful to laypersons with little or advanced knowledge of the subject matter. This book would also serve as a resource for nursing and other health care professions students. It would be useful in public, academic, and hospital libraries with consumer health collections." — *E-Streams, Jul '02*

Alternative Medicine Sourcebook, 2nd Edition

Basic Consumer Health Information about Alternative and Complementary Medical Practices, Including Acupuncture, Chiropractic, Herbal Medicine, Homeopathy, Naturopathic Medicine, Mind-Body Interventions, Ayurveda, and Other Non-Western Medical Traditions

Along with Facts about such Specific Therapies as Massage Therapy, Aromatherapy, Qigong, Hypnosis, Prayer, Dance, and Art Therapies, a Glossary, and Resources for Further Information

Edited by Dawn D. Matthews. 618 pages. 2002. 0-7808-0605-0. $78.

ALSO AVAILABLE: *Alternative Medicine Sourcebook, 1st Edition.* Edited by Allan R. Cook. 737 pages. 1999. 0-7808-0200-4. $78.

"Recommended for public, high school, and academic libraries that have consumer health collections. Hospital libraries that also serve the public will find this to be a useful resource." — *E-Streams, Feb '03*

"Recommended reference source."
— *Booklist, American Library Association, Jan '03*

"An important alternate health reference."
— *MBR Bookwatch, Oct '02*

"A great addition to the reference collection of every type of library." — *American Reference Books Annual, 2000*

Alzheimer's Disease Sourcebook, 3rd Edition

Basic Consumer Health Information about Alzheimer's Disease, Other Dementias, and Related Disorders, Including Multi-Infarct Dementia, AIDS Dementia Complex, Dementia with Lewy Bodies, Huntington's Disease, Wernicke-Korsakoff Syndrome (Alcohol-Reated Dementia), Delirium, and Confusional States

Along with Information for People Newly Diagnosed with Alzheimer's Disease and Caregivers, Reports Detailing Current Research Efforts in Prevention, Diagnosis, and Treatment, Facts about Long-Term Care Issues, and Listings of Sources for Additional Information

Edited by Karen Bellenir. 645 pages. 2003. 0-7808-0666-2. $78.

ALSO AVAILABLE: *Alzheimer's, Stroke & 29 Other Neurological Disorders Sourcebook, 1st Edition.* Edited by Frank E. Bair. 579 pages. 1993. 1-55888-748-2. $78.

ALSO AVAILABLE: *Alzheimer's Disease Sourcebook, 2nd Edition.* Edited by Karen Bellenir. 524 pages. 1999. 0-7808-0223-3. $78.

"Provides a wealth of useful information not otherwise available in one place. This resource is recommended for all types of libraries."
— *American Reference Books Annual, 2000*

"Recommended reference source."
— *Booklist, American Library Association, Oct '99*

SEE ALSO *Brain Disorders Sourcebook*

Arthritis Sourcebook

Basic Consumer Health Information about Specific Forms of Arthritis and Related Disorders, Including Rheumatoid Arthritis, Osteoarthritis, Gout, Polymyalgia Rheumatica, Psoriatic Arthritis, Spondyloarthropathies, Juvenile Rheumatoid Arthritis, and Juvenile Ankylosing Spondylitis

Along with Information about Medical, Surgical, and Alternative Treatment Options, and Including Strategies for Coping with Pain, Fatigue, and Stress

Edited by Allan R. Cook. 550 pages. 1998. 0-7808-0201-2. $78.

". . . accessible to the layperson."
— *Reference and Research Book News, Feb '99*

Asthma Sourcebook

Basic Consumer Health Information about Asthma, Including Symptoms, Traditional and Nontraditional Remedies, Treatment Advances, Quality-of-Life Aids, Medical Research Updates, and the Role of Allergies, Exercise, Age, the Environment, and Genetics in the Development of Asthma

Along with Statistical Data, a Glossary, and Directories of Support Groups, and Other Resources for Further Information

Edited by Annemarie S. Muth. 628 pages. 2000. 0-7808-0381-7. $78.

"A worthwhile reference acquisition for public libraries and academic medical libraries whose readers desire a quick introduction to the wide range of asthma information." —*Choice, Association of College & Research Libraries, Jun '01*

"Recommended reference source." —*Booklist, American Library Association, Feb '01*

"Highly recommended." —*The Bookwatch, Jan '01*

"There is much good information for patients and their families who deal with asthma daily." —*American Medical Writers Association Journal, Winter '01*

"This informative text is recommended for consumer health collections in public, secondary school, and community college libraries and the libraries of universities with a large undergraduate population." —*American Reference Books Annual, 2001*

Attention Deficit Disorder Sourcebook

Basic Consumer Health Information about Attention Deficit/Hyperactivity Disorder in Children and Adults, Including Facts about Causes, Symptoms, Diagnostic Criteria, and Treatment Options Such as Medications, Behavior Therapy, Coaching, and Homeopathy

Along with Reports on Current Research Initiatives, Legal Issues, and Government Regulations, and Featuring a Glossary of Related Terms, Internet Resources, and a List of Additional Reading Material

Edited by Dawn D. Matthews. 470 pages. 2002. 0-7808-0624-7. $78.

"Recommended reference source." —*Booklist, American Library Association, Jan '03*

"This book is recommended for all school libraries and the reference or consumer health sections of public libraries." —*American Reference Books Annual, 2003*

Back & Neck Disorders Sourcebook

Basic Information about Disorders and Injuries of the Spinal Cord and Vertebrae, Including Facts on Chiropractic Treatment, Surgical Interventions, Paralysis, and Rehabilitation

Along with Advice for Preventing Back Trouble

Edited by Karen Bellenir. 548 pages. 1997. 0-7808-0202-0. $78.

"The strength of this work is its basic, easy-to-read format. Recommended." —*Reference and User Services Quarterly, American Library Association, Winter '97*

Blood & Circulatory Disorders Sourcebook

Basic Information about Blood and Its Components, Anemias, Leukemias, Bleeding Disorders, and Circulatory Disorders, Including Aplastic Anemia, Thalassemia, Sickle-Cell Disease, Hemochromatosis, Hemophilia, Von Willebrand Disease, and Vascular Diseases

Along with a Special Section on Blood Transfusions and Blood Supply Safety, a Glossary, and Source Listings for Further Help and Information

Edited by Karen Bellenir and Linda M. Shin. 554 pages. 1998. 0-7808-0203-9. $78.

"Recommended reference source." —*Booklist, American Library Association, Feb '99*

"An important reference sourcebook written in simple language for everyday, non-technical users." —*Reviewer's Bookwatch, Jan '99*

Brain Disorders Sourcebook

Basic Consumer Health Information about Strokes, Epilepsy, Amyotrophic Lateral Sclerosis (ALS/Lou Gehrig's Disease), Parkinson's Disease, Brain Tumors, Cerebral Palsy, Headache, Tourette Syndrome, and More

Along with Statistical Data, Treatment and Rehabilitation Options, Coping Strategies, Reports on Current Research Initiatives, a Glossary, and Resource Listings for Additional Help and Information

Edited by Karen Bellenir. 481 pages. 1999. 0-7808-0229-2. $78.

"Belongs on the shelves of any library with a consumer health collection." —*E-Streams, Mar '00*

"Recommended reference source." —*Booklist, American Library Association, Oct '99*

SEE ALSO Alzheimer's Disease Sourcebook

Breast Cancer Sourcebook

Basic Consumer Health Information about Breast Cancer, Including Diagnostic Methods, Treatment Options, Alternative Therapies, Self-Help Information, Related Health Concerns, Statistical and Demographic Data, and Facts for Men with Breast Cancer

Along with Reports on Current Research Initiatives, a Glossary of Related Medical Terms, and a Directory of Sources for Further Help and Information

Edited by Edward J. Prucha and Karen Bellenir. 580 pages. 2001. 0-7808-0244-6. $78.

"It would be a useful reference book in a library or on loan to women in a support group." —*Cancer Forum, Mar '03*

"Recommended reference source." —*Booklist, American Library Association, Jan '02*

"This reference source is highly recommended. It is quite informative, comprehensive and detailed in nature, and yet it offers practical advice in easy-to-read language. It could be thought of as the 'bible' of breast cancer for the consumer." —*E-Streams, Jan '02*

"The broad range of topics covered in lay language make the *Breast Cancer Sourcebook* an excellent addition to public and consumer health library collections." —*American Reference Books Annual 2002*

"From the pros and cons of different screening methods and results to treatment options, *Breast Cancer Sourcebook* provides the latest information on the subject." —*Library Bookwatch, Dec '01*

"This thoroughgoing, very readable reference covers all aspects of breast health and cancer. . . . Readers will find much to consider here. Recommended for all public and patient health collections." —*Library Journal, Sep '01*

SEE ALSO *Cancer Sourcebook for Women, Women's Health Concerns Sourcebook*

■

Breastfeeding Sourcebook

Basic Consumer Health Information about the Benefits of Breastmilk, Preparing to Breastfeed, Breastfeeding as a Baby Grows, Nutrition, and More, Including Information on Special Situations and Concerns Such as Mastitis, Illness, Medications, Allergies, Multiple Births, Prematurity, Special Needs, and Adoption

Along with a Glossary and Resources for Additional Help and Information

Edited by Jenni Lynn Colson. 388 pages. 2002. 0-7808-0332-9. $78.

SEE ALSO *Pregnancy & Birth Sourcebook*

"Particularly useful is the information about professional lactation services and chapters on breastfeeding when returning to work. . . . *Breastfeeding Sourcebook* will be useful for public libraries, consumer health libraries, and technical schools offering nurse assistant training, especially in areas where Internet access is problematic." —*American Reference Books Annual, 2003*

■

Burns Sourcebook

Basic Consumer Health Information about Various Types of Burns and Scalds, Including Flame, Heat, Cold, Electrical, Chemical, and Sun Burns

Along with Information on Short-Term and Long-Term Treatments, Tissue Reconstruction, Plastic Surgery, Prevention Suggestions, and First Aid

Edited by Allan R. Cook. 604 pages. 1999. 0-7808-0204-7. $78.

"This is an exceptional addition to the series and is highly recommended for all consumer health collections, hospital libraries, and academic medical centers." —*E-Streams, Mar '00*

"This key reference guide is an invaluable addition to all health care and public libraries in confronting this ongoing health issue." —*American Reference Books Annual, 2000*

"Recommended reference source." —*Booklist, American Library Association, Dec '99*

SEE ALSO *Skin Disorders Sourcebook*

■

Cancer Sourcebook, 4th Edition

Basic Consumer Health Information about Major Forms and Stages of Cancer, Featuring Facts about Head and Neck Cancers, Lung Cancers, Gastrointestinal Cancers, Genitourinary Cancers, Lymphomas, Blood Cell Cancers, Endocrine Cancers, Skin Cancers, Bone Cancers, Sarcomas, and Others, and Including Information about Cancer Treatments and Therapies, Identifying and Reducing Cancer Risks, and Strategies for Coping with Cancer and the Side Effects of Treatment

Along with a Cancer Glossary, Statistical and Demographic Data, and a Directory of Sources for Additional Help and Information

Edited by Karen Bellenir. 1,119 pages. 2003. 0-7808-0633-6. $78.

ALSO AVAILABLE: *Cancer Sourcebook, 1st Edition.* Edited by Frank E. Bair. 932 pages. 1990. 1-55888-888-8. $78.

New Cancer Sourcebook, 2nd Edition. Edited by Allan R. Cook. 1,313 pages. 1996. 0-7808-0041-9. $78.

Cancer Sourcebook, 3rd Edition. Edited by Edward J. Prucha. 1,069 pages. 2000. 0-7808-0227-6. $78.

"This title is recommended for health sciences and public libraries with consumer health collections." —*E-Streams, Feb '01*

". . . can be effectively used by cancer patients and their families who are looking for answers in a language they can understand. Public and hospital libraries should have it on their shelves." —*American Reference Books Annual, 2001*

"Recommended reference source." —*Booklist, American Library Association, Dec '00*

Cited in *Reference Sources for Small and Medium-Sized Libraries, American Library Association, 1999*

"The amount of factual and useful information is extensive. The writing is very clear, geared to general readers. Recommended for all levels." —*Choice, Association of College & Research Libraries, Jan '97*

SEE ALSO *Breast Cancer Sourcebook, Cancer Sourcebook for Women, Pediatric Cancer Sourcebook, Prostate Cancer Sourcebook*

Cancer Sourcebook for Women, 2nd Edition

Basic Consumer Health Information about Gynecologic Cancers and Related Concerns, Including Cervical Cancer, Endometrial Cancer, Gestational Trophoblastic Tumor, Ovarian Cancer, Uterine Cancer, Vaginal Cancer, Vulvar Cancer, Breast Cancer, and Common Non-Cancerous Uterine Conditions, with Facts about Cancer Risk Factors, Screening and Prevention, Treatment Options, and Reports on Current Research Initiatives

Along with a Glossary of Cancer Terms and a Directory of Resources for Additional Help and Information

Edited by Karen Bellenir. 604 pages. 2002. 0-7808-0226-8. $78.

ALSO AVAILABLE: *Cancer Sourcebook for Women, 1st Edition.* Edited by Allan R. Cook and Peter D. Dresser. 524 pages. 1996. 0-7808-0076-1. $78.

"An excellent addition to collections in public, consumer health, and women's health libraries."
— *American Reference Books Annual, 2003*

"Overall, the information is excellent, and complex topics are clearly explained. As a reference book for the consumer it is a valuable resource to assist them to make informed decisions about cancer and its treatments." — *Cancer Forum, Nov '02*

"Highly recommended for academic and medical reference collections." — *Library Bookwatch, Sep '02*

"This is a highly recommended book for any public or consumer library, being reader friendly and containing accurate and helpful information."
— *E-Streams, Aug '02*

"Recommended reference source."
— *Booklist, American Library Association, Jul '02*

SEE ALSO *Breast Cancer Sourcebook, Women's Health Concerns Sourcebook*

Cardiovascular Diseases & Disorders Sourcebook, 1st Edition

SEE *Heart Diseases & Disorders Sourcebook, 2nd Edition*

Caregiving Sourcebook

Basic Consumer Health Information for Caregivers, Including a Profile of Caregivers, Caregiving Responsibilities and Concerns, Tips for Specific Conditions, Care Environments, and the Effects of Caregiving

Along with Facts about Legal Issues, Financial Information, and Future Planning, a Glossary, and a Listing of Additional Resources

Edited by Joyce Brennfleck Shannon. 600 pages. 2001. 0-7808-0331-0. $78.

"Essential for most collections."
— *Library Journal, Apr 1, 2002*

"An ideal addition to the reference collection of any public library. Health sciences information professionals may also want to acquire the *Caregiving Sourcebook* for their hospital or academic library for use as a ready reference tool by health care workers interested in aging and caregiving." — *E-Streams, Jan '02*

"Recommended reference source."
— *Booklist, American Library Association, Oct '01*

Childhood Diseases & Disorders Sourcebook

Basic Consumer Health Information about Medical Problems Often Encountered in Pre-Adolescent Children, Including Respiratory Tract Ailments, Ear Infections, Sore Throats, Disorders of the Skin and Scalp, Digestive and Genitourinary Diseases, Infectious Diseases, Inflammatory Disorders, Chronic Physical and Developmental Disorders, Allergies, and More

Along with Information about Diagnostic Tests, Common Childhood Surgeries, and Frequently Used Medications, with a Glossary of Important Terms and Resource Directory

Edited by Chad T. Kimball. 662 pages. 2003. 0-7808-0458-9. $78.

Colds, Flu & Other Common Ailments Sourcebook

Basic Consumer Health Information about Common Ailments and Injuries, Including Colds, Coughs, the Flu, Sinus Problems, Headaches, Fever, Nausea and Vomiting, Menstrual Cramps, Diarrhea, Constipation, Hemorrhoids, Back Pain, Dandruff, Dry and Itchy Skin, Cuts, Scrapes, Sprains, Bruises, and More

Along with Information about Prevention, Self-Care, Choosing a Doctor, Over-the-Counter Medications, Folk Remedies, and Alternative Therapies, and Including a Glossary of Important Terms and a Directory of Resources for Further Help and Information

Edited by Chad T. Kimball. 638 pages. 2001. 0-7808-0435-X. $78.

"A good starting point for research on common illnesses. It will be a useful addition to public and consumer health library collections."
— *American Reference Books Annual 2002*

"Will prove valuable to any library seeking to maintain a current, comprehensive reference collection of health resources. . . . Excellent reference."
— *The Bookwatch, Aug '01*

"Recommended reference source."
— *Booklist, American Library Association, July '01*

Communication Disorders Sourcebook

Basic Information about Deafness and Hearing Loss, Speech and Language Disorders, Voice Disorders, Balance and Vestibular Disorders, and Disorders of Smell, Taste, and Touch

Edited by Linda M. Ross. 533 pages. 1996. 0-7808-0077-X. $78.

"This is skillfully edited and is a welcome resource for the layperson. It should be found in every public and medical library." —*Booklist Health Sciences Supplement, American Library Association, Oct '97*

Congenital Disorders Sourcebook

Basic Information about Disorders Acquired during Gestation, Including Spina Bifida, Hydrocephalus, Cerebral Palsy, Heart Defects, Craniofacial Abnormalities, Fetal Alcohol Syndrome, and More

Along with Current Treatment Options and Statistical Data

Edited by Karen Bellenir. 607 pages. 1997. 0-7808-0205-5. $78.

"Recommended reference source."
—*Booklist, American Library Association, Oct '97*

SEE ALSO *Pregnancy & Birth Sourcebook*

Consumer Issues in Health Care Sourcebook

Basic Information about Health Care Fundamentals and Related Consumer Issues, Including Exams and Screening Tests, Physician Specialties, Choosing a Doctor, Using Prescription and Over-the-Counter Medications Safely, Avoiding Health Scams, Managing Common Health Risks in the Home, Care Options for Chronically or Terminally Ill Patients, and a List of Resources for Obtaining Help and Further Information

Edited by Karen Bellenir. 618 pages. 1998. 0-7808-0221-7. $78.

"Both public and academic libraries will want to have a copy in their collection for readers who are interested in self-education on health issues."
—*American Reference Books Annual, 2000*

"The editor has researched the literature from government agencies and others, saving readers the time and effort of having to do the research themselves. Recommended for public libraries."
—*Reference and User Services Quarterly, American Library Association, Spring '99*

"Recommended reference source."
—*Booklist, American Library Association, Dec '98*

Contagious & Non-Contagious Infectious Diseases Sourcebook

Basic Information about Contagious Diseases like Measles, Polio, Hepatitis B, and Infectious Mononucleosis, and Non-Contagious Infectious Diseases like Tetanus and Toxic Shock Syndrome, and Diseases Occurring as Secondary Infections Such as Shingles and Reye Syndrome

Along with Vaccination, Prevention, and Treatment Information, and a Section Describing Emerging Infectious Disease Threats

Edited by Karen Bellenir and Peter D. Dresser. 566 pages. 1996. 0-7808-0075-3. $78.

Death & Dying Sourcebook

Basic Consumer Health Information for the Layperson about End-of-Life Care and Related Ethical and Legal Issues, Including Chief Causes of Death, Autopsies, Pain Management for the Terminally Ill, Life Support Systems, Insurance, Euthanasia, Assisted Suicide, Hospice Programs, Living Wills, Funeral Planning, Counseling, Mourning, Organ Donation, and Physician Training

Along with Statistical Data, a Glossary, and Listings of Sources for Further Help and Information

Edited by Annemarie S. Muth. 641 pages. 1999. 0-7808-0230-6. $78.

"Public libraries, medical libraries, and academic libraries will all find this sourcebook a useful addition to their collections."
—*American Reference Books Annual, 2001*

"An extremely useful resource for those concerned with death and dying in the United States."
—*Respiratory Care, Nov '00*

"Recommended reference source."
—*Booklist, American Library Association, Aug '00*

"This book is a definite must for all those involved in end-of-life care." —*Doody's Review Service, 2000*

Dental Care & Oral Health Sourcebook, 2nd Edition

Basic Consumer Health Information about Dental Care, Including Oral Hygiene, Dental Visits, Pain Management, Cavities, Crowns, Bridges, Dental Implants, and Fillings, and Other Oral Health Concerns, Such as Gum Disease, Bad Breath, Dry Mouth, Genetic and Developmental Abnormalities, Oral Cancers, Orthodontics, and Temporomandibular Disorders

Along with Updates on Current Research in Oral Health, a Glossary, a Directory of Dental and Oral Health Organizations, and Resources for People with Dental and Oral Health Disorders

Edited by Amy L. Sutton. 609 pages. 2003. 0-7808-0634-4. $78.

Depression Sourcebook

Basic Consumer Health Information about Unipolar Depression, Bipolar Disorder, Postpartum Depression, Seasonal Affective Disorder, and Other Types of Depression in Children, Adolescents, Women, Men, the Elderly, and Other Selected Populations

Along with Facts about Causes, Risk Factors, Diagnostic Criteria, Treatment Options, Coping Strategies, Suicide Prevention, a Glossary, and a Directory of Sources for Additional Help and Information

Edited by Karen Belleni. 602 pages. 2002. 0-7808-0611-5. $78.

Diabetes Sourcebook, 3rd Edition

Basic Consumer Health Information about Type 1 Diabetes (Insulin-Dependent or Juvenile-Onset Diabetes), Type 2 Diabetes (Noninsulin-Dependent or Adult-Onset Diabetes), Gestational Diabetes, Impaired Glucose Tolerance (IGT), and Related Complications, Such as Amputation, Eye Disease, Gum Disease, Nerve Damage, and End-Stage Renal Disease, Including Facts about Insulin, Oral Diabetes Medications, Blood Sugar Testing, and the Role of Exercise and Nutrition in the Control of Diabetes

Along with a Glossary and Resources for Further Help and Information

Edited by Dawn D. Matthews. 622 pages. 2003. 0-7808-0629-8. $78.

ALSO AVAILABLE: Diabetes Sourcebook, 1st Edition. Edited by Karen Bellenir and Peter D. Dresser. 827 pages. 1994. 1-55888-751-2. $78.

Diabetes Sourcebook, 2nd Edition. Edited by Karen Bellenir. 688 pages. 1998. 0-7808-0224-1. $78.

Diet & Nutrition Sourcebook, 2nd Edition

Basic Consumer Health Information about Dietary Guidelines, Recommended Daily Intake Values, Vitamins, Minerals, Fiber, Fat, Weight Control, Dietary Supplements, and Food Additives

Along with Special Sections on Nutrition Needs throughout Life and Nutrition for People with Such Specific Medical Concerns as Allergies, High Blood Cholesterol, Hypertension, Diabetes, Celiac Disease, Seizure Disorders, Phenylketonuria (PKU), Cancer, and Eating Disorders, and Including Reports on Current Nutrition Research and Source Listings for Additional Help and Information

Edited by Karen Bellenir. 650 pages. 1999. 0-7808-0228-4. $78.

ALSO AVAILABLE: Diet & Nutrition Sourcebook, 1st Edition. Edited by Dan R. Harris. 662 pages. 1996. 0-7808-0084-2. $78.

SEE ALSO Digestive Diseases & Disorders Sourcebook, Eating Disorders Sourcebook, Gastrointestinal Diseases & Disorders Sourcebook, Vegetarian Sourcebook

Digestive Diseases & Disorders Sourcebook

Basic Consumer Health Information about Diseases and Disorders that Impact the Upper and Lower Digestive System, Including Celiac Disease, Constipation,

Crohn's Disease, Cyclic Vomiting Syndrome, Diarrhea, Diverticulosis and Diverticulitis, Gallstones, Heartburn, Hemorrhoids, Hernias, Indigestion (Dyspepsia), Irritable Bowel Syndrome, Lactose Intolerance, Ulcers, and More

Along with Information about Medications and Other Treatments, Tips for Maintaining a Healthy Digestive Tract, a Glossary, and Directory of Digestive Diseases Organizations

Edited by Karen Bellenir. 335 pages. 2000. 0-7808-0327-2. $78.

"This title would be an excellent addition to all public or patient-research libraries."
—American Reference Books Annual, 2001

"This title is recommended for public, hospital, and health sciences libraries with consumer health collections."
—E-Streams, Jul-Aug '00

"Recommended reference source."
—Booklist, American Library Association, May '00

SEE ALSO Diet & Nutrition Sourcebook, Eating Disorders Sourcebook, Gastrointestinal Diseases & Disorders Sourcebook

Disabilities Sourcebook

Basic Consumer Health Information about Physical and Psychiatric Disabilities, Including Descriptions of Major Causes of Disability, Assistive and Adaptive Aids, Workplace Issues, and Accessibility Concerns

Along with Information about the Americans with Disabilities Act, a Glossary, and Resources for Additional Help and Information

Edited by Dawn D. Matthews. 616 pages. 2000. 0-7808-0389-2. $78.

"It is a must for libraries with a consumer health section."
—American Reference Books Annual 2002

"A much needed addition to the Omnigraphics Health Reference Series. A current reference work to provide people with disabilities, their families, caregivers or those who work with them, a broad range of information in one volume, has not been available until now. . . . It is recommended for all public and academic library reference collections."
—E-Streams, May '01

"An excellent source book in easy-to-read format covering many current topics; highly recommended for all libraries."
—Choice, Association of College and Research Libraries, Jan '01

"Recommended reference source."
—Booklist, American Library Association, Jul '00

Domestic Violence & Child Abuse Sourcebook

Basic Consumer Health Information about Spousal/ Partner, Child, Sibling, Parent, and Elder Abuse, Covering Physical, Emotional, and Sexual Abuse, Teen Dating Violence, and Stalking; Includes Information

about Hotlines, Safe Houses, Safety Plans, and Other Resources for Support and Assistance, Community Initiatives, and Reports on Current Directions in Research and Treatment

Along with a Glossary, Sources for Further Reading, and Governmental and Non-Governmental Organizations Contact Information

Edited by Helene Henderson. 1,064 pages. 2001. 0-7808-0235-7. $78.

"Interested lay persons should find the book extremely beneficial. . . . A copy of Domestic Violence and Child Abuse Sourcebook should be in every public library in the United States."
—Social Science & Medicine, No. 56, 2003

"This is important information. The Web has many resources but this sourcebook fills an important societal need. I am not aware of any other resources of this type."
—Doody's Review Service, Sep '01

"Recommended for all libraries, scholars, and practitioners."
—Choice, Association of College & Research Libraries, Jul '01

"Recommended reference source."
—Booklist, American Library Association, Apr '01

"Important pick for college-level health reference libraries."
—The Bookwatch, Mar '01

"Because this problem is so widespread and because this book includes a lot of issues within one volume, this work is recommended for all public libraries."
—American Reference Books Annual, 2001

Drug Abuse Sourcebook

Basic Consumer Health Information about Illicit Substances of Abuse and the Diversion of Prescription Medications, Including Depressants, Hallucinogens, Inhalants, Marijuana, Narcotics, Stimulants, and Anabolic Steroids

Along with Facts about Related Health Risks, Treatment Issues, and Substance Abuse Prevention Programs, a Glossary of Terms, Statistical Data, and Directories of Hotline Services, Self-Help Groups, and Organizations Able to Provide Further Information

Edited by Karen Bellenir. 629 pages. 2000. 0-7808-0242-X. $78.

"Containing a wealth of information . . . . This resource belongs in libraries that serve a lower-division undergraduate or community college clientele as well as the general public."
—Choice, Association of College and Research Libraries, Jun '01

"Recommended reference source."
—Booklist, American Library Association, Feb '01

"Highly recommended."
—The Bookwatch, Jan '01

"Even though there is a plethora of books on drug abuse, this volume is recommended for school, public, and college libraries."
—American Reference Books Annual, 2001

SEE ALSO Alcoholism Sourcebook, Substance Abuse Sourcebook

Ear, Nose & Throat Disorders Sourcebook

Basic Information about Disorders of the Ears, Nose, Sinus Cavities, Pharynx, and Larynx, Including Ear Infections, Tinnitus, Vestibular Disorders, Allergic and Non-Allergic Rhinitis, Sore Throats, Tonsillitis, and Cancers That Affect the Ears, Nose, Sinuses, and Throat

Along with Reports on Current Research Initiatives, a Glossary of Related Medical Terms, and a Directory of Sources for Further Help and Information

Edited by Karen Bellenir and Linda M. Shin. 576 pages. 1998. 0-7808-0206-3. $78.

"Overall, this sourcebook is helpful for the consumer seeking information on ENT issues. It is recommended for public libraries."
—American Reference Books Annual, 1999

"Recommended reference source."
—Booklist, American Library Association, Dec '98

■

Eating Disorders Sourcebook

Basic Consumer Health Information about Eating Disorders, Including Information about Anorexia Nervosa, Bulimia Nervosa, Binge Eating, Body Dysmorphic Disorder, Pica, Laxative Abuse, and Night Eating Syndrome

Along with Information about Causes, Adverse Effects, and Treatment and Prevention Issues, and Featuring a Section on Concerns Specific to Children and Adolescents, a Glossary, and Resources for Further Help and Information

Edited by Dawn D. Matthews. 322 pages. 2001. 0-7808-0335-3. $78.

"Recommended for health science libraries that are open to the public, as well as hospital libraries. This book is a good resource for the consumer who is concerned about eating disorders." *— E-Streams, Mar '02*

"This volume is another convenient collection of excerpted articles. Recommended for school and public library patrons; lower-division undergraduates; and two-year technical program students." *— Choice, Association of College & Research Libraries, Jan '02*

"Recommended reference source." *— Booklist, American Library Association, Oct '01*

SEE ALSO *Diet & Nutrition Sourcebook, Digestive Diseases & Disorders Sourcebook, Gastrointestinal Diseases & Disorders Sourcebook*

■

Emergency Medical Services Sourcebook

Basic Consumer Health Information about Preventing, Preparing for, and Managing Emergency Situations, When and Who to Call for Help, What to Expect in the Emergency Room, the Emergency Medical Team, Patient Issues, and Current Topics in Emergency Medicine

Along with Statistical Data, a Glossary, and Sources of Additional Help and Information

Edited by Jenni Lynn Colson. 494 pages. 2002. 0-7808-0420-1. $78.

"Handy and convenient for home, public, school, and college libraries. Recommended."
— Choice, Association of College and Research Libraries, Apr '03

"This reference can provide the consumer with answers to most questions about emergency care in the United States, or it will direct them to a resource where the answer can be found."
—American Reference Books Annual, 2003

"Recommended reference source."
— Booklist, American Library Association, Feb '03

■

Endocrine & Metabolic Disorders Sourcebook

Basic Information for the Layperson about Pancreatic and Insulin-Related Disorders Such as Pancreatitis, Diabetes, and Hypoglycemia; Adrenal Gland Disorders Such as Cushing's Syndrome, Addison's Disease, and Congenital Adrenal Hyperplasia; Pituitary Gland Disorders Such as Growth Hormone Deficiency, Acromegaly, and Pituitary Tumors; Thyroid Disorders Such as Hypothyroidism, Graves' Disease, Hashimoto's Disease, and Goiter; Hyperparathyroidism; and Other Diseases and Syndromes of Hormone Imbalance or Metabolic Dysfunction

Along with Reports on Current Research Initiatives

Edited by Linda M. Shin. 574 pages. 1998. 0-7808-0207-1. $78.

"Omnigraphics has produced another needed resource for health information consumers."
—American Reference Books Annual, 2000

"Recommended reference source."
— Booklist, American Library Association, Dec '98

■

Environmental Health Sourcebook, 2nd Edition

Basic Consumer Health Information about the Environment and Its Effect on Human Health, Including the Effects of Air Pollution, Water Pollution, Hazardous Chemicals, Food Hazards, Radiation Hazards, Biological Agents, Household Hazards, Such as Radon, Asbestos, Carbon Monoxide, and Mold, and Information about Associated Diseases and Disorders, Including Cancer, Allergies, Respiratory Problems, and Skin Disorders

Along with Information about Environmental Concerns for Specific Populations, a Glossary of Related Terms, and Resources for Further Help and Information

Edited by Dawn D. Matthews. 673 pages. 2003. 0-7808-0632-8. $78.

ALSO AVAILABLE: *Environmentally Induced Disorders Sourcebook, 1st Edition. Edited by Allan R. Cook. 620 pages. 1997. 0-7808-0083-4. $78.*

Environmentally Induced Disorders Sourcebook, 1st Edition

SEE *Environmental Health Sourcebook, 2nd Edition*

Ethnic Diseases Sourcebook

Basic Consumer Health Information for Ethnic and Racial Minority Groups in the United States, Including General Health Indicators and Behaviors, Ethnic Diseases, Genetic Testing, the Impact of Chronic Diseases, Women's Health, Mental Health Issues, and Preventive Health Care Services

Along with a Glossary and a Listing of Additional Resources

Edited by Joyce Brennfleck Shannon. 664 pages. 2001. 0-7808-0336-1. $78.

Eye Care Sourcebook, 2nd Edition

Basic Consumer Health Information about Eye Care and Eye Disorders, Including Facts about the Diag-

nosis, Prevention, and Treatment of Common Refractive Problems Such as Myopia, Hyperopia, Astigmatism, and Presbyopia, and Eye Diseases, Including Glaucoma, Cataract, Age-Related Macular Degeneration, and Diabetic Retinopathy

Along with a Section on Vision Correction and Refractive Surgeries, Including LASIK and LASEK, a Glossary, and Directories of Resources for Additional Help and Information

Edited by Amy L. Sutton. 543 pages. 2003. 0-7808-0635-2. $78.

ALSO AVAILABLE: *Ophthalmic Disorders Sourcebook, 1st Edition.* Edited by Linda M. Ross. 631 pages. 1996. 0-7808-0081-8. $78.

Family Planning Sourcebook

Basic Consumer Health Information about Planning for Pregnancy and Contraception, Including Traditional Methods, Barrier Methods, Hormonal Methods, Permanent Methods, Future Methods, Emergency Contraception, and Birth Control Choices for Women at Each Stage of Life

Along with Statistics, a Glossary, and Sources of Additional Information

Edited by Amy Marcaccio Keyzer. 520 pages. 2001. 0-7808-0379-5. $78.

SEE ALSO *Pregnancy & Birth Sourcebook*

Fitness & Exercise Sourcebook, 2nd Edition

Basic Consumer Health Information about the Fundamentals of Fitness and Exercise, Including How to Begin and Maintain a Fitness Program, Fitness as a Lifestyle, the Link between Fitness and Diet, Advice for Specific Groups of People, Exercise as It Relates to Specific Medical Conditions, and Recent Research in Fitness and Exercise

Along with a Glossary of Important Terms and Resources for Additional Help and Information

Edited by Kristen M. Gledhill. 646 pages. 2001. 0-7808-0334-5. $78.

"This work is recommended for all general reference collections."
— *American Reference Books Annual 2002*

"Highly recommended for public, consumer, and school grades fourth through college."
— *E-Streams, Nov '01*

"Recommended reference source." — *Booklist, American Library Association, Oct '01*

"The information appears quite comprehensive and is considered reliable. . . . This second edition is a welcomed addition to the series."
— *Doody's Review Service, Sep '01*

"This reference is a valuable choice for those who desire a broad source of information on exercise, fitness, and chronic-disease prevention through a healthy lifestyle." — *American Medical Writers Association Journal, Fall '01*

"Will prove valuable to any library seeking to maintain a current, comprehensive reference collection of health resources. . . . Excellent reference."
— *The Bookwatch, Aug '01*

Food & Animal Borne Diseases Sourcebook

Basic Information about Diseases That Can Be Spread to Humans through the Ingestion of Contaminated Food or Water or by Contact with Infected Animals and Insects, Such as Botulism, E. Coli, Hepatitis A, Trichinosis, Lyme Disease, and Rabies

Along with Information Regarding Prevention and Treatment Methods, and Including a Special Section for International Travelers Describing Diseases Such as Cholera, Malaria, Travelers' Diarrhea, and Yellow Fever, and Offering Recommendations for Avoiding Illness

Edited by Karen Bellenir and Peter D. Dresser. 535 pages. 1995. 0-7808-0033-8. $78.

"Targeting general readers and providing them with a single, comprehensive source of information on selected topics, this book continues, with the excellent caliber of its predecessors, to catalog topical information on health matters of general interest. Readable and thorough, this valuable resource is highly recommended for all libraries."
— *Academic Library Book Review, Summer '96*

"A comprehensive collection of authoritative information." — *Emergency Medical Services, Oct '95*

Food Safety Sourcebook

Basic Consumer Health Information about the Safe Handling of Meat, Poultry, Seafood, Eggs, Fruit Juices, and Other Food Items, and Facts about Pesticides, Drinking Water, Food Safety Overseas, and the Onset, Duration, and Symptoms of Foodborne Illnesses,

Including Types of Pathogenic Bacteria, Parasitic Protozoa, Worms, Viruses, and Natural Toxins

Along with the Role of the Consumer, the Food Handler, and the Government in Food Safety; a Glossary, and Resources for Additional Help and Information

Edited by Dawn D. Matthews. 339 pages. 1999. 0-7808-0326-4. $78.

"This book is recommended for public libraries and universities with home economic and food science programs." — *E-Streams, Nov '00*

"Recommended reference source."
— *Booklist, American Library Association, May '00*

"This book takes the complex issues of food safety and foodborne pathogens and presents them in an easily understood manner. [It does] an excellent job of covering a large and often confusing topic."
— *American Reference Books Annual, 2000*

Forensic Medicine Sourcebook

Basic Consumer Information for the Layperson about Forensic Medicine, Including Crime Scene Investigation, Evidence Collection and Analysis, Expert Testimony, Computer-Aided Criminal Identification, Digital Imaging in the Courtroom, DNA Profiling, Accident Reconstruction, Autopsies, Ballistics, Drugs and Explosives Detection, Latent Fingerprints, Product Tampering, and Questioned Document Examination

Along with Statistical Data, a Glossary of Forensics Terminology, and Listings of Sources for Further Help and Information

Edited by Annemarie S. Muth. 574 pages. 1999. 0-7808-0232-2. $78.

"Given the expected widespread interest in its content and its easy to read style, this book is recommended for most public and all college and university libraries."
— *E-Streams, Feb '01*

"Recommended for public libraries."
— *Reference & User Services Quarterly, American Library Association, Spring 2000*

"Recommended reference source."
— *Booklist, American Library Association, Feb '00*

"A wealth of information, useful statistics, references are up-to-date and extremely complete. This wonderful collection of data will help students who are interested in a career in any type of forensic field. It is a great resource for attorneys who need information about types of expert witnesses needed in a particular case. It also offers useful information for fiction and nonfiction writers whose work involves a crime. A fascinating compilation. All levels." — *Choice, Association of College and Research Libraries, Jan 2000*

"There are several items that make this book attractive to consumers who are seeking certain forensic data. . . . This is a useful current source for those seeking general forensic medical answers."
— *American Reference Books Annual, 2000*

Gastrointestinal Diseases & Disorders Sourcebook

Basic Information about Gastroesophageal Reflux Disease (Heartburn), Ulcers, Diverticulosis, Irritable Bowel Syndrome, Crohn's Disease, Ulcerative Colitis, Diarrhea, Constipation, Lactose Intolerance, Hemorrhoids, Hepatitis, Cirrhosis, and Other Digestive Problems, Featuring Statistics, Descriptions of Symptoms, and Current Treatment Methods of Interest for Persons Living with Upper and Lower Gastrointestinal Maladies

Edited by Linda M. Ross. 413 pages. 1996. 0-7808-0078-8. $78.

". . . very readable form. The successful editorial work that brought this material together into a useful and understandable reference makes accessible to all readers information that can help them more effectively understand and obtain help for digestive tract problems."
— *Choice, Association of College & Research Libraries, Feb '97*

SEE ALSO *Diet & Nutrition Sourcebook, Digestive Diseases & Disorders, Eating Disorders Sourcebook*

Genetic Disorders Sourcebook, 2nd Edition

Basic Consumer Health Information about Hereditary Diseases and Disorders, Including Cystic Fibrosis, Down Syndrome, Hemophilia, Huntington's Disease, Sickle Cell Anemia, and More; Facts about Genes, Gene Research and Therapy, Genetic Screening, Ethics of Gene Testing, Genetic Counseling, and Advice on Coping and Caring

Along with a Glossary of Genetic Terminology and a Resource List for Help, Support, and Further Information

Edited by Kathy Massimini. 768 pages. 2001. 0-7808-0241-1. $78.

ALSO AVAILABLE: *Genetic Disorders Sourcebook, 1st Edition*. Edited by Karen Bellenir. 642 pages. 1996. 0-7808-0034-6. $78.

"Recommended for public libraries and medical and hospital libraries with consumer health collections."
— *E-Streams, May '01*

"Recommended reference source."
— *Booklist, American Library Association, Apr '01*

"Important pick for college-level health reference libraries." — *The Bookwatch, Mar '01*

"Provides essential medical information to both the general public and those diagnosed with a serious or fatal genetic disease or disorder." —*Choice, Association of College and Research Libraries, Jan '97*

Head Trauma Sourcebook

Basic Information for the Layperson about Open-Head and Closed-Head Injuries, Treatment Advances, Recovery, and Rehabilitation

Along with Reports on Current Research Initiatives

Edited by Karen Bellenir. 414 pages. 1997. 0-7808-0208-X. $78.

Headache Sourcebook

Basic Consumer Health Information about Migraine, Tension, Cluster, Rebound and Other Types of Headaches, with Facts about the Cause and Prevention of Headaches, the Effects of Stress and the Environment, Headaches during Pregnancy and Menopause, and Childhood Headaches

Along with a Glossary and Other Resources for Additional Help and Information

Edited by Dawn D. Matthews. 362 pages. 2002. 0-7808-0337-X. $78.

"Highly recommended for academic and medical reference collections." — *Library Bookwatch, Sep '02*

Health Insurance Sourcebook

Basic Information about Managed Care Organizations, Traditional Fee-for-Service Insurance, Insurance Portability and Pre-Existing Conditions Clauses, Medicare, Medicaid, Social Security, and Military Health Care

Along with Information about Insurance Fraud

Edited by Wendy Wilcox. 530 pages. 1997. 0-7808-0222-5. $78.

"Particularly useful because it brings much of this information together in one volume. This book will be a handy reference source in the health sciences library, hospital library, college and university library, and medium to large public library."
— *Medical Reference Services Quarterly, Fall '98*

Awarded "Books of the Year Award"
— *American Journal of Nursing, 1997*

"The layout of the book is particularly helpful as it provides easy access to reference material. A most useful addition to the vast amount of information about health insurance. The use of data from U.S. government agencies is most commendable. Useful in a library or learning center for healthcare professional students."
— *Doody's Health Sciences Book Reviews, Nov '97*

Health Reference Series Cumulative Index 1999

A Comprehensive Index to the Individual Volumes of the Health Reference Series, Including a Subject Index, Name Index, Organization Index, and Publication Index

Along with a Master List of Acronyms and Abbreviations

Edited by Edward J. Prucha, Anne Holmes, and Robert Rudnick. 990 pages. 2000. 0-7808-0382-5. $78.

"This volume will be most helpful in libraries that have a relatively complete collection of the Health Reference Series." —*American Reference Books Annual, 2001*

"Essential for collections that hold any of the numerous *Health Reference Series* titles." —*Choice, Association of College and Research Libraries, Nov '00*

Healthy Aging Sourcebook

Basic Consumer Health Information about Maintaining Health through the Aging Process, Including Advice on Nutrition, Exercise, and Sleep, Help in Making Decisions about Midlife Issues and Retirement, and Guidance Concerning Practical and Informed Choices in Health Consumerism

Along with Data Concerning the Theories of Aging, Different Experiences in Aging by Minority Groups, and Facts about Aging Now and Aging in the Future; and Featuring a Glossary, a Guide to Consumer Help, Additional Suggested Reading, and Practical Resource Directory

Edited by Jenifer Swanson. 536 pages. 1999. 0-7808-0390-6. $78.

"Recommended reference source." —*Booklist, American Library Association, Feb '00*

SEE ALSO *Physical & Mental Issues in Aging Sourcebook*

Healthy Children Sourcebook

Basic Consumer Health Information about the Physical and Mental Development of Children between the Ages of 3 and 12, Including Routine Health Care, Preventative Health Services, Safety and First Aid, Healthy Sleep, Dental Care, Nutrition, and Fitness, and Featuring Parenting Tips on Such Topics as Bedwetting, Choosing Day Care, Monitoring TV and Other Media, and Establishing a Foundation for Substance Abuse Prevention

Along with a Glossary of Commonly Used Pediatric Terms and Resources for Additional Help and Information.

Edited by Chad T. Kimball. 647 pages. 2003. 0-7808-0247-0. $78.

Healthy Heart Sourcebook for Women

Basic Consumer Health Information about Cardiac Issues Specific to Women, Including Facts about Major Risk Factors and Prevention, Treatment and Control Strategies, and Important Dietary Issues

Along with a Special Section Regarding the Pros and Cons of Hormone Replacement Therapy and Its Impact on Heart Health, and Additional Help, Including Recipes, a Glossary, and a Directory of Resources

Edited by Dawn D. Matthews. 336 pages. 2000. 0-7808-0329-9. $78.

"A good reference source and recommended for all public, academic, medical, and hospital libraries." —*Medical Reference Services Quarterly, Summer '01*

"Because of the lack of information specific to women on this topic, this book is recommended for public libraries and consumer libraries." —*American Reference Books Annual, 2001*

"Contains very important information about coronary artery disease that all women should know. The information is current and presented in an easy-to-read format. The book will make a good addition to any library." —*American Medical Writers Association Journal, Summer '00*

"Important, basic reference." —*Reviewer's Bookwatch, Jul '00*

SEE ALSO *Heart Diseases & Disorders Sourcebook, Women's Health Concerns Sourcebook*

Heart Diseases & Disorders Sourcebook, 2nd Edition

Basic Consumer Health Information about Heart Attacks, Angina, Rhythm Disorders, Heart Failure, Valve Disease, Congenital Heart Disorders, and More, Including Descriptions of Surgical Procedures and Other Interventions, Medications, Cardiac Rehabilitation, Risk Identification, and Prevention Tips

Along with Statistical Data, Reports on Current Research Initiatives, a Glossary of Cardiovascular Terms, and Resource Directory

Edited by Karen Bellenir. 612 pages. 2000. 0-7808-0238-1. $78.

ALSO AVAILABLE: *Cardiovascular Diseases & Disorders Sourcebook, 1st Edition.* Edited by Karen Bellenir and Peter D. Dresser. 683 pages. 1995. 0-7808-0032-X. $78.

"This work stands out as an imminently accessible resource for the general public. It is recommended for the reference and circulating shelves of school, public, and academic libraries." —*American Reference Books Annual, 2001*

"Recommended reference source." —*Booklist, American Library Association, Dec '00*

"Provides comprehensive coverage of matters related to the heart. This title is recommended for health sciences and public libraries with consumer health collections." —*E-Streams, Oct '00*

SEE ALSO *Healthy Heart Sourcebook for Women*

Household Safety Sourcebook

Basic Consumer Health Information about Household Safety, Including Information about Poisons, Chemicals, Fire, and Water Hazards in the Home

Along with Advice about the Safe Use of Home Maintenance Equipment, Choosing Toys and Nursery Furni-

ture, *Holiday and Recreation Safety, a Glossary, and Resources for Further Help and Information*

Edited by Dawn D. Matthews. 606 pages. 2002. 0-7808-0338-8. $78.

"This work will be useful in public libraries with large consumer health and wellness departments."
— *American Reference Books Annual, 2003*

"As a sourcebook on household safety this book meets its mark. It is encyclopedic in scope and covers a wide range of safety issues that are commonly seen in the home."
— *E-Streams, Jul '02*

Immune System Disorders Sourcebook

Basic Information about Lupus, Multiple Sclerosis, Guillain-Barré Syndrome, Chronic Granulomatous Disease, and More

Along with Statistical and Demographic Data and Reports on Current Research Initiatives

Edited by Allan R. Cook. 608 pages. 1997. 0-7808-0209-8. $78.

Infant & Toddler Health Sourcebook

Basic Consumer Health Information about the Physical and Mental Development of Newborns, Infants, and Toddlers, Including Neonatal Concerns, Nutrition Recommendations, Immunization Schedules, Common Pediatric Disorders, Assessments and Milestones, Safety Tips, and Advice for Parents and Other Caregivers

Along with a Glossary of Terms and Resource Listings for Additional Help

Edited by Jenifer Swanson. 585 pages. 2000. 0-7808-0246-2. $78.

"As a reference for the general public, this would be useful in any library."
— *E-Streams, May '01*

"Recommended reference source."
— *Booklist, American Library Association, Feb '01*

"This is a good source for general use."
— *American Reference Books Annual, 2001*

Injury & Trauma Sourcebook

Basic Consumer Health Information about the Impact of Injury, the Diagnosis and Treatment of Common and Traumatic Injuries, Emergency Care, and Specific Injuries Related to Home, Community, Workplace, Transportation, and Recreation

Along with Guidelines for Injury Prevention, a Glossary, and a Directory of Additional Resources

Edited by Joyce Brennfleck Shannon. 696 pages. 2002. 0-7808-0421-X. $78.

"This publication is the most comprehensive work of its kind about injury and trauma."
— *American Reference Books Annual, 2003*

"This sourcebook provides concise, easily readable, basic health information about injuries. . . . This book is well organized and an easy to use reference resource suitable for hospital, health sciences and public libraries with consumer health collections."
— *E-Streams, Nov '02*

"Practitioners should be aware of guides such as this in order to facilitate their use by patients and their families."
— *Doody's Health Sciences Book Review Journal, Sep-Oct '02*

"Recommended reference source."
— *Booklist, American Library Association, Sep '02*

"Highly recommended for academic and medical reference collections."
— *Library Bookwatch, Sep '02*

Kidney & Urinary Tract Diseases & Disorders Sourcebook

Basic Information about Kidney Stones, Urinary Incontinence, Bladder Disease, End Stage Renal Disease, Dialysis, and More

Along with Statistical and Demographic Data and Reports on Current Research Initiatives

Edited by Linda M. Ross. 602 pages. 1997. 0-7808-0079-6. $78.

Learning Disabilities Sourcebook, 2nd Edition

Basic Consumer Health Information about Learning Disabilities, Including Dyslexia, Developmental Speech and Language Disabilities, Non-Verbal Learning Disorders, Developmental Arithmetic Disorder, Developmental Writing Disorder, and Other Conditions That Impede Learning Such as Attention Deficit/ Hyperactivity Disorder, Brain Injury, Hearing Impairment, Klinefelter Syndrome, Dyspraxia, and Tourette Syndrome

Along with Facts about Educational Issues and Assistive Technology, Coping Strategies, a Glossary of Related Terms, and Resources for Further Help and Information

Edited by Dawn D. Matthews. 621 pages. 2003. 0-7808-0626-3. $78.

ALSO AVAILABLE: Learning Disabilities Sourcebook, 1st Edition. Edited by Linda M. Shin. 579 pages. 1998. 0-7808-0210-1. $78.

"Teachers as well as consumers will find this an essential guide to understanding various syndromes and their latest treatments. [An] invaluable reference for public and school library collections alike."
— *Library Bookwatch, Apr '03*

Named "Outstanding Reference Book of 1999."
— *New York Public Library, Feb 2000*

"An excellent candidate for inclusion in a public library reference section. It's a great source of information. Teachers will also find the book useful. Definitely worth reading."
— *Journal of Adolescent & Adult Literacy, Feb 2000*

"Readable . . . provides a solid base of information regarding successful techniques used with individuals who have learning disabilities, as well as practical suggestions for educators and family members. Clear language, concise descriptions, and pertinent information for contacting multiple resources add to the strength of this book as a useful tool." — *Choice, Association of College and Research Libraries, Feb '99*

"Recommended reference source."
— *Booklist, American Library Association, Sep '98*

"A useful resource for libraries and for those who don't have the time to identify and locate the individual publications." — *Disability Resources Monthly, Sep '98*

Leukemia Sourcebook

Basic Consumer Health Information about Adult and Childhood Leukemias, Including Acute Lymphocytic Leukemia (ALL), Chronic Lymphocytic Leukemia (CLL), Acute Myelogenous Leukemia (AML), Chronic Myelogenous Leukemia (CML), and Hairy Cell Leukemia, and Treatments Such as Chemotherapy, Radiation Therapy, Peripheral Blood Stem Cell and Marrow Transplantation, and Immunotherapy

Along with Tips for Life During and After Treatment, a Glossary, and Directories of Additional Resources

Edited by Joyce Brennfleck Shannon. 587 pages. 2003. 0-7808-0627-1. $78.

Liver Disorders Sourcebook

Basic Consumer Health Information about the Liver and How It Works; Liver Diseases, Including Cancer, Cirrhosis, Hepatitis, and Toxic and Drug Related Diseases; Tips for Maintaining a Healthy Liver; Laboratory Tests, Radiology Tests, and Facts about Liver Transplantation

Along with a Section on Support Groups, a Glossary, and Resource Listings

Edited by Joyce Brennfleck Shannon. 591 pages. 2000. 0-7808-0383-3. $78.

"A valuable resource."
— *American Reference Books Annual, 2001*

"This title is recommended for health sciences and public libraries with consumer health collections."
— *E-Streams, Oct '00*

"Recommended reference source."
— *Booklist, American Library Association, Jun '00*

Lung Disorders Sourcebook

Basic Consumer Health Information about Emphysema, Pneumonia, Tuberculosis, Asthma, Cystic Fibrosis, and Other Lung Disorders, Including Facts about Diagnostic Procedures, Treatment Strategies, Disease Prevention Efforts, and Such Risk Factors as Smoking, Air Pollution, and Exposure to Asbestos, Radon, and Other Agents

Along with a Glossary and Resources for Additional Help and Information

Edited by Dawn D. Matthews. 678 pages. 2002. 0-7808-0339-6. $78.

"This title is a great addition for public and school libraries because it provides concise health information on the lungs."
— *American Reference Books Annual, 2003*

"Highly recommended for academic and medical reference collections." — *Library Bookwatch, Sep '02*

Medical Tests Sourcebook

Basic Consumer Health Information about Medical Tests, Including Periodic Health Exams, General Screening Tests, Tests You Can Do at Home, Findings of the U.S. Preventive Services Task Force, X-ray and Radiology Tests, Electrical Tests, Tests of Blood and Other Body Fluids and Tissues, Scope Tests, Lung Tests, Genetic Tests, Pregnancy Tests, Newborn Screening Tests, Sexually Transmitted Disease Tests, and Computer Aided Diagnoses

Along with a Section on Paying for Medical Tests, a Glossary, and Resource Listings

Edited by Joyce Brennfleck Shannon. 691 pages. 1999. 0-7808-0243-8. $78.

"Recommended for hospital and health sciences libraries with consumer health collections."
— *E-Streams, Mar '00*

"This is an overall excellent reference with a wealth of general knowledge that may aid those who are reluctant to get vital tests performed."
— *Today's Librarian, Jan 2000*

"A valuable reference guide."
— *American Reference Books Annual, 2000*

Men's Health Concerns Sourcebook

Basic Information about Health Issues That Affect Men, Featuring Facts about the Top Causes of Death in Men, Including Heart Disease, Stroke, Cancers, Prostate Disorders, Chronic Obstructive Pulmonary Disease, Pneumonia and Influenza, Human Immunodeficiency Virus and Acquired Immune Deficiency Syndrome, Diabetes Mellitus, Stress, Suicide, Accidents and Homicides; and Facts about Common Concerns for Men, Including Impotence, Contraception, Circumcision, Sleep Disorders, Snoring, Hair Loss, Diet, Nutrition, Exercise, Kidney and Urological Disorders, and Backaches

Edited by Allan R. Cook. 738 pages. 1998. 0-7808-0212-8. $78.

"This comprehensive resource and the series are highly recommended."
— *American Reference Books Annual, 2000*

"Recommended reference source."
— *Booklist, American Library Association, Dec '98*

Mental Health Disorders Sourcebook, 2nd Edition

Basic Consumer Health Information about Anxiety Disorders, Depression and Other Mood Disorders, Eating Disorders, Personality Disorders, Schizophrenia, and More, Including Disease Descriptions, Treatment Options, and Reports on Current Research Initiatives

Along with Statistical Data, Tips for Maintaining Mental Health, a Glossary, and Directory of Sources for Additional Help and Information

Edited by Karen Bellenir. 605 pages. 2000. 0-7808-0240-3. $78.

ALSO AVAILABLE: *Mental Health Disorders Sourcebook, 1st Edition.* Edited by Karen Bellenir. 548 pages. 1995. 0-7808-0040-0. $78.

"Well organized and well written."
— *American Reference Books Annual, 2001*

"Recommended reference source."
— *Booklist, American Library Association, Jun '00*

Mental Retardation Sourcebook

Basic Consumer Health Information about Mental Retardation and Its Causes, Including Down Syndrome, Fetal Alcohol Syndrome, Fragile X Syndrome, Genetic Conditions, Injury, and Environmental Sources

Along with Preventive Strategies, Parenting Issues, Educational Implications, Health Care Needs, Employment and Economic Matters, Legal Issues, a Glossary, and a Resource Listing for Additional Help and Information

Edited by Joyce Brennfleck Shannon. 642 pages. 2000. 0-7808-0377-9. $78.

"Public libraries will find the book useful for reference and as a beginning research point for students, parents, and caregivers."
— *American Reference Books Annual, 2001*

"The strength of this work is that it compiles many basic fact sheets and addresses for further information in one volume. It is intended and suitable for the general public. This sourcebook is relevant to any collection providing health information to the general public."
— *E-Streams, Nov '00*

"From preventing retardation to parenting and family challenges, this covers health, social and legal issues and will prove an invaluable overview."
— *Reviewer's Bookwatch, Jul '00*

Movement Disorders Sourcebook

Basic Consumer Health Information about Neurological Movement Disorders, Including Essential Tremor, Parkinson's Disease, Dystonia, Cerebral Palsy, Huntington's Disease, Myasthenia Gravis, Multiple Sclerosis, and Other Early-Onset and Adult-Onset Movement Disorders, Their Symptoms and Causes, Diagnostic Tests, and Treatments

Along with Mobility and Assistive Technology Infor-

mation, a Glossary, and a Directory of Additional Resources*

Edited by Joyce Brennfleck Shannon. 655 pages. 2003. 0-7808-0628-X. $78.

Obesity Sourcebook

Basic Consumer Health Information about Diseases and Other Problems Associated with Obesity, and Including Facts about Risk Factors, Prevention Issues, and Management Approaches

Along with Statistical and Demographic Data, Information about Special Populations, Research Updates, a Glossary, and Source Listings for Further Help and Information

Edited by Wilma Caldwell and Chad T. Kimball. 376 pages. 2001. 0-7808-0333-7. $78.

"The book synthesizes the reliable medical literature on obesity into one easy-to-read and useful resource for the general public."
— *American Reference Books Annual 2002*

"This is a very useful resource book for the lay public."
— *Doody's Review Service, Nov '01*

"Well suited for the health reference collection of a public library or an academic health science library that serves the general population." — *E-Streams, Sep '01*

"Recommended reference source."
— *Booklist, American Library Association, Apr '01*

" Recommended pick both for specialty health library collections and any general consumer health reference collection." — *The Bookwatch, Apr '01*

Ophthalmic Disorders Sourcebook, 1st Edition

SEE Eye Care Sourcebook, 2nd Edition

Oral Health Sourcebook

SEE Dental Care & Oral Health Sourcebook, 2nd Edition

Osteoporosis Sourcebook

Basic Consumer Health Information about Primary and Secondary Osteoporosis and Juvenile Osteoporosis and Related Conditions, Including Fibrous Dysplasia, Gaucher Disease, Hyperthyroidism, Hypophosphatasia, Myeloma, Osteopetrosis, Osteogenesis Imperfecta, and Paget's Disease

Along with Information about Risk Factors, Treatments, Traditional and Non-Traditional Pain Management, a Glossary of Related Terms, and a Directory of Resources

Edited by Allan R. Cook. 584 pages. 2001. 0-7808-0239-X. $78.

"This would be a book to be kept in a staff or patient library. The targeted audience is the layperson, but the therapist who needs a quick bit of information on a particular topic will also find the book useful."
— *Physical Therapy, Jan '02*

"This resource is recommended as a great reference source for public, health, and academic libraries, and is another triumph for the editors of Omnigraphics."
— *American Reference Books Annual 2002*

"Recommended for all public libraries and general health collections, especially those supporting patient education or consumer health programs."
— *E-Streams, Nov '01*

"Will prove valuable to any library seeking to maintain a current, comprehensive reference collection of health resources. . . . From prevention to treatment and associated conditions, this provides an excellent survey."
— *The Bookwatch, Aug '01*

"Recommended reference source."
— *Booklist, American Library Association, July '01*

SEE ALSO *Women's Health Concerns Sourcebook*

▪

Pain Sourcebook, 2nd Edition

Basic Consumer Health Information about Specific Forms of Acute and Chronic Pain, Including Muscle and Skeletal Pain, Nerve Pain, Cancer Pain, and Disorders Characterized by Pain, Such as Fibromyalgia, Shingles, Angina, Arthritis, and Headaches

Along with Information about Pain Medications and Management Techniques, Complementary and Alternative Pain Relief Options, Tips for People Living with Chronic Pain, a Glossary, and a Directory of Sources for Further Information

Edited by Karen Bellenir. 670 pages. 2002. 0-7808-0612-3. $78.

ALSO AVAILABLE: *Pain Sourcebook, 1st Edition.* Edited by Allan R. Cook. 667 pages. 1997. 0-7808-0213-6. $78.

"A source of valuable information. . . . This book offers help to nonmedical people who need information about pain and pain management. It is also an excellent reference for those who participate in patient education."
— *Doody's Review Service, Sep '02*

"The text is readable, easily understood, and well indexed. This excellent volume belongs in all patient education libraries, consumer health sections of public libraries, and many personal collections."
— *American Reference Books Annual, 1999*

"A beneficial reference." — *Booklist Health Sciences Supplement, American Library Association, Oct '98*

"The information is basic in terms of scholarship and is appropriate for general readers. Written in journalistic style . . . intended for non-professionals. Quite thorough in its coverage of different pain conditions and summarizes the latest clinical information regarding pain treatment." — *Choice, Association of College and Research Libraries, Jun '98*

"Recommended reference source."
— *Booklist, American Library Association, Mar '98*

Pediatric Cancer Sourcebook

Basic Consumer Health Information about Leukemias, Brain Tumors, Sarcomas, Lymphomas, and Other Cancers in Infants, Children, and Adolescents, Including Descriptions of Cancers, Treatments, and Coping Strategies

Along with Suggestions for Parents, Caregivers, and Concerned Relatives, a Glossary of Cancer Terms, and Resource Listings

Edited by Edward J. Prucha. 587 pages. 1999. 0-7808-0245-4. $78.

"An excellent source of information. Recommended for public, hospital, and health science libraries with consumer health collections." — *E-Streams, Jun '00*

"Recommended reference source."
— *Booklist, American Library Association, Feb '00*

"A valuable addition to all libraries specializing in health services and many public libraries."
— *American Reference Books Annual, 2000*

▪

Physical & Mental Issues in Aging Sourcebook

Basic Consumer Health Information on Physical and Mental Disorders Associated with the Aging Process, Including Concerns about Cardiovascular Disease, Pulmonary Disease, Oral Health, Digestive Disorders, Musculoskeletal and Skin Disorders, Metabolic Changes, Sexual and Reproductive Issues, and Changes in Vision, Hearing, and Other Senses

Along with Data about Longevity and Causes of Death, Information on Acute and Chronic Pain, Descriptions of Mental Concerns, a Glossary of Terms, and Resource Listings for Additional Help

Edited by Jenifer Swanson. 660 pages. 1999. 0-7808-0233-0. $78.

"This is a treasure of health information for the layperson." — *Choice Health Sciences Supplement, Association of College & Research Libraries, May 2000*

"Recommended for public libraries."
— *American Reference Books Annual, 2000*

"Recommended reference source."
— *Booklist, American Library Association, Oct '99*

SEE ALSO *Healthy Aging Sourcebook*

▪

Podiatry Sourcebook

Basic Consumer Health Information about Foot Conditions, Diseases, and Injuries, Including Bunions, Corns, Calluses, Athlete's Foot, Plantar Warts, Hammertoes and Clawtoes, Clubfoot, Heel Pain, Gout, and More

Along with Facts about Foot Care, Disease Prevention, Foot Safety, Choosing a Foot Care Specialist, a Glossary of Terms, and Resource Listings for Additional Information

Edited by M. Lisa Weatherford. 380 pages. 2001. 0-7808-0215-2. $78.

"There is a lot of information presented here on a topic that is usually only covered sparingly in most larger comprehensive medical encyclopedias."
— *American Reference Books Annual 2002*

∎

Pregnancy & Birth Sourcebook

Basic Information about Planning for Pregnancy, Maternal Health, Fetal Growth and Development, Labor and Delivery, Postpartum and Perinatal Care, Pregnancy in Mothers with Special Concerns, and Disorders of Pregnancy, Including Genetic Counseling, Nutrition and Exercise, Obstetrical Tests, Pregnancy Discomfort, Multiple Births, Cesarean Sections, Medical Testing of Newborns, Breastfeeding, Gestational Diabetes, and Ectopic Pregnancy

Edited by Heather E. Aldred. 737 pages. 1997. 0-7808-0216-0. $78.

"A well-organized handbook. Recommended."
— *Choice, Association of College and Research Libraries, Apr '98*

"Recommended reference source."
— *Booklist, American Library Association, Mar '98*

"Recommended for public libraries."
— *American Reference Books Annual, 1998*

SEE ALSO *Congenital Disorders Sourcebook, Family Planning Sourcebook*

∎

Prostate Cancer Sourcebook

Basic Consumer Health Information about Prostate Cancer, Including Information about the Associated Risk Factors, Detection, Diagnosis, and Treatment of Prostate Cancer

Along with Information on Non-Malignant Prostate Conditions, and Featuring a Section Listing Support and Treatment Centers and a Glossary of Related Terms

Edited by Dawn D. Matthews. 358 pages. 2001. 0-7808-0324-8. $78.

"Recommended reference source."
— *Booklist, American Library Association, Jan '02*

"A valuable resource for health care consumers seeking information on the subject. . . .All text is written in a clear, easy-to-understand language that avoids technical jargon. Any library that collects consumer health resources would strengthen their collection with the addition of the *Prostate Cancer Sourcebook*."
— *American Reference Books Annual 2002*

∎

Public Health Sourcebook

Basic Information about Government Health Agencies, Including National Health Statistics and Trends, Healthy People 2000 Program Goals and Objectives, the Centers for Disease Control and Prevention, the

Food and Drug Administration, and the National Institutes of Health

Along with Full Contact Information for Each Agency

Edited by Wendy Wilcox. 698 pages. 1998. 0-7808-0220-9. $78.

"Recommended reference source."
— *Booklist, American Library Association, Sep '98*

"This consumer guide provides welcome assistance in navigating the maze of federal health agencies and their data on public health concerns."
— *SciTech Book News, Sep '98*

∎

Reconstructive & Cosmetic Surgery Sourcebook

Basic Consumer Health Information on Cosmetic and Reconstructive Plastic Surgery, Including Statistical Information about Different Surgical Procedures, Things to Consider Prior to Surgery, Plastic Surgery Techniques and Tools, Emotional and Psychological Considerations, and Procedure-Specific Information

Along with a Glossary of Terms and a Listing of Resources for Additional Help and Information

Edited by M. Lisa Weatherford. 374 pages. 2001. 0-7808-0214-4. $78.

"An excellent reference that addresses cosmetic and medically necessary reconstructive surgeries. . . . The style of the prose is calm and reassuring, discussing the many positive outcomes now available due to advances in surgical techniques."
— *American Reference Books Annual 2002*

"Recommended for health science libraries that are open to the public, as well as hospital libraries that are open to the patients. This book is a good resource for the consumer interested in plastic surgery."
— *E-Streams, Dec '01*

"Recommended reference source."
— *Booklist, American Library Association, July '01*

∎

Rehabilitation Sourcebook

Basic Consumer Health Information about Rehabilitation for People Recovering from Heart Surgery, Spinal Cord Injury, Stroke, Orthopedic Impairments, Amputation, Pulmonary Impairments, Traumatic Injury, and More, Including Physical Therapy, Occupational Therapy, Speech/ Language Therapy, Massage Therapy, Dance Therapy, Art Therapy, and Recreational Therapy

Along with Information on Assistive and Adaptive Devices, a Glossary, and Resources for Additional Help and Information

Edited by Dawn D. Matthews. 531 pages. 1999. 0-7808-0236-5. $78.

"This is an excellent resource for public library reference and health collections."
— *American Reference Books Annual, 2001*

"Recommended reference source."
— *Booklist, American Library Association, May '00*

Respiratory Diseases & Disorders Sourcebook

Basic Information about Respiratory Diseases and Disorders, Including Asthma, Cystic Fibrosis, Pneumonia, the Common Cold, Influenza, and Others, Featuring Facts about the Respiratory System, Statistical and Demographic Data, Treatments, Self-Help Management Suggestions, and Current Research Initiatives

Edited by Allan R. Cook and Peter D. Dresser. 771 pages. 1995. 0-7808-0037-0. $78.

"Designed for the layperson and for patients and their families coping with respiratory illness. . . . an extensive array of information on diagnosis, treatment, management, and prevention of respiratory illnesses for the general reader." *— Choice, Association of College and Research Libraries, Jun '96*

"A highly recommended text for all collections. It is a comforting reminder of the power of knowledge that good books carry between their covers."
— Academic Library Book Review, Spring '96

"A comprehensive collection of authoritative information presented in a nontechnical, humanitarian style for patients, families, and caregivers."
— Association of Operating Room Nurses, Sep/Oct '95

SEE ALSO *Lung Disorders Sourcebook*

Sexually Transmitted Diseases Sourcebook, 2nd Edition

Basic Consumer Health Information about Sexually Transmitted Diseases, Including Information on the Diagnosis and Treatment of Chlamydia, Gonorrhea, Hepatitis, Herpes, HIV, Mononucleosis, Syphilis, and Others

Along with Information on Prevention, Such as Condom Use, Vaccines, and STD Education; And Featuring a Section on Issues Related to Youth and Adolescents, a Glossary, and Resources for Additional Help and Information

Edited by Dawn D. Matthews. 538 pages. 2001. 0-7808-0249-7. $78.

ALSO AVAILABLE: *Sexually Transmitted Diseases Sourcebook, 1st Edition.* Edited by Linda M. Ross. 550 pages. 1997. 0-7808-0217-9. $78.

"Recommended for consumer health collections in public libraries, and secondary school and community college libraries."
— American Reference Books Annual 2002

"Every school and public library should have a copy of this comprehensive and user-friendly reference book."
— Choice, Association of College & Research Libraries, Sep '01

"This is a highly recommended book. This is an especially important book for all school and public libraries." *— AIDS Book Review Journal, Jul-Aug '01*

"Recommended reference source."
— Booklist, American Library Association, Apr '01

"Recommended pick both for specialty health library collections and any general consumer health reference collection." *— The Bookwatch, Apr '01*

Skin Disorders Sourcebook

Basic Information about Common Skin and Scalp Conditions Caused by Aging, Allergies, Immune Reactions, Sun Exposure, Infectious Organisms, Parasites, Cosmetics, and Skin Traumas, Including Abrasions, Cuts, and Pressure Sores

Along with Information on Prevention and Treatment

Edited by Allan R. Cook. 647 pages. 1997. 0-7808-0080-X. $78.

". . . comprehensive, easily read reference book."
— Doody's Health Sciences Book Reviews, Oct '97

SEE ALSO *Burns Sourcebook*

Sleep Disorders Sourcebook

Basic Consumer Health Information about Sleep and Its Disorders, Including Insomnia, Sleepwalking, Sleep Apnea, Restless Leg Syndrome, and Narcolepsy

Along with Data about Shiftwork and Its Effects, Information on the Societal Costs of Sleep Deprivation, Descriptions of Treatment Options, a Glossary of Terms, and Resource Listings for Additional Help

Edited by Jenifer Swanson. 439 pages. 1998. 0-7808-0234-9. $78.

"This text will complement any home or medical library. It is user-friendly and ideal for the adult reader."
— American Reference Books Annual, 2000

"A useful resource that provides accurate, relevant, and accessible information on sleep to the general public. Health care providers who deal with sleep disorders patients may also find it helpful in being prepared to answer some of the questions patients ask."
— Respiratory Care, Jul '99

"Recommended reference source."
— Booklist, American Library Association, Feb '99

Sports Injuries Sourcebook, 2nd Edition

Basic Consumer Health Information about the Diagnosis, Treatment, and Rehabilitation of Common Sports-Related Injuries in Children and Adults

Along with Suggestions for Conditioning and Training, Information and Prevention Tips for Injuries Frequently Associated with Specific Sports and Special Populations, a Glossary, and a Directory of Additional Resources

Edited by Joyce Brennfleck Shannon. 614 pages. 2002. 0-7808-0604-2. $78.

ALSO AVAILABLE: *Sports Injuries Sourcebook, 1st Edition.* Edited by Heather E. Aldred. 624 pages. 1999. 0-7808-0218-7. $78.

Stress-Related Disorders Sourcebook

Basic Consumer Health Information about Stress and Stress-Related Disorders, Including Stress Origins and Signals, Environmental Stress at Work and Home, Mental and Emotional Stress Associated with Depression, Post-Traumatic Stress Disorder, Panic Disorder, Suicide, and the Physical Effects of Stress on the Cardiovascular, Immune, and Nervous Systems

Along with Stress Management Techniques, a Glossary, and a Listing of Additional Resources

Edited by Joyce Brennfleck Shannon. 610 pages. 2002. 0-7808-0560-7. $78.

Stroke Sourcebook

Basic Consumer Health Information about Stroke, Including Ischemic, Hemorrhagic, Transient Ischemic Attack (TIA), and Pediatric Stroke, Stroke Triggers and Risks, Diagnostic Tests, Treatments, and Rehabilitation Information

Along with Stroke Prevention Guidelines, Legal and Financial Information, a Glossary, and a Directory of Additional Resources

Edited by Joyce Brennfleck Shannon. 606 pages. 2003. 0-7808-0630-1. $78.

Substance Abuse Sourcebook

Basic Health-Related Information about the Abuse of Legal and Illegal Substances Such as Alcohol, Tobacco, Prescription Drugs, Marijuana, Cocaine, and Heroin; and Including Facts about Substance Abuse Prevention Strategies, Intervention Methods, Treatment and Recovery Programs, and a Section Addressing the Special Problems Related to Substance Abuse during Pregnancy

Edited by Karen Bellenir. 573 pages. 1996. 0-7808-0038-9. $78.

SEE ALSO Alcoholism Sourcebook, Drug Abuse Sourcebook

Surgery Sourcebook

Basic Consumer Health Information about Inpatient and Outpatient Surgeries, Including Cardiac, Vascular, Orthopedic, Ocular, Reconstructive, Cosmetic, Gynecologic, and Ear, Nose, and Throat Procedures and More

Along with Information about Operating Room Policies and Instruments, Laser Surgery Techniques, Hospital Errors, Statistical Data, a Glossary, and Listings of Sources for Further Help and Information

Edited by Annemarie S. Muth and Karen Bellenir. 596 pages. 2002. 0-7808-0380-9. $78.

Transplantation Sourcebook

Basic Consumer Health Information about Organ and Tissue Transplantation, Including Physical and Financial Preparations, Procedures and Issues Relating to Specific Solid Organ and Tissue Transplants, Rehabilitation, Pediatric Transplant Information, the Future of Transplantation, and Organ and Tissue Donation

Along with a Glossary and Listings of Additional Resources

Edited by Joyce Brennfleck Shannon. 628 pages. 2002. 0-7808-0322-1. $78.

Traveler's Health Sourcebook

Basic Consumer Health Information for Travelers, Including Physical and Medical Preparations, Transportation Health and Safety, Essential Information about Food and Water, Sun Exposure, Insect and Snake Bites, Camping and Wilderness Medicine, and Travel with Physical or Medical Disabilities

Along with International Travel Tips, Vaccination Recommendations, Geographical Health Issues, Disease Risks, a Glossary, and a Listing of Additional Resources

Edited by Joyce Brennfleck Shannon. 613 pages. 2000. 0-7808-0384-1. $78.

"Recommended reference source."
— *Booklist, American Library Association, Feb '01*

"This book is recommended for any public library, any travel collection, and especially any collection for the physically disabled."
— *American Reference Books Annual, 2001*

■

Vegetarian Sourcebook

Basic Consumer Health Information about Vegetarian Diets, Lifestyle, and Philosophy, Including Definitions of Vegetarianism and Veganism, Tips about Adopting Vegetarianism, Creating a Vegetarian Pantry, and Meeting Nutritional Needs of Vegetarians, with Facts Regarding Vegetarianism's Effect on Pregnant and Lactating Women, Children, Athletes, and Senior Citizens

Along with a Glossary of Commonly Used Vegetarian Terms and Resources for Additional Help and Information

Edited by Chad T. Kimball. 360 pages. 2002. 0-7808-0439-2. $78.

"Organizes into one concise volume the answers to the most common questions concerning vegetarian diets and lifestyles. This title is recommended for public and secondary school libraries." — *E-Streams, Apr '03*

"Invaluable reference for public and school library collections alike." — *Library Bookwatch, Apr '03*

"The articles in this volume are easy to read and come from authoritative sources. The book does not necessarily support the vegetarian diet but instead provides the pros and cons of this important decision. The *Vegetarian Sourcebook* is recommended for public libraries and consumer health libraries."
— *American Reference Books Annual, 2003*

■

Women's Health Concerns Sourcebook

Basic Information about Health Issues That Affect Women, Featuring Facts about Menstruation and Other Gynecological Concerns, Including Endometriosis, Fibroids, Menopause, and Vaginitis; Reproductive Concerns, Including Birth Control, Infertility, and Abortion; and Facts about Additional Physical, Emotional, and Mental Health Concerns Prevalent among Women Such as Osteoporosis, Urinary Tract Disorders, Eating Disorders, and Depression

Along with Tips for Maintaining a Healthy Lifestyle

Edited by Heather E. Aldred. 567 pages. 1997. 0-7808-0219-5. $78.

"Handy compilation. There is an impressive range of diseases, devices, disorders, procedures, and other phys-

ical and emotional issues covered . . . well organized, illustrated, and indexed."** — *Choice, Association of College and Research Libraries, Jan '98*

SEE ALSO *Breast Cancer Sourcebook, Cancer Sourcebook for Women, Healthy Heart Sourcebook for Women, Osteoporosis Sourcebook*

■

Workplace Health & Safety Sourcebook

Basic Consumer Health Information about Workplace Health and Safety, Including the Effect of Workplace Hazards on the Lungs, Skin, Heart, Ears, Eyes, Brain, Reproductive Organs, Musculoskeletal System, and Other Organs and Body Parts

Along with Information about Occupational Cancer, Personal Protective Equipment, Toxic and Hazardous Chemicals, Child Labor, Stress, and Workplace Violence

Edited by Chad T. Kimball. 626 pages. 2000. 0-7808-0231-4. $78.

"As a reference for the general public, this would be useful in any library." — *E-Streams, Jun '01*

"Provides helpful information for primary care physicians and other caregivers interested in occupational medicine. . . . General readers; professionals."
— *Choice, Association of College & Research Libraries, May '01*

"Recommended reference source."
— *Booklist, American Library Association, Feb '01*

"Highly recommended." — *The Bookwatch, Jan '01*

■

Worldwide Health Sourcebook

Basic Information about Global Health Issues, Including Malnutrition, Reproductive Health, Disease Dispersion and Prevention, Emerging Diseases, Risky Health Behaviors, and the Leading Causes of Death

Along with Global Health Concerns for Children, Women, and the Elderly, Mental Health Issues, Research and Technology Advancements, and Economic, Environmental, and Political Health Implications, a Glossary, and a Resource Listing for Additional Help and Information

Edited by Joyce Brennfleck Shannon. 614 pages. 2001. 0-7808-0330-2. $78.

"Named an Outstanding Academic Title."
— *Choice, Association of College & Research Libraries, Jan '02*

"Yet another handy but also unique compilation in the extensive Health Reference Series, this is a useful work because many of the international publications reprinted or excerpted are not readily available. Highly recommended." — *Choice, Association of College & Research Libraries, Nov '01*

"Recommended reference source."
— *Booklist, American Library Association, Oct '01*

643

Teen Health Series

Helping Young Adults Understand, Manage, and Avoid Serious Illness

Diet Information for Teens

Health Tips about Diet and Nutrition

Including Facts about Nutrients, Dietary Guidelines, Breakfasts, School Lunches, Snacks, Party Food, Weight Control, Eating Disorders, and More

Edited by Karen Bellenir. 399 pages. 2001. 0-7808-0441-4. $58.

"Full of helpful insights and facts throughout the book. ... An excellent resource to be placed in public libraries or even in personal collections."
—*American Reference Books Annual 2002*

"Recommended for middle and high school libraries and media centers as well as academic libraries that educate future teachers of teenagers. It is also a suitable addition to health science libraries that serve patrons who are interested in teen health promotion and education."
—*E-Streams, Oct '01*

"This comprehensive book would be beneficial to collections that need information about nutrition, dietary guidelines, meal planning, and weight control. ... This reference is so easy to use that its purchase is recommended."
—*The Book Report, Sep-Oct '01*

"This book is written in an easy to understand format describing issues that many teens face every day, and then provides thoughtful explanations so that teens can make informed decisions. This is an interesting book that provides important facts and information for today's teens."
—*Doody's Health Sciences Book Review Journal, Jul-Aug '01*

"A comprehensive compendium of diet and nutrition. The information is presented in a straightforward, plain-spoken manner. This title will be useful to those working on reports on a variety of topics, as well as to general readers concerned about their dietary health."
—*School Library Journal, Jun '01*

◼

Drug Information for Teens

Health Tips about the Physical and Mental Effects of Substance Abuse

Including Facts about Alcohol, Anabolic Steroids, Club Drugs, Cocaine, Depressants, Hallucinogens, Herbal Products, Inhalants, Marijuana, Narcotics, Stimulants, Tobacco, and More

Edited by Karen Bellenir. 452 pages. 2002. 0-7808-0444-9. $58.

"The chapters are quick to make a connection to their teenage reading audience. The prose is straightforward and the book lends itself to spot reading. It should be useful both for practical information and for research, and it is suitable for public and school libraries."
—*American Reference Books Annual, 2003*

"Recommended reference source."
—*Booklist, American Library Association, Feb '03*

"This is an excellent resource for teens and their parents. Education about drugs and substances is key to discouraging teen drug abuse and this book provides this much needed information in a way that is interesting and factual."
—*Doody's Review Service, Dec '02*

◼

Mental Health Information for Teens

Health Tips about Mental Health and Mental Illness

Including Facts about Anxiety, Depression, Suicide, Eating Disorders, Obsessive-Compulsive Disorders, Panic Attacks, Phobias, Schizophrenia, and More

Edited by Karen Bellenir. 406 pages. 2001. 0-7808-0442-2. $58.

"In both language and approach, this user-friendly entry in the *Teen Health Series* is on target for teens needing information on mental health concerns."
—*Booklist, American Library Association, Jan '02*

"Readers will find the material accessible and informative, with the shaded notes, facts, and embedded glossary insets adding appropriately to the already interesting and succinct presentation."
—*School Library Journal, Jan '02*

"This title is highly recommended for any library that serves adolescents and parents/caregivers of adolescents."
—*E-Streams, Jan '02*

"Recommended for high school libraries and young adult collections in public libraries. Both health professionals and teenagers will find this book useful."
—*American Reference Books Annual 2002*

"This is a nice book written to enlighten the society, primarily teenagers, about common teen mental health issues. It is highly recommended to teachers and parents as well as adolescents."
—*Doody's Review Service, Dec '01*

◼

Sexual Health Information for Teens

Health Tips about Sexual Development, Human Reproduction, and Sexually Transmitted Diseases

Including Facts about Puberty, Reproductive Health, Chlamydia, Human Papillomavirus, Pelvic Inflam-

matory Disease, Herpes, AIDS, Contraception, Pregnancy, and More

Edited by Deborah A. Stanley. 391 pages. 2003. 0-7808-0445-7. $58.

Skin Health Information For Teens

Health Tips about Dermatological Concerns and Skin Cancer Risks

Including Facts about Acne, Warts, Hives, and Other Conditions and Lifestyle Choices, Such as Tanning, Tattooing, and Piercing, That Affect the Skin, Nails, Scalp, and Hair

Edited by Robert Aquinas McNally. 430 pages. 2003. 0-7808-0446-5. $58.

Sports Injuries Information For Teens

Health Tips about Sports Injuries and Injury Protection

Including Facts about Specific Injuries, Emergency Treatment, Rehabilitation, Sports Safety, Competition Stress, Fitness, Sports Nutrition, Steroid Risks, and More

Edited by Joyce Brennfleck Shannon. 425 pages. 2003. 0-7808-0447-3. $58.